CANCER MORTALITY AND MORBIDITY STATISTICS

Gann Monograph on Cancer Research

The "Gann Monograph on Cancer Research" series is promoted by the Japanese Cancer Association. This semiannual series of monographs was initiated in 1966 by the late Dr. Tomizo Yoshida (1903–1973) and is now published jointly by Japan Scientific Societies Press, Tokyo and CRC Press, Boca Raton. Each volume consists of collected contributions on current topics in cancer problems and allied research fields. The planning for each volume is done by the Monograph Committee of the Japanese Cancer Association, with the final approval of the Board of Directors. It is hoped that the series will serve as an important source of information in the field of cancer research.

The publication of these monographs owes much to the financial support given by the late Professor Kazushige Higuchi, the Jikei University School of Medicine.

Japanese Cancer Association

JAPANESE CANCER ASSOCIATION

Gann Monograph on Cancer Research No. 41

CANCER MORTALITY AND MORBIDITY STATISTICS

JAPAN AND THE WORLD-1994

Edited by SUKETAMI TOMINAGA
KUNIO AOKI
ISABURO FUJIMOTO
MINORU KURIHARA

JAPAN SCIENTIFIC SOCIETIES PRESS, Tokyo
CRC PRESS, Boca Raton Ann Arbor London Tokyo

February 1994

Published jointly by
JAPAN SCIENTIFIC SOCIETIES PRESS
2-10 Hongo, 6-chome, Bunkyo-ku, Tokyo 113, Japan
ISBN 4-7622-7758-4

and

CRC PRESS
2000 Corporate Blvd., N.W., Boca Raton, FL 33431, U.S.A.
ISBN 0-8493-7748-X

Library of Congress Cataloging-in-Publication Data

Cancer mortality and morbidity statistics: Japan and the world. 1994/
edited by Suketami Tominaga—[et al.].
p. cm.—(Gann monograph on cancer research; no. 41)
Includes bibliographical references and index.
ISBN 0-8493-7748-X
1. Cancer—Japan—Mortality—Statistics. 2. Cancer—Mortality—Statistics. 3. Japan—Statistics. Medical.
I. Tominaga, Suketami.
II. Series.
[DNLM: 1. Neoplasms—mortality. 2. Neoplasms—mortality—Japan. 3. Neoplasms—epidemiology—statistics. 4. Japan. 5. Neoplasms—epidemiology—Japan—statistics. W3 GA163 no. 41 1994/QZ 16 C215 1994]
RC279. J3C36 1994
615. 5'999—dc20
DNLM/DLC
for Library of Congress 93-35677
CIP

Distributed in all areas outside Japan and Asia between Pakistan and Korea by CRC Press.

Printed in Japan

PREFACE

Cancer is one of the major causes of deaths in most developed countries. In Japan it has been the leading cause since 1981 and continues to increase. In most developing countries the number of cancer deaths has also been rising while deaths due to infectious and parasitic diseases have been declining.

Cancer statistics are useful to know the magnitude of the problem in populations and to evaluate the effects of control measures. Analyses of these statistics often provide etiological clues and suggest methods for countermeasures to prevent the disease. This makes the recording of information on cancer mortality and morbidity by epidemiologists and public health workers valuable, and to clinicians and researchers it may provide clues to biological derivation and/or impact.

The 1981 "Cancer Mortality and Morbidity Statistics-Japan and the World" (Gann Monograph on Cancer Research, No. 26) was up-to-date at the time it was published, but in the more than 10 years that have passed since then many other statistics have been gathered. This new monograph contains the most recent cancer statistics available for Japan and the rest of the world.

In 1992 Drs. Kunio Aoki, Minoru Kurihara, Norihiko Hayakawa, and Sadao Suzuki employed then the most recent cancer mortality statistics for their monograph published by UICC (International Union Against Cancer) "Death Rates for Malignant Neoplasms for Selected Sites by Sex and Five-Year Age Groups in 33 Countries 1953–57 to 1983–87". We have extracted some of their data, updated it and have prepared illustrations to help readers understand the trends indicated by the statistics. This volume offers figures on cancer mortality in Japan through 1990 and cancer incidence in Japan through 1989. The 1981 Gann Monograph covered through 1978 and 1975, respectively.

The editors of this monograph hope that the publication will make a substantial contribution to cancer researchers and cancer control programs in Japan and throughout the world. They wish to acknowledge the support and assistance of the Statistics and Information Department of the Minister's Secretariat of the Ministry of Health and Welfare of Japan, and the Dissemination of Statistical Information Office of the World Health Organization.

January 1993 Suketami TOMINAGA

CONTENTS

CANCER MORTALITY IN JAPAN (1950–1990)

Tetsuo KUROISHI,[*1] Kaoru HIROSE,[*1] Kazuo TAJIMA,[*1]
and Suketami TOMINAGA[*2]
*Division of Epidemiology,[*1] Aichi Cancer Center Research Institute[*2]*

Cancer mortality statistics in Japan (1950–1990) were calculated from the *"Vital Statistics, Japan"* series published annually by the Statistics and Information Department, Minister's Secretariat, Ministry of Health and Welfare and from data edited from magnetic tape copies of *"Vital Statistics"* with the official permission of the Management and Coordination Agency.

This report includes the following cancer mortality statistics in Japan:

1) The number of deaths from malignant neoplasms by site, its proportion of all malignant neoplasms and the death rates in Japan (1990).
2) The number of deaths, the death rates and the average age at death from malignant neoplasms by site in Japan (1950–1990).
3) Age- and sex-specific mortality rates by site in Japan (1950, 1955, 1960, 1965, 1970, 1975, 1980, 1985, and 1990).
4) Age-adjusted death rates for cancer by site for cities and counties in Japan (1970, 1980, and 1990).
5) Standardized mortality ratio (SMR) of cancer by site in Japan by prefecture (1990).

This report was prepared to update data on "Cancer Mortality in Japan" last published in 1981 in *"Cancer Mortality and Morbidity Statistics—Japan and the World" Gann Monograph on Cancer Research No. 26* (*2*).

Cancer mortality statistics for 1950–1990 were taken from the *"Vital Statistics, Japan"* series (*3*) which is published annually by the Statistics and Information Department, Minister's Secretariat, Ministry of Health and Welfare. Mortality statistics for 1970, 1980, and 1990 for cities and counties and those for 1990 by prefecture were based on fundamental data edited from magnetic tape copies of *"Vital Statistics"* provided by the Ministry of Health and Welfare after obtaining official permission from the Management and Coordination Agency.

The Statistics and Information Department, Minister's Secretariat, Ministry of Health and Welfare of Japan recommended use of the 'model' population for the year 1985 in Japan (Table A and Fig. A) as a standard population for calculation of age-adjusted death rates (*1*), and this 1985 model population was employed for the age-adjusted death rates by site for 1950–1990, and for those by site for cities and counties in Japan for 1970, 1980, and 1990. For the sake of comparison, age-adjusted death rates by site in Japan for the year 1990 were calculated both by this 1985 model population and by Segi-Doll's World Population as the standard population (Table A and Fig. A).

[*1,*2] 1-1 Kanokoden, Chikusa-ku, Nagoya 464, Japan (黒石哲生，広瀬加緒瑠，田島和雄，富永祐民).

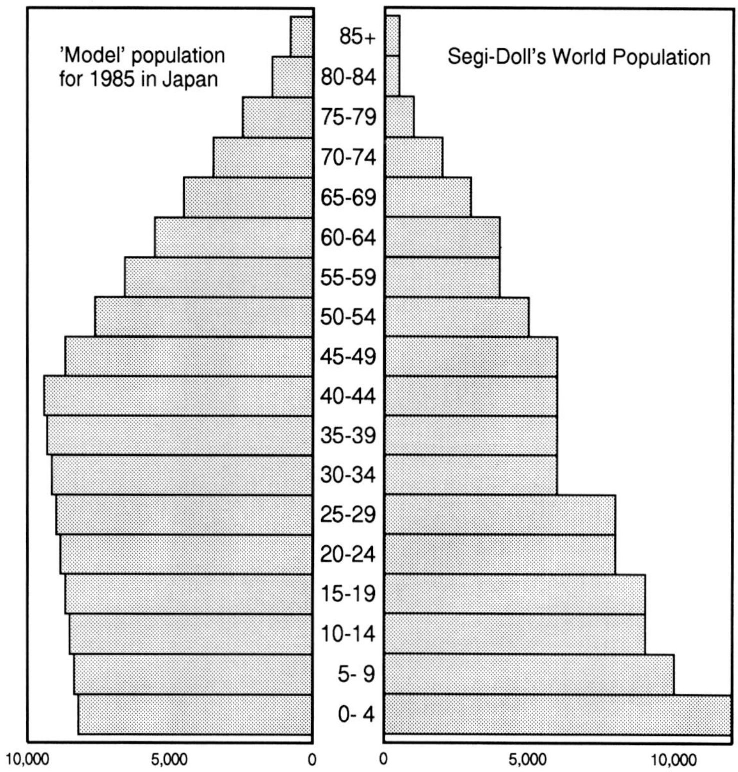

FIG. A. Standard population

TABLE A. Standard Population

Age group in years	'Model' population for 1985 in Japan in thousands	Segi-Doll's World Population
0–4	8,180	12,000
5–9	8,338	10,000
10–14	8,497	9,000
15–19	8,655	9,000
20–24	8,814	8,000
25–29	8,972	8,000
30–34	9,130	6,000
35–39	9,289	6,000
40–44	9,400	6,000
45–49	8,651	6,000
50–54	7,616	5,000
55–59	6,581	4,000
60–64	5,546	4,000
65–69	4,511	3,000
70–74	3,476	2,000
75–79	2,441	1,000
80–84	1,406	500
85 and over	784	500
Total	120,287	100,000

Number of Deaths from Malignant Neoplasms by Site, Its Proportion of All Malignant Neoplasms and the Death Rates in Japan (1990)

The number of deaths from malignant neoplasms by sex and site and the proportion of all malignant neoplasms in Japan for 1990 are shown in Table I-1. In 1990 there were 130,395 male cancer deaths and 87,018 female cancer deaths in Japan, accounting for 29.4% and 23.1% of all deaths, respectively. Major cancers which rank top to seventh in proportion among all malignant neoplasms for both sexes are shown in Fig. 1.

The crude and age-adjusted death rates per 100,000 population from malignant neoplasms by sex and site in Japan for 1990 are shown in Table I-2. As stated, two kinds of age-adjusted death rates per 100,000 population were calculated. The first (ADR1 in Table I-2) is standardized on the age distribution of Segi-Doll's World Population, and the second (ADR2 in Table I-2) is standardized on the age distribution of the 'model' population for the year 1985 in Japan.

Number of Deaths, Death Rates, and Average Age at Death from Malignant Neoplasms by Site in Japan (1950–1990)

The number of deaths, the crude and age-adjusted death rates, and the average age at death from malignant neoplasms by site in Japan for 1950–1990 are given in Tables II-1 to II-21. The age-adjusted death rates are standardized on the age distribution of the 'model' population for the year 1985 in Japan. Trends in this rate and the average age at death for cancer of major sites are illustrated in Fig. 2-1 and Fig. 2-2, respectively.

The contents of Tables II-1 to II-21 are as follows:

	Site of cancer	ICD		
		7th revision	8th revision	9th revision
Table II-1	All sites	140–205	140–209	140–208
Table II-2	Buccal cavity and pharynx	140–148	140–149	140–149
Table II-3	Esophagus	150	150	150
Table II-4	Stomach	151	151	151
Table II-5	Colon	153	153	153
Table II-6	Rectum	154	154	154
Table II-7	Liver	155.0, 156	155, 197.7,197.8	155
Table II-8	Biliary passages	155.1	156	156
Table II-9	Pancreas	157	157	157
Table II-10	Larynx	161	161	161
Table II-11	Trachea, bronchus, and lung	162, 163	162	162
Table II-12	Bone	196	170	170
Table II-13	Skin	190, 191	172, 173	172, 173
Table II-14	Breast	170	174	174
Table II-15	Uterus	171–174	180–182	179–182
Table II-16	Ovary	175a	183.0	183.0
Table II-17	Prostate	177	185	185
Table II-18	Urinary bladder	181a	188	188
Table II-19	Kidney	180	189.0, 189.1	189.0, 189.1
Table II-20	Lymphatic tissue	200–205	200–203, 208–209	200–203
Table II-21	Leukemia	204	204–207	204–208

ICD: International Classification of Diseases.

Age- and Sex-Specific Mortality Rates by Site in Japan (Each 5 Years from 1950–1990)

The age- and sex-specific mortality rates by site in Japan for 1950, 1955, 1960, 1965, 1970, 1975, 1980, 1985, and 1990 are given in Tables III-1 to III-21, and illustrated by age group (A) and by birth-year cohort (B) in Figs. 3-1 to 3-21. The contents of these tables and figures are as follows:

		Site of cancer	ICD (9th revision)
Table III-1	Fig. 3-1	All sites	140–208
Table III-2	Fig. 3-2	Buccal cavity and pharynx	140–149
Table III-3	Fig. 3-3	Esophagus	150
Table III-4	Fig. 3-4	Stomach	151
Table III-5	Fig. 3-5	Colon	153
Table III-6	Fig. 3-6	Rectum	154
Table III-7	Fig. 3-7	Liver	155
Table III-8	Fig. 3-8	Biliary passages	156
Table III-9	Fig. 3-9	Pancreas	157
Table III-10	Fig. 3-10	Larynx	161
Table III-11	Fig. 3-11	Trachea, bronchus, and lung	162
Table III-12	Fig. 3-12	Bone	170
Table III-13	Fig. 3-13	Skin	172, 173
Table III-14	Fig. 3-14	Breast	174
Table III-15	Fig. 3-15	Uterus	179–182
Table III-16	Fig. 3-16	Ovary	183.0
Table III-17	Fig. 3-17	Prostate	185
Table III-18	Fig. 3-18	Urinary bladder	188
Table III-19	Fig. 3-19	Kidney	189.0, 189.1
Table III-20	Fig. 3-20	Lymphatic tissue	200–203
Table III-21	Fig. 3-21	Leukemia	204–208

Age-Adjusted Death Rates for Cancer by Site for Cities and Counties in Japan (1970, 1980, and 1990)

The age-adjusted death rates for cancer by site for 10 large cities (Sapporo, Tokyo, Yokohama, Kawasaki, Nagoya, Kyoto, Osaka, Kobe, Kitakyushu, and Fukuoka), all other cities and counties in Japan for 1970, 1980, and 1990 are given by sex in Tables IV-1, IV-2, and IV-3 for the three respective years. The report of population census of Japan contains only total population (including foreigners) of each city by age (*4*). Thus we calculated the age-adjusted death rates based on this

		Site of cancer	ICD (8th revision)	ICD (9th revision)
Fig. 4-1	A	All sites	140–209	140–208
	B	Buccal cavity and pharynx	140–149	140–149
	C	Esophagus	150	150
Fig. 4-2	A	Stomach	151	151
	B	Colon	153	153
	C	Rectum	154	154

		Site of cancer	ICD (8th revision)	ICD (9th revision)
Fig. 4-3	A	Liver	155, 197.7, 197.8	155
	B	Biliary passages	156	156
	C	Pancreas	157	157
Fig. 4-4	A	Larynx	161	161
	B	Trachea, bronchus, and lung	162	162
	C	Bone	170	170
Fig. 4-5	A	Skin	172, 173	172, 173
	B	Breast	174	174
	C	Uterus	180–182	179–182
Fig. 4-6	A	Ovary	183.0	183.0
	B	Prostate	185	185
	C	Urinary bladder	188	188
Fig. 4-7	A	Kidney	189.0, 189.1	189.0, 189.1
	B	Lymphatic tissue	200–203, 208–209	200–203
	C	Leukemia	204–207	204–208

total population. Trends in the age-adjusted death rate for the cities and counties are illustrated in Figs. 4-1 to 4-7. The contents of these figures are as follows:

Standardized Mortality Ratio (SMR) of Cancer by Site by Prefecture (1990)

The SMR of cancer by site in Japan for 1990 was calculated for each prefecture. Locations of each prefecture and 10 large cities are shown in Fig. B. Maps of distri-

			Site of cancer	ICD (9th revision)
Table V-1	Fig. 5-1	A	All sites	140–208
		B	Buccal cavity and pharynx	140–149
Table V-2	Fig. 5-2	A	Esophagus	150
		B	Stomach	151
Table V-3	Fig. 5-3	A	Colon	153
		B	Rectum	154
Table V-4	Fig. 5-4	A	Liver	155
		B	Biliary passages	156
Table V-5	Fig. 5-5	A	Pancreas	157
		B	Larynx	161
Table V-6	Fig. 5-6	A	Trachea, bronchus, and lung	162
		B	Bone	170
Table V-7	Fig. 5-7	A	Skin	172, 173
		B	Breast	174
Table V-8	Fig. 5-8	A	Uterus	179–182
		B	Ovary	183.0
Table V-9	Fig. 5-9	A	Prostate	185
		B	Urinary bladder	188
Table V-10	Fig. 5-10	A	Kidney	189.0, 189.1
		B	Lymphatic tissue	200–203
Table V-11	Fig. 5-11	A	Leukemia	204–208

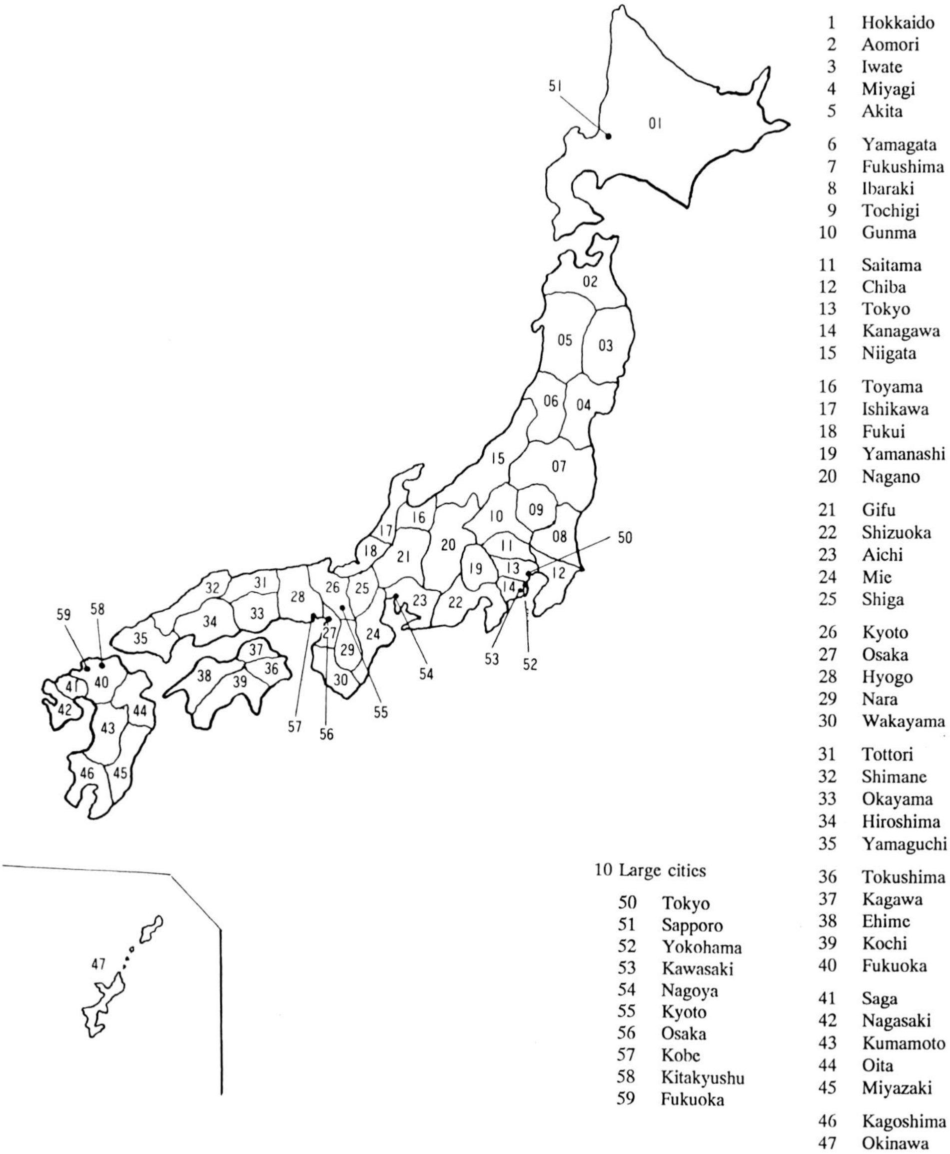

FIG. B. Map of 47 prefectures and 10 large cities in Japan

bution of SMR are shown in Figs. 5-1 to 5-11. SMRs of cancer by prefecture are given in Tables V-1 to V-11. The contents of these tables and figures are as follows:

Acknowledgments

We would like to thank the Statistics and Information Department, Ministry of Health and Welfare of Japan for providing us magnetic tape copies of *"Vital Statis-*

tics" with the official permission of the Management and Coordination Agency. We also thank Miss E. Nakamura for her excellent technical assistance in drawing the maps and making the tables by computer.

REFERENCES

1. Abe, Y., Onodera, M., Kamiya, K., Saito, F., and Matsue, T. On the revision of the age-adjusted death rate. *Kousei no Shihyo*, **38**(5), 12–16 (1991) (in Japanese).
2. Kuroishi, T., Tominaga, S., Hirose, K., Aoki K., and Segi, M. Cancer mortality in Japan. *In* "Cancer Mortality and Morbidity Statistics—Japan and World," Gann Monograph on Cancer Research, No. 26, eds. M. Segi, S. Tominaga, K. Aoki, and I. Fujimoto, pp. 1–91 (1981). Japan Scientific Societies Press, Tokyo.
3. Statistics and Information Department, Minister's Secretariat, Ministry of Health and Welfare. Vital Statistics 1950–1990 Japan (1950–1990). Kousei Tokei Kyokai, Tokyo (in Japanese).
4. Statistics Bureau, Management and Coordination Agency. 1990 population census of Japan, Vol. 1 and Vol. 2 (1991). Nihon Tokei Kyokai, Tokyo (in Japanese).

TABLE I-1. Number of Deaths from Malignant Neoplasms by Site and

ICD (9th revision)	Site of malignant neoplasm	Male		Female	
		No.	%	No.	%
140–208	All sites	130,395	100.0	87,018	100.0
140–149	Buccal cavity and pharynx	1,866	1.4	741	0.9
140–145	Buccal cavity	984	0.8	531	0.6
140	Lip	6	0.0	7	0.0
141	Tongue	440	0.3	255	0.3
142	Salivary gland	173	0.1	74	0.1
143	Gum	103	0.1	80	0.1
144	Floor of mouth	114	0.1	21	0.0
145	Other and unspecified parts of mouth	148	0.1	94	0.1
146	Oropharynx	191	0.1	33	0.0
147	Nasopharynx	179	0.1	65	0.1
148	Hypopharynx	396	0.3	73	0.1
149	Other and ill-defined sites within the lip, oral cavity, and pharynx	116	0.1	39	0.0
150–159	Digestive organs and peritoneum	79,977	61.3	49,980	57.4
150	Esophagus	6,004	4.6	1,270	1.5
151	Stomach	29,909	22.9	17,562	20.2
152	Small intestine, including duodenum	285	0.2	206	0.2
153	Colon	7,791	6.0	7,718	8.9
154	Rectum, rectosigmoid junction, and anus	5,569	4.3	3,701	4.3
155	Liver and intrahepatic bile ducts	17,786	13.6	6,447	7.4
156	Gallbladder and extrahepatic bile ducts	5,069	3.9	6,802	7.8
157	Pancreas	7,317	5.6	6,001	6.9
158	Retroperitoneum and peritoneum	167	0.1	171	0.2
159	Other and ill-defined sites within the digestive organs and peritoneum	80	0.1	102	0.1
160–165	Respiratory and intrathoracic organs	28,485	21.8	10,170	11.7
160	Nasal cavities, middle ear, and accessory sinuses	495	0.4	306	0.4
161	Larynx	770	0.6	77	0.1
162	Trachea, bronchus, and lung	26,872	20.6	9,614	11.0
163	Pleura	115	0.1	52	0.1
164	Thymus, heart, and mediastinum	233	0.2	120	0.1
165	Other and ill-defined sites within the respiratory system and intrathoracic organs	0	0.0	1	0.0
170–175	Bone, connective tissue, skin, and breast	1,009	0.8	6,618	7.6
170	Bone and articular cartilage	265	0.2	190	0.2
171	Connective tissue and other soft tissue	329	0.3	276	0.3
172, 173	Skin	381	0.3	304	0.3
172	Malignant melanoma of skin	191	0.1	144	0.2
173	Skin (other)	190	0.1	160	0.2
174	Female breast			5,848	6.7
175	Male breast	34	0.0		

ICD: International Classification of Diseases.

Its Proportion of All Malignant Neoplasmis in Japan (1990)

ICD (9th revision)	Site of malignant neoplasm	Male		Female	
		No.	%	No.	%
179–189	Genito-urinary organs	7,823	6.0	10,072	11.6
179–184	Female genital organs			8,136	9.3
179–182	Uterus			4,600	5.3
179	Uterus, part unspecified			2,131	2.4
180	Cervix uteri			1,875	2.2
181	Placenta			27	0.0
182	Body of uterus			567	0.7
183	Ovary and other uterine adnexa			3,330	3.8
183.0	Ovary			3,279	3.8
184	Other and unspecified female genital organs			206	0.2
185–187	Male genital organs	3,704	2.8		
185	Prostate	3,460	2.7		
186	Testis	124	0.1		
187	Penis and other male genital organs	120	0.1		
188	Bladder	2,110	1.6	938	1.1
189	Kidney and other and unspecified urinary organs	2,009	1.5	998	1.1
189.0, 189.1	Kidney	1,763	1.4	850	1.0
190–199	Other and unspecified sites	3,751	2.9	3,929	4.5
190	Eye	17	0.0	10	0.0
191	Brain	652	0.5	504	0.6
192	Other and unspecified parts of nervous system	33	0.0	38	0.0
193	Thyroid gland	306	0.2	688	0.8
194	Other endocrine glands and related structures	124	0.1	81	0.1
195	Other and ill-defined sites	259	0.2	291	0.3
196	Lymph nodes specified as secondary and unspecified	0	0.0	0	0.0
197	Respiratory and digestive systems specified as secondary	0	0.0	0	0.0
198	Other sites, specified as secondary	0	0.0	0	0.0
199	Without specification of site	2,360	1.8	2,317	2.7
200–208	Lymphatic and hematopoietic tissue	7,484	5.7	5,508	6.3
200–202	Lymphoid tissue	3,173	2.4	2,097	2.4
200	Lymphosarcoma and reticulosarcoma	17	0.0	12	0.0
201	Hodgkin's disease	87	0.1	42	0.0
202	Other neoplasm of lymphoid and histiocytic tissue	3,069	2.4	2,043	2.3
203	Multiple myeloma and immunoproliferative neoplasms	1,086	0.8	1,003	1.2
204–208	Leukemia	3,225	2.5	2,408	2.8
204	Lymphoid leukemia	809	0.6	648	0.7
205	Myeloid leukemia	1,648	1.3	1,188	1.4
206	Monocytic leukemia	55	0.0	51	0.1
207	Other specified leukemia	45	0.0	26	0.0
208	Leukemia of unspecified cell type	668	0.5	495	0.6

TABLE I-2. Death Rates from Malignant Neoplasms

ICD (9th revision)	Site of malignant neoplasm	Male			Female		
		CDR	ADR1	ADR2	CDR	ADR1	ADR2
140–208	All sites	217.2	150.5	216.3	139.5	76.1	107.9
140–149	Buccal cavity and pharynx	3.1	2.2	3.0	1.2	0.7	0.9
140–145	Buccal cavity	1.6	1.2	1.6	0.9	0.5	0.6
140	Lip	0.0	0.0	0.0	0.0	0.0	0.0
141	Tongue	0.7	0.5	0.7	0.4	0.2	0.3
142	Salivary gland	0.3	0.2	0.3	0.1	0.1	0.1
143	Gum	0.2	0.1	0.2	0.1	0.1	0.1
144	Floor of mouth	0.2	0.1	0.2	0.0	0.0	0.0
145	Other and unspecified parts of mouth	0.3	0.2	0.3	0.2	0.1	0.1
146	Oropharynx	0.3	0.2	0.3	0.1	0.0	0.0
147	Nasopharynx	0.3	0.2	0.3	0.1	0.1	0.1
148	Hypopharynx	0.7	0.5	0.6	0.1	0.1	0.1
149	Other and ill-defined sites within the lip, oral cavity, and pharynx	0.2	0.1	0.2	0.1	0.0	0.1
150–159	Digestive organs and peritoneum	133.2	92.2	131.8	80.1	41.7	60.6
150	Esophagus	10.0	7.0	9.9	2.0	1.0	1.5
151	Stomach	49.8	34.3	49.7	28.2	15.0	21.6
152	Small intestine, including duodenum	0.5	0.3	0.5	0.3	0.2	0.3
153	Colon	13.0	8.9	12.9	12.4	6.5	9.4
154	Rectum, rectosigmoid junction, and anus	9.3	6.4	9.2	5.9	3.2	4.6
155	Liver and intrahepatic bile ducts	29.6	20.9	28.5	10.3	5.5	7.8
156	Gallbladder and extrahepatic bile ducts	8.4	5.7	8.5	10.9	5.3	8.0
157	Pancreas	12.2	8.4	12.2	9.6	4.8	7.2
158	Retroperitoneum and peritoneum	0.3	0.2	0.3	0.3	0.2	0.2
159	Other and ill-defined sites within the digestive organs and peritoneum	0.1	0.1	0.1	0.2	0.1	0.1
160–165	Respiratory and intrathoracic organs	47.5	32.2	47.8	16.3	8.4	12.3
160	Nasal cavities, middle ear, and accessory sinuses	0.8	0.6	0.8	0.5	0.3	0.4
161	Larynx	1.3	0.9	1.3	0.1	0.1	0.1
162	Trachea, bronchus, and lung	44.8	30.4	45.2	15.4	7.9	11.6
163	Pleura	0.2	0.1	0.2	0.1	0.1	0.1
164	Thymus, heart, and mediastinum	0.4	0.3	0.4	0.2	0.1	0.2
165	Other and ill-defined sites within the respiratory system and intrathoracic organs	0.0	0.0	0.0	0.0	0.0	0.0
170–175	Bone, connective tissue, skin, and breast	1.7	1.3	1.7	10.6	7.1	9.2
170	Bone and articular cartilage	0.4	0.4	0.4	0.3	0.2	0.3
171	Connective tissue and other soft tissue	0.6	0.4	0.6	0.4	0.3	0.4
172, 173	Skin	0.6	0.5	0.6	0.5	0.3	0.4
172	Malignant melanoma of skin	0.3	0.2	0.3	0.2	0.1	0.2
173	Skin (other)	0.3	0.2	0.3	0.3	0.1	0.2
174	Female breast				9.4	6.3	8.2
175	Male breast	0.1	0.0	0.1			

CDR : crude death rate per 100,000 population.
ADR1 : age-adjusted death rate per 100,000 population standardized on the age distribution of the 'world' population.
ADR2 : age-adjusted death rate per 100,000 population standardized on the age distribution of the 'model' population for the year 1985 in Japan.

by Site in Japan (1990)

ICD (9th revision)	Site of malignant neoplasm	Male			Female		
		CDR	ADR1	ADR2	CDR	ADR1	ADR2
179–189	Genito-urinary organs	13.0	8.8	13.3	16.2	9.3	12.9
179–184	Female genital organs				13.0	7.7	10.6
179–182	Uterus				7.4	4.2	5.9
179	Uterus, part unspecified				3.4	1.8	2.6
180	Cervix uteri				3.0	1.8	2.5
181	Placenta				0.0	0.0	0.0
182	Body of uterus				0.9	0.6	0.7
183	Ovary and other uterine adnexa				5.3	3.4	4.5
183.0	Ovary				5.3	3.3	4.4
184	Other and unspecified female genital organs				0.3	0.2	0.3
185–187	Male genital organs	6.2	4.1	6.4			
185	Prostate	5.8	3.7	6.0			
186	Testis	0.2	0.2	0.2			
187	Penis and other male genital organs	0.2	0.1	0.2			
188	Bladder	3.5	2.4	3.6	1.5	0.7	1.0
189	Kidney and other and unspecified urinary organs	3.4	2.3	3.3	1.6	0.9	1.2
189.0, 189.1	Kidney	2.9	2.0	2.9	1.4	0.7	1.0
190–199	Other and unspecified sites	6.3	4.6	6.3	6.3	3.5	4.8
190	Eye	0.0	0.0	0.0	0.0	0.0	0.0
191	Brain	1.1	0.9	1.1	0.8	0.6	0.7
192	Other and unspecified parts of nervous system	0.1	0.0	0.1	0.1	0.0	0.1
193	Thyroid gland	0.5	0.4	0.5	1.1	0.6	0.8
194	Other endocrine glands and related structures	0.2	0.2	0.2	0.1	0.2	0.1
195	Other and ill-defined sites	0.4	0.3	0.4	0.5	0.3	0.4
196	Lymph nodes specified as secondary and unspecified	0.0	0.0	0.0	0.0	0.0	0.0
197	Respiratory and digestive systems specified as secondary	0.0	0.0	0.0	0.0	0.0	0.0
198	Other sites, specified as secondary	0.0	0.0	0.0	0.0	0.0	0.0
199	Without specification of site	3.9	2.7	4.0	3.7	1.9	2.8
200–208	Lymphatic and hematopoietic tissue	12.5	9.3	12.4	8.8	5.5	7.2
200–202	Lymphoid tissue	5.3	3.8	5.3	3.4	1.9	2.7
200	Lymphosarcoma and reticulosarcoma	0.0	0.0	0.0	0.0	0.0	0.0
201	Hodgkin's disease	0.1	0.1	0.1	0.1	0.0	0.1
202	Other neoplasm of lymphoid and histiocytic tissue	5.1	3.7	5.1	3.3	1.9	2.6
203	Multiple myeloma and immunoproliferative neoplasms	1.8	1.2	1.8	1.6	0.8	1.2
204–208	Leukemia	5.4	4.3	5.3	3.9	2.8	3.4
204	Lymphoid leukemia	1.4	1.2	1.3	1.0	0.8	0.9
205	Myeloid leukemia	2.8	2.1	2.7	1.9	1.3	1.7
206	Monocytic leukemia	0.1	0.1	0.1	0.1	0.1	0.1
207	Other specified leukemia	0.1	0.1	0.1	0.0	0.0	0.0
208	Leukemia of unspecified cell type	1.1	0.8	1.1	0.8	0.5	0.7

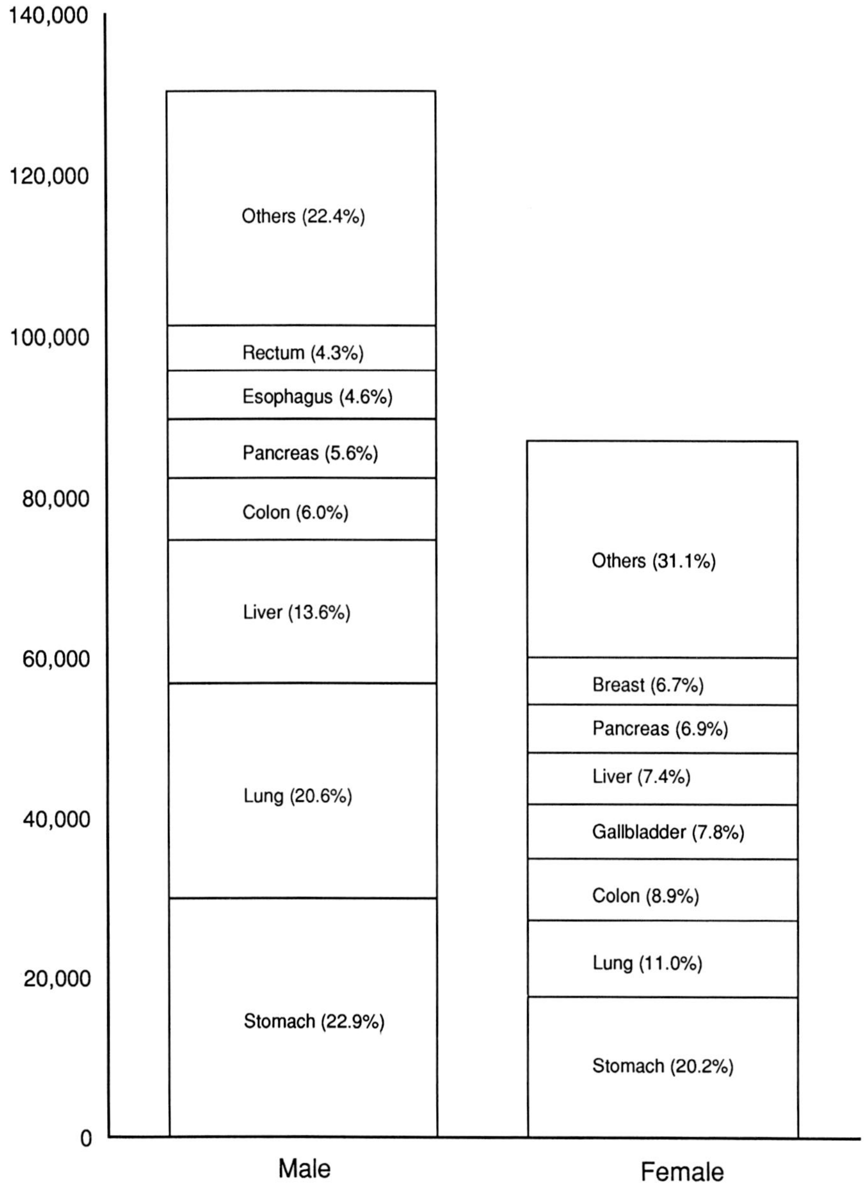

FIG. 1. Number of deaths from malignant neoplasms and its proportion of all malignant neoplasms for major sites by sex in Japan (1990)

TABLE II-1. Cancer Mortality Statistics in Japan (1950–1990)
Cancer of all sites (ICD, 9th revision: 140–208)

Year	No. of deaths		Crude death rate per 100,000		Age-adjusted death rate per 100,000[a]		Average age at death in years	
	Male	Female	Male	Female	Male	Female	Male	Female
1950	32,670	31,758	80.1	74.9	148.2	121.4	59.6	57.7
1951	33,872	32,482	81.6	75.4	150.3	122.4	59.8	58.1
1952	35,845	33,643	85.1	77.0	155.7	123.9	59.9	58.4
1953	37,386	34,192	87.5	77.2	160.1	122.7	60.1	58.4
1954	39,703	35,606	91.6	79.3	166.1	124.7	60.2	58.6
1955	41,223	36,498	94.0	80.4	167.9	125.4	60.4	59.2
1956	43,628	38,251	98.4	83.3	174.7	128.5	60.6	59.3
1957	44,777	38,378	100.0	82.9	175.7	126.0	60.9	59.2
1958	47,237	40,658	104.4	86.9	182.7	130.7	61.1	59.6
1959	49,215	42,071	107.7	89.0	186.0	132.3	61.3	59.8
1960	50,898	42,875	110.9	90.2	188.3	132.0	61.5	60.1
1961	52,254	44,188	112.9	92.1	188.8	132.3	61.7	60.2
1962	53,499	44,725	114.4	92.3	188.0	130.6	61.7	60.2
1963	55,567	45,859	117.7	93.7	192.6	131.2	61.8	60.3
1964	57,705	46,619	120.9	94.3	195.9	130.0	62.1	60.5
1965	58,899	47,637	122.1	95.2	195.6	130.3	62.2	60.7
1966	60,803	49,002	125.0	97.2	197.3	130.5	62.5	60.8
1967	62,308	50,285	127.4	99.1	197.9	130.8	62.6	61.2
1968	64,244	51,218	129.8	99.8	200.0	129.7	62.9	61.4
1969	66,270	52,289	132.3	100.7	202.1	129.1	63.2	61.7
1970	67,074	52,903	132.6	100.7	199.2	126.9	63.2	61.8
1971	68,399	54,451	133.5	102.5	198.2	126.5	63.5	62.1
1972	71,298	56,001	137.5	103.9	202.3	126.4	63.7	62.3
1973	73,401	57,563	138.5	104.5	201.9	125.2	64.1	62.7
1974	75,456	58,295	139.7	104.0	202.0	123.0	64.3	63.0
1975	76,922	59,461	140.6	105.2	198.9	121.1	64.3	63.1
1976	79,995	60,898	144.6	106.7	202.0	120.7	64.5	63.5
1977	83,088	62,684	148.7	108.8	203.4	120.0	64.8	64.0
1978	85,630	64,706	151.9	111.3	203.8	120.0	65.1	64.3
1979	90,136	66,525	158.6	113.5	208.6	119.6	65.4	64.8
1980	93,501	68,263	163.5	115.5	210.9	118.8	65.6	65.2
1981	96,524	69,875	167.4	117.3	211.6	117.8	65.9	65.5
1982	99,114	71,016	170.7	118.5	210.7	115.7	66.2	66.0
1983	103,330	72,876	176.8	120.8	213.3	114.9	66.4	66.3
1984	107,175	75,105	182.3	123.7	215.0	114.6	66.7	66.7
1985	110,660	77,054	187.2	125.9	214.8	113.1	67.0	67.2
1986	113,589	78,065	191.1	126.9	213.8	110.9	67.1	67.6
1987	119,161	80,402	199.5	130.1	216.9	110.1	67.4	68.0
1988	122,015	83,455	203.5	134.5	215.5	110.5	67.8	68.4
1989	127,211	85,414	211.4	137.1	217.8	109.4	67.9	68.7
1990	130,395	87,018	217.2	139.5	216.3	107.9	68.1	69.2

[a] Standardized on the age distribution of the model population for the year 1985 in Japan.

TABLE II-2. Cancer Mortality Statistics in Japan (1950–1990)
Cancer of the buccal cavity and pharynx (ICD, 9th revision: 140–149)

Year	No. of deaths		Crude death rate per 100,000		Age-adjusted death rate per 100,000[a]		Average age at death in years	
	Male	Female	Male	Female	Male	Female	Male	Female
1950	432	267	1.1	0.6	2.1	1.1	59.0	60.9
1951	409	235	1.0	0.6	2.0	0.9	60.8	59.7
1952	427	217	1.0	0.5	1.9	0.9	61.1	61.9
1953	468	237	1.1	0.5	2.0	0.9	59.1	59.6
1954	410	246	1.0	0.6	1.8	0.9	60.2	60.1
1955	414	236	0.9	0.5	1.7	0.9	60.4	61.7
1956	413	238	0.9	0.5	1.7	0.8	60.4	59.6
1957	430	285	1.0	0.6	1.8	1.0	60.8	61.0
1958	443	252	1.0	0.5	1.7	0.8	60.9	63.4
1959	509	280	1.1	0.6	2.0	0.9	60.7	61.5
1960	484	277	1.1	0.6	1.8	0.9	60.9	61.4
1961	522	263	1.1	0.6	1.9	0.8	61.8	61.1
1962	498	287	1.1	0.6	1.7	0.9	60.5	61.9
1963	592	296	1.3	0.6	2.0	0.9	59.7	62.4
1964	580	331	1.2	0.7	2.0	0.9	61.7	61.8
1965	561	333	1.2	0.7	1.9	0.9	61.9	62.5
1966	579	321	1.2	0.6	1.9	0.9	60.7	62.3
1967	640	337	1.3	0.7	2.0	0.9	61.4	62.4
1968	675	362	1.4	0.7	2.1	0.9	61.3	62.7
1969	695	384	1.4	0.7	2.1	1.0	62.2	62.3
1970	738	374	1.5	0.7	2.2	0.9	61.7	62.3
1971	813	374	1.6	0.7	2.3	0.9	61.6	63.1
1972	786	371	1.5	0.7	2.2	0.8	62.1	62.8
1973	784	429	1.5	0.8	2.1	0.9	62.1	63.7
1974	874	424	1.6	0.8	2.3	0.9	62.4	64.1
1975	943	505	1.7	0.9	2.4	1.0	62.5	63.9
1976	1,012	466	1.8	0.8	2.5	0.9	61.9	65.2
1977	1,007	478	1.8	0.8	2.4	0.9	62.3	63.6
1978	1,052	499	1.9	0.9	2.4	0.9	62.2	64.8
1979	1,218	588	2.1	1.0	2.8	1.1	62.6	65.4
1980	1,233	592	2.2	1.0	2.7	1.0	62.8	66.4
1981	1,320	528	2.3	0.9	2.8	0.9	63.6	66.2
1982	1,283	593	2.2	1.0	2.7	1.0	63.4	66.2
1983	1,408	584	2.4	1.0	2.8	0.9	63.4	66.8
1984	1,450	598	2.5	1.0	2.9	0.9	64.0	67.3
1985	1,462	627	2.5	1.0	2.8	0.9	63.9	68.1
1986	1,611	633	2.7	1.0	3.0	0.9	63.6	68.3
1987	1,643	650	2.8	1.1	2.9	0.9	64.3	68.0
1988	1,787	659	3.0	1.1	3.1	0.9	64.3	68.3
1989	1,755	691	2.9	1.1	2.9	0.9	64.4	68.2
1990	1,866	741	3.1	1.2	3.0	0.9	64.4	69.5

[a] Standardized on the age distribution of the model population for the year 1985 in Japan.

TABLE II-3. Cancer Mortality Statistics in Japan (1950–1990)
Cancer of the esophagus (ICD, 9th revision: 150)

Year	No. of deaths		Crude death rate per 100,000		Age-adjusted death rate per 100,000[a]		Average age at death in years	
	Male	Female	Male	Female	Male	Female	Male	Female
1950	1,961	802	4.8	1.9	9.5	3.2	63.9	63.3
1951	1,899	785	4.6	1.8	9.1	3.2	64.2	63.8
1952	2,070	845	4.9	1.9	9.6	3.3	64.3	64.0
1953	2,101	875	4.9	2.0	9.7	3.3	64.4	64.1
1954	2,155	849	5.0	1.9	9.8	3.1	65.1	64.6
1955	2,102	871	4.8	1.9	9.3	3.2	65.4	65.8
1956	2,272	962	5.1	2.1	9.9	3.4	65.6	65.6
1957	2,297	931	5.1	2.0	9.6	3.3	65.1	65.7
1958	2,329	965	5.2	2.1	9.7	3.3	65.6	66.2
1959	2,412	950	5.3	2.0	9.8	3.2	65.9	65.6
1960	2,472	995	5.4	2.1	9.6	3.3	65.5	67.3
1961	2,675	1,041	5.8	2.2	10.2	3.3	66.0	66.5
1962	2,683	994	5.7	2.1	9.9	3.1	66.0	66.7
1963	2,797	1,018	5.9	2.1	10.2	3.1	65.9	66.8
1964	2,931	1,102	6.1	2.2	10.5	3.3	66.4	67.3
1965	2,870	1,088	6.0	2.2	10.1	3.2	66.5	67.8
1966	3,076	1,090	6.3	2.2	10.5	3.1	66.8	68.3
1967	3,180	1,164	6.5	2.3	10.6	3.2	66.8	68.4
1968	3,447	1,183	7.0	2.3	11.2	3.2	66.7	69.1
1969	3,526	1,225	7.0	2.4	11.2	3.2	67.1	69.2
1970	3,673	1,150	7.3	2.2	11.4	2.9	67.2	68.7
1971	3,737	1,263	7.3	2.4	11.3	3.1	67.4	68.9
1972	3,739	1,182	7.2	2.2	11.0	2.8	67.3	69.7
1973	3,903	1,207	7.4	2.2	11.1	2.7	67.7	69.7
1974	3,946	1,262	7.3	2.3	10.9	2.8	67.6	70.4
1975	3,862	1,135	7.1	2.0	10.3	2.4	67.4	70.2
1976	3,924	1,166	7.1	2.0	10.1	2.4	67.2	70.9
1977	4,057	1,184	7.3	2.1	10.2	2.3	67.9	71.7
1978	4,130	1,195	7.3	2.1	10.1	2.3	67.8	71.8
1979	4,347	1,132	7.7	1.9	10.3	2.1	68.0	71.8
1980	4,490	1,243	7.9	2.1	10.3	2.2	68.1	71.7
1981	4,454	1,184	7.7	2.0	9.9	2.0	67.8	72.1
1982	4,646	1,208	8.0	2.0	10.0	1.9	67.7	71.8
1983	4,776	1,220	8.2	2.0	9.9	1.9	67.8	73.0
1984	4,791	1,167	8.2	1.9	9.6	1.7	67.7	73.4
1985	5,046	1,151	8.5	1.9	9.8	1.6	67.4	73.4
1986	5,202	1,183	8.8	1.9	9.7	1.6	67.4	73.4
1987	5,573	1,127	9.3	1.8	10.1	1.5	67.7	72.9
1988	5,625	1,199	9.4	1.9	9.9	1.5	67.7	73.9
1989	5,798	1,243	9.6	2.0	9.8	1.5	67.4	74.4
1990	6,004	1,270	10.0	2.0	9.9	1.5	67.4	73.4

[a] Standardized on the age distribution of the model population for the year 1985 in Japan.

TABLE II-4. Cancer Mortality Statistics in Japan (1950–1990)
Cancer of the stomach (ICD, 9th revision: 151)

Year	No. of deaths		Crude death rate per 100,000		Age-adjusted death rate per 100,000[a]		Average age at death in years	
	Male	Female	Male	Female	Male	Female	Male	Female
1950	19,023	12,188	46.6	28.8	87.3	48.0	61.1	60.9
1951	19,865	12,491	47.9	29.0	89.1	48.4	61.2	61.3
1952	20,814	13,101	49.4	30.0	91.8	49.7	61.4	61.7
1953	21,347	13,418	49.9	30.3	92.8	49.4	61.7	61.3
1954	22,116	13,875	51.0	30.9	93.8	50.0	61.9	61.6
1955	22,899	14,407	52.2	31.7	94.4	50.8	62.0	62.0
1956	23,642	15,081	53.3	32.9	95.9	51.8	62.2	61.9
1957	24,380	15,104	54.5	32.6	96.9	50.7	62.4	61.7
1958	25,151	15,598	55.6	33.3	98.3	51.3	62.6	62.1
1959	25,757	16,127	56.4	34.1	98.5	51.9	62.8	62.4
1960	26,283	16,467	57.3	34.6	98.5	51.8	62.9	62.5
1961	26,469	16,772	57.2	35.0	96.7	51.2	63.2	62.4
1962	26,585	16,918	56.9	34.9	94.5	50.4	63.2	62.5
1963	27,284	17,252	57.8	35.3	95.9	50.3	63.3	62.4
1964	28,219	17,474	59.1	35.3	96.8	49.5	63.4	62.4
1965	28,636	17,749	59.4	35.5	96.0	49.4	63.6	62.7
1966	28,923	17,849	59.5	35.4	94.7	48.3	63.9	62.7
1967	29,160	18,505	59.6	36.5	93.5	48.8	63.9	62.9
1968	30,043	19,257	60.7	37.5	94.5	49.4	64.2	63.1
1969	30,322	19,216	60.5	37.0	93.4	47.9	64.5	63.2
1970	29,653	19,170	58.6	36.5	88.9	46.5	64.5	63.4
1971	29,882	19,563	58.3	36.8	87.4	45.8	64.8	63.5
1972	30,380	19,563	58.6	36.3	87.1	44.5	65.0	63.8
1973	30,603	20,075	57.7	36.5	85.0	44.0	65.2	64.2
1974	30,599	19,791	56.7	35.3	82.7	42.1	65.4	64.5
1975	30,403	19,454	55.6	34.4	79.4	39.8	65.5	64.3
1976	30,537	19,555	55.2	34.3	77.6	38.9	65.6	64.6
1977	30,326	19,806	54.3	34.4	74.9	38.0	65.9	65.0
1978	30,136	19,428	53.5	33.4	72.3	36.1	66.0	65.2
1979	30,777	19,843	54.2	33.9	71.8	35.7	66.3	65.7
1980	30,845	19,598	53.9	33.2	69.9	34.1	66.5	66.0
1981	30,876	19,258	53.6	32.3	68.0	32.4	66.7	66.2
1982	30,036	18,977	51.7	31.7	64.1	30.9	66.8	66.5
1983	30,591	18,775	52.4	31.1	63.3	29.5	66.9	66.7
1984	30,876	18,909	52.5	31.1	62.2	28.8	67.3	67.2
1985	30,146	18,756	51.0	30.7	58.7	27.4	67.6	67.8
1986	30,127	18,139	50.7	29.5	56.9	25.7	67.7	68.0
1987	30,237	18,103	50.6	29.3	55.3	24.7	68.1	68.4
1988	30,009	17,995	50.1	29.0	53.1	23.7	68.2	68.9
1989	30,271	17,954	50.3	28.8	51.9	22.9	68.5	69.1
1990	29,909	17,562	49.8	28.2	49.7	21.6	68.6	69.7

[a] Standardized on the age distribution of the model population for the year 1985 in Japan.

TABLE II-5. Cancer Mortality Statistics in Japan (1950–1990)
Cancer of the colon (ICD, 9th revision: 153)

Year	No. of deaths		Crude death rate per 100,000		Age-adjusted death rate per 100,000[a]		Average age at death in years	
	Male	Female	Male	Female	Male	Female	Male	Female
1950	620	837	1.5	2.0	2.9	3.3	60.4	62.1
1951	663	797	1.6	1.9	3.0	3.1	60.4	61.7
1952	606	828	1.4	1.9	2.7	3.1	60.5	62.0
1953	608	808	1.4	1.8	2.6	3.0	60.4	62.9
1954	644	862	1.5	1.9	2.8	3.1	60.6	62.3
1955	723	905	1.7	2.0	3.1	3.2	61.3	62.9
1956	772	946	1.7	2.1	3.2	3.3	62.5	63.6
1957	783	967	1.8	2.1	3.1	3.3	61.5	63.7
1958	815	1,090	1.8	2.3	3.3	3.6	61.6	64.0
1959	867	1,131	1.9	2.4	3.5	3.7	62.4	64.2
1960	910	1,129	2.0	2.4	3.6	3.6	62.6	64.2
1961	968	1,246	2.1	2.6	3.7	3.9	62.4	64.8
1962	1,047	1,296	2.2	2.7	3.8	3.9	62.6	64.1
1963	1,057	1,325	2.2	2.7	3.8	3.9	62.1	64.5
1964	1,250	1,420	2.6	2.9	4.3	4.1	61.4	64.3
1965	1,272	1,532	2.6	3.1	4.3	4.3	61.8	64.5
1966	1,349	1,654	2.8	3.3	4.5	4.6	62.1	64.8
1967	1,445	1,729	3.0	3.4	4.6	4.7	61.9	65.2
1968	1,580	1,819	3.2	3.5	5.0	4.7	62.5	64.8
1969	1,666	2,036	3.3	3.9	5.1	5.2	62.1	65.5
1970	1,766	2,052	3.5	3.9	5.2	5.0	62.3	65.2
1971	1,931	2,230	3.8	4.2	5.7	5.3	63.3	65.9
1972	2,089	2,360	4.0	4.4	6.0	5.4	63.6	65.5
1973	2,322	2,669	4.4	4.9	6.4	5.9	63.9	65.5
1974	2,508	2,761	4.6	4.9	6.7	5.9	64.3	65.9
1975	2,662	2,911	4.9	5.2	7.0	6.0	64.4	65.7
1976	2,901	3,214	5.2	5.6	7.4	6.4	64.9	66.4
1977	3,105	3,355	5.6	5.8	7.7	6.5	65.0	66.9
1978	3,353	3,763	6.0	6.5	8.0	7.0	65.3	67.0
1979	3,553	3,772	6.3	6.4	8.2	6.8	65.7	67.4
1980	3,842	4,090	6.7	6.9	8.7	7.1	66.2	67.5
1981	4,168	4,462	7.2	7.5	9.2	7.5	66.6	68.3
1982	4,494	4,729	7.7	7.9	9.7	7.7	66.6	68.1
1983	4,763	4,983	8.2	8.3	9.9	7.8	67.1	68.6
1984	5,196	5,350	8.8	8.8	10.5	8.1	67.3	69.0
1985	5,522	5,703	9.3	9.3	10.8	8.3	67.8	69.0
1986	5,895	5,983	9.9	9.7	11.2	8.4	68.0	69.5
1987	6,453	6,255	10.8	10.1	11.8	8.4	68.2	69.9
1988	6,747	6,893	11.3	11.1	12.0	9.0	68.2	70.4
1989	7,274	7,371	12.1	11.8	12.5	9.3	68.5	70.5
1990	7,791	7,718	13.0	12.4	12.9	9.4	68.8	71.0

[a] Standardized on the age distribution of the model population for the year 1985 in Japan.

TABLE II-6. Cancer Mortality Statistics in Japan (1950–1990)
Cancer of the rectum (ICD, 9th revision: 154)

Year	No. of deaths		Crude death rate per 100,000		Age-adjusted death rate per 100,000[a]		Average age at death in years	
	Male	Female	Male	Female	Male	Female	Male	Female
1950	1,199	1,072	2.9	2.5	5.7	4.2	61.2	59.6
1951	1,251	1,101	3.0	2.6	5.9	4.3	61.8	60.9
1952	1,236	1,163	2.9	2.7	5.6	4.4	61.8	61.6
1953	1,239	1,144	2.9	2.6	5.7	4.3	62.1	61.8
1954	1,351	1,207	3.1	2.7	6.1	4.4	62.6	62.0
1955	1,356	1,255	3.1	2.8	6.0	4.5	63.3	62.3
1956	1,439	1,297	3.2	2.8	6.1	4.5	63.3	63.0
1957	1,456	1,360	3.3	2.9	6.1	4.6	63.2	62.7
1958	1,500	1,417	3.3	3.0	6.2	4.7	63.7	62.9
1959	1,615	1,467	3.5	3.1	6.4	4.7	63.1	62.9
1960	1,480	1,518	3.2	3.2	5.9	4.8	64.7	63.9
1961	1,677	1,589	3.6	3.3	6.4	4.9	63.9	63.7
1962	1,679	1,579	3.6	3.3	6.2	4.8	63.3	63.9
1963	1,839	1,628	3.9	3.3	6.7	4.8	63.7	63.5
1964	1,868	1,653	3.9	3.3	6.7	4.8	63.9	64.1
1965	1,993	1,803	4.1	3.6	7.0	5.1	64.1	63.8
1966	1,961	1,879	4.0	3.7	6.7	5.1	64.2	63.1
1967	2,146	1,978	4.4	3.9	7.1	5.3	63.8	63.8
1968	2,266	2,128	4.6	4.2	7.4	5.5	64.4	64.8
1969	2,417	2,165	4.8	4.2	7.6	5.4	64.2	64.1
1970	2,555	2,162	5.1	4.1	7.8	5.3	63.7	64.3
1971	2,611	2,355	5.1	4.4	7.7	5.5	63.9	64.0
1972	2,692	2,374	5.2	4.4	7.8	5.4	64.1	64.7
1973	2,964	2,542	5.6	4.6	8.4	5.6	65.2	65.2
1974	3,178	2,739	5.9	4.9	8.7	5.9	65.1	65.4
1975	3,148	2,756	5.8	4.9	8.3	5.7	65.0	65.5
1976	3,324	2,694	6.0	4.7	8.6	5.4	65.8	66.2
1977	3,493	2,780	6.3	4.8	8.6	5.4	65.3	65.9
1978	3,504	2,898	6.2	5.0	8.5	5.4	65.6	66.3
1979	3,838	3,070	6.8	5.2	9.0	5.5	65.9	66.8
1980	3,933	2,984	6.9	5.1	9.0	5.2	66.2	67.1
1981	4,123	3,156	7.2	5.3	9.1	5.3	66.5	67.7
1982	4,131	3,153	7.1	5.3	8.9	5.1	67.0	68.0
1983	4,299	3,319	7.4	5.5	8.9	5.2	66.6	68.1
1984	4,477	3,343	7.6	5.5	9.0	5.1	66.7	67.7
1985	4,643	3,291	7.9	5.4	9.0	4.8	66.8	68.6
1986	4,732	3,420	8.0	5.6	8.9	4.8	66.7	68.5
1987	4,884	3,484	8.2	5.6	8.8	4.7	66.9	69.2
1988	5,070	3,589	8.5	5.8	8.9	4.7	67.1	68.8
1989	5,352	3,666	8.9	5.9	9.1	4.7	67.2	69.3
1990	5,569	3,701	9.3	5.9	9.2	4.6	67.4	69.6

[a] Standardized on the age distribution of the model population for the year 1985 in Japan.

TABLE II-7. Cancer Mortality Statistics in Japan (1950–1990)
Cancer of the liver (ICD, 9th revision: 155)

Year	No. of deaths		Crude death rate per 100,000		Age-adjusted death rate per 100,000[a]		Average age at death in years	
	Male	Female	Male	Female	Male	Female	Male	Female
1950								
1951								
1952								
1953								
1954								
1955								
1956								
1957								
1958	4,806	3,485	10.6	7.5	19.0	11.7	62.6	64.2
1959	4,878	3,534	10.7	7.5	18.7	11.6	62.7	64.5
1960	5,204	3,613	11.3	7.6	19.5	11.6	62.7	64.8
1961	5,064	3,530	10.9	7.4	18.6	11.0	62.8	64.9
1962	5,175	3,454	11.1	7.1	18.5	10.5	62.9	65.1
1963	5,190	3,516	11.0	7.2	18.3	10.5	63.0	64.9
1964	5,194	3,497	10.9	7.1	17.9	10.2	62.9	65.2
1965	5,006	3,497	10.4	7.0	17.0	9.9	63.3	65.0
1966	5,341	3,566	11.0	7.1	17.6	9.9	63.3	65.4
1967	5,320	3,449	10.9	6.8	16.9	9.3	62.9	65.9
1968	5,468	3,544	11.1	6.9	17.2	9.3	63.4	65.7
1969	5,838	3,635	11.7	7.0	18.0	9.3	63.5	66.1
1970	5,908	3,608	11.7	6.9	17.7	8.9	63.5	66.0
1971	6,038	3,723	11.8	7.0	17.5	8.9	63.5	66.2
1972	6,100	3,688	11.8	6.8	17.3	8.5	63.4	66.5
1973	6,333	3,699	12.0	6.7	17.3	8.2	63.4	66.2
1974	6,443	3,673	11.9	6.6	17.1	7.9	63.5	67.0
1975	6,795	3,793	12.4	6.7	17.4	7.8	63.4	66.8
1976	7,520	3,972	13.6	7.0	18.7	8.0	63.3	67.4
1977	7,937	4,062	14.2	7.1	19.0	7.9	63.2	67.7
1978	8,743	4,308	15.5	7.4	20.3	8.0	63.1	67.9
1979	9,198	4,225	16.2	7.2	20.8	7.6	63.3	68.3
1980	9,741	4,227	17.0	7.2	21.3	7.4	63.1	68.8
1981	10,332	4,515	17.9	7.6	21.9	7.6	63.1	68.8
1982	11,278	4,582	19.4	7.6	23.1	7.4	63.1	69.2
1983	12,160	4,726	20.8	7.8	24.2	7.4	63.7	69.2
1984	12,906	4,915	22.0	8.1	25.0	7.4	63.5	70.0
1985	13,780	5,192	23.3	8.5	25.8	7.5	63.4	69.7
1986	14,574	5,288	24.5	8.6	26.4	7.4	63.7	70.1
1987	15,624	5,560	26.2	9.0	27.4	7.5	63.8	70.6
1988	16,238	5,830	27.1	9.4	27.7	7.6	64.2	70.7
1989	17,040	6,045	28.3	9.7	28.2	7.6	64.4	70.9
1990	17,786	6,447	29.6	10.3	28.5	7.8	64.7	71.4

[a] Standardized on the age distribution of the model population for the year 1985 in Japan.

TABLE II-8. Cancer Mortality Statistics in Japan (1950–1990)
Cancer of the biliary passages (ICD, 9th revision: 156)

Year	No. of deaths		Crude death rate per 100,000		Age-adjusted death rate per 100,000[a]		Average age at death in years	
	Male	Female	Male	Female	Male	Female	Male	Female
1950								
1951								
1952								
1953								
1954								
1955								
1956								
1957								
1958	427	493	0.9	1.1	1.7	1.7	64.0	63.7
1959	483	543	1.1	1.2	1.8	1.8	62.3	64.5
1960	556	588	1.2	1.2	2.1	1.9	63.7	63.9
1961	609	747	1.3	1.6	2.3	2.3	64.5	65.1
1962	677	831	1.5	1.7	2.5	2.5	64.4	65.0
1963	742	932	1.6	1.9	2.6	2.8	64.2	64.8
1964	870	1,049	1.8	2.1	3.0	3.0	64.5	65.2
1965	991	1,050	2.1	2.1	3.4	3.0	64.7	65.4
1966	993	1,271	2.0	2.5	3.3	3.5	65.1	65.1
1967	1,083	1,411	2.2	2.8	3.6	3.8	65.5	65.7
1968	1,139	1,436	2.3	2.8	3.7	3.7	65.8	65.4
1969	1,252	1,519	2.5	2.9	3.9	3.9	65.2	66.0
1970	1,340	1,764	2.7	3.4	4.1	4.3	65.6	65.6
1971	1,420	1,912	2.8	3.6	4.3	4.6	66.2	66.7
1972	1,626	2,124	3.1	3.9	4.8	4.9	66.7	66.5
1973	1,674	2,254	3.2	4.1	4.8	5.0	67.1	66.8
1974	1,750	2,326	3.2	4.2	4.8	5.0	66.8	67.0
1975	1,905	2,579	3.5	4.6	5.1	5.3	67.1	67.5
1976	2,101	2,806	3.8	4.9	5.4	5.6	67.2	67.7
1977	2,267	3,087	4.1	5.4	5.7	6.0	67.5	67.7
1978	2,350	3,261	4.2	5.6	5.8	6.1	68.0	68.2
1979	2,488	3,505	4.4	6.0	5.9	6.3	68.4	69.0
1980	2,791	3,808	4.9	6.4	6.5	6.6	68.6	69.1
1981	2,961	4,095	5.1	6.9	6.6	6.9	68.6	69.2
1982	3,148	4,370	5.4	7.3	6.8	7.1	69.0	70.1
1983	3,405	4,763	5.8	7.9	7.2	7.4	69.4	70.4
1984	3,634	5,168	6.2	8.5	7.5	7.8	69.9	70.6
1985	3,949	5,521	6.7	9.0	7.9	7.9	70.4	71.4
1986	4,201	5,680	7.1	9.2	8.1	7.9	70.4	71.7
1987	4,502	6,185	7.5	10.0	8.4	8.2	70.6	72.3
1988	4,655	6,445	7.8	10.4	8.4	8.2	71.1	72.5
1989	5,034	6,571	8.4	10.6	8.8	8.1	71.2	73.0
1990	5,069	6,802	8.4	10.9	8.5	8.0	71.2	73.7

[a] Standardized on the age distribution of the model population for the year 1985 in Japan.

TABLE II-9. Cancer Mortality Statistics in Japan (1950–1990)
Cancer of the pancreas (ICD, 9th revision: 157)

Year	No. of deaths		Crude death rate per 100,000		Age-adjusted death rate per 100,000[a]		Average age at death in years	
	Male	Female	Male	Female	Male	Female	Male	Female
1950	328	198	0.8	0.5	1.4	0.8	56.0	56.4
1951	318	265	0.8	0.6	1.3	1.0	56.6	57.0
1952	364	286	0.9	0.7	1.5	1.0	57.8	56.8
1953	509	359	1.2	0.8	2.0	1.3	57.6	57.5
1954	570	448	1.3	1.0	2.2	1.6	58.1	58.8
1955	625	477	1.4	1.1	2.4	1.6	58.8	59.0
1956	719	576	1.6	1.3	2.7	1.9	59.3	59.2
1957	851	626	1.9	1.4	3.1	2.1	58.7	59.5
1958	909	711	2.0	1.5	3.4	2.3	60.1	60.3
1959	975	800	2.1	1.7	3.5	2.5	60.3	60.0
1960	1,150	825	2.5	1.7	4.1	2.6	60.4	60.8
1961	1,220	859	2.6	1.8	4.2	2.6	61.0	61.9
1962	1,353	977	2.9	2.0	4.5	2.9	60.8	61.6
1963	1,376	1,058	2.9	2.2	4.6	3.1	61.1	62.5
1964	1,613	1,173	3.4	2.4	5.3	3.3	61.9	62.3
1965	1,748	1,318	3.6	2.6	5.6	3.6	61.9	62.1
1966	1,845	1,410	3.8	2.8	5.7	3.8	61.5	62.8
1967	2,087	1,498	4.3	3.0	6.4	4.0	62.3	63.3
1968	2,257	1,543	4.6	3.0	6.8	3.9	62.1	63.4
1969	2,385	1,698	4.8	3.3	7.1	4.3	63.0	64.3
1970	2,549	1,850	5.0	3.5	7.4	4.5	63.0	63.9
1971	2,670	1,870	5.2	3.5	7.6	4.4	63.5	64.5
1972	2,857	2,073	5.5	3.9	8.0	4.7	63.7	64.3
1973	2,948	2,140	5.6	3.9	8.0	4.7	64.0	64.9
1974	3,139	2,263	5.8	4.0	8.3	4.8	64.1	65.8
1975	3,155	2,480	5.8	4.4	8.1	5.1	64.4	65.7
1976	3,430	2,499	6.2	4.4	8.6	5.0	64.8	66.1
1977	3,688	2,657	6.6	4.6	8.9	5.1	64.8	66.3
1978	3,894	2,913	6.9	5.0	9.2	5.4	65.0	67.0
1979	4,147	3,063	7.3	5.2	9.5	5.5	65.4	67.3
1980	4,483	3,352	7.8	5.7	10.0	5.8	65.4	67.9
1981	4,764	3,488	8.3	5.9	10.4	5.9	66.0	68.4
1982	5,033	3,743	8.7	6.2	10.7	6.1	66.7	68.8
1983	5,229	4,032	9.0	6.7	10.7	6.3	66.6	69.3
1984	5,389	4,096	9.2	6.7	10.8	6.2	67.1	69.8
1985	5,953	4,488	10.1	7.3	11.5	6.5	67.3	70.2
1986	6,273	4,893	10.6	8.0	11.8	6.8	67.8	71.4
1987	6,829	5,196	11.4	8.4	12.5	6.9	68.1	71.5
1988	6,906	5,649	11.5	9.1	12.2	7.2	68.6	72.2
1989	7,251	5,737	12.1	9.2	12.4	7.1	68.5	72.4
1990	7,317	6,001	12.2	9.6	12.2	7.2	68.6	72.6

[a] Standardized on the age distribution of the model population for the year 1985 in Japan.

TABLE II-10. Cancer Mortality Statistics in Japan (1950–1990)
Cancer of the larynx (ICD, 9th revision: 161)

Year	No. of deaths		Crude death rate per 100,000		Age-adjusted death rate per 100,000[a]		Average age at death in years	
	Male	Female	Male	Female	Male	Female	Male	Female
1950	575	225	1.4	0.5	2.7	0.9	62.0	60.7
1951	487	155	1.2	0.4	2.3	0.6	63.3	61.3
1952	556	194	1.3	0.4	2.5	0.7	62.7	62.0
1953	583	179	1.4	0.4	2.6	0.7	63.8	62.4
1954	539	188	1.2	0.4	2.4	0.7	64.4	64.9
1955	536	181	1.2	0.4	2.3	0.7	64.1	64.3
1956	556	199	1.3	0.4	2.4	0.7	65.2	62.6
1957	564	187	1.3	0.4	2.4	0.7	64.9	64.0
1958	537	175	1.2	0.4	2.2	0.6	65.3	66.4
1959	546	182	1.2	0.4	2.2	0.6	64.8	66.7
1960	557	181	1.2	0.4	2.2	0.6	65.4	65.9
1961	615	160	1.3	0.3	2.3	0.5	66.0	65.6
1962	569	164	1.2	0.3	2.1	0.5	65.7	65.1
1963	561	168	1.2	0.3	2.0	0.5	66.1	65.6
1964	608	146	1.3	0.3	2.2	0.4	66.8	65.3
1965	624	168	1.3	0.3	2.2	0.5	67.1	66.9
1966	665	168	1.4	0.3	2.3	0.5	66.9	68.5
1967	643	178	1.3	0.4	2.2	0.5	67.6	67.6
1968	643	148	1.3	0.3	2.1	0.4	67.5	68.0
1969	673	149	1.3	0.3	2.2	0.4	68.2	67.7
1970	773	170	1.5	0.3	2.5	0.4	68.2	66.1
1971	718	140	1.4	0.3	2.1	0.3	67.6	68.8
1972	763	144	1.5	0.3	2.3	0.3	68.4	70.0
1973	746	134	1.4	0.2	2.1	0.3	68.2	67.5
1974	818	148	1.5	0.3	2.3	0.3	68.0	68.3
1975	738	124	1.4	0.2	2.0	0.3	69.2	70.8
1976	751	146	1.4	0.3	2.0	0.3	69.0	71.3
1977	742	127	1.3	0.2	1.9	0.3	68.8	69.7
1978	766	107	1.4	0.2	1.9	0.2	69.6	72.8
1979	748	111	1.3	0.2	1.8	0.2	69.1	72.4
1980	736	130	1.3	0.2	1.7	0.2	70.2	70.9
1981	729	120	1.3	0.2	1.7	0.2	69.7	73.0
1982	736	106	1.3	0.2	1.6	0.2	70.8	72.8
1983	716	91	1.2	0.2	1.5	0.1	70.7	73.1
1984	785	87	1.3	0.1	1.6	0.1	70.3	72.3
1985	747	88	1.3	0.1	1.5	0.1	70.2	71.7
1986	740	66	1.2	0.1	1.4	0.1	70.4	72.1
1987	729	87	1.2	0.1	1.3	0.1	70.4	74.2
1988	760	96	1.3	0.2	1.4	0.1	70.6	73.8
1989	752	90	1.3	0.1	1.3	0.1	70.8	75.2
1990	770	77	1.3	0.1	1.3	0.1	70.3	75.0

[a] Standardized on the age distribution of the model population for the year 1985 in Japan.

TABLE II-11. Cancer Mortality Statistics in Japan (1950–1990)
Cancer of the trachea, bronchus, and lung (ICD, 9th revision: 162)

Year	No. of deaths		Crude death rate per 100,000		Age-adjusted death rate per 100,000[a]		Average age at death in years	
	Male	Female	Male	Female	Male	Female	Male	Female
1950	789	330	1.9	0.8	3.6	1.3	61.7	58.9
1951	809	387	2.0	0.9	3.6	1.5	60.8	60.2
1952	1,084	496	2.6	1.1	4.6	1.8	60.0	58.7
1953	1,234	518	2.9	1.2	5.2	1.9	60.3	59.1
1954	1,599	685	3.7	1.5	6.5	2.4	61.0	58.9
1955	1,893	818	4.3	1.8	7.8	2.8	62.4	59.3
1956	2,318	999	5.2	2.2	9.3	3.4	62.5	60.4
1957	2,568	1,085	5.7	2.3	10.0	3.6	62.5	61.0
1958	2,919	1,352	6.5	2.9	11.3	4.4	63.1	61.0
1959	3,329	1,410	7.3	3.0	12.6	4.5	63.3	61.6
1960	3,638	1,533	7.9	3.2	13.6	4.8	63.6	62.0
1961	3,932	1,766	8.5	3.7	14.3	5.4	63.7	61.6
1962	4,336	1,891	9.3	3.9	15.3	5.6	63.7	62.3
1963	4,768	1,968	10.1	4.0	16.5	5.8	64.1	63.0
1964	5,067	2,105	10.6	4.3	17.3	6.0	64.3	62.9
1965	5,404	2,321	11.2	4.6	18.1	6.5	64.7	63.2
1966	5,857	2,508	12.0	5.0	19.1	6.8	64.9	63.5
1967	6,296	2,566	12.9	5.1	20.2	6.8	65.2	63.0
1968	6,666	2,699	13.5	5.3	20.9	6.9	65.4	63.8
1969	7,209	2,924	14.4	5.6	22.2	7.3	65.7	64.2
1970	7,502	2,987	14.8	5.7	22.5	7.3	65.9	64.6
1971	8,042	3,087	15.7	5.8	23.6	7.3	66.2	64.7
1972	8,837	3,453	17.0	6.4	25.4	7.9	66.5	65.2
1973	9,256	3,600	17.5	6.5	25.9	7.9	66.9	65.7
1974	9,986	3,730	18.5	6.7	27.1	8.0	67.1	66.0
1975	10,711	4,048	19.6	7.2	28.1	8.3	67.2	66.0
1976	11,440	4,429	20.7	7.8	29.6	8.9	67.6	66.8
1977	12,542	4,693	22.5	8.1	31.3	9.1	67.8	67.0
1978	13,417	5,113	23.8	8.8	32.5	9.5	68.2	67.5
1979	14,600	5,323	25.7	9.1	34.5	9.6	68.5	67.8
1980	15,438	5,856	27.0	9.9	35.5	10.2	68.6	68.3
1981	16,638	6,161	28.9	10.4	37.2	10.4	68.9	68.5
1982	17,555	6,661	30.2	11.1	38.0	10.8	69.1	69.0
1983	18,644	7,007	31.9	11.6	39.3	11.0	69.4	69.5
1984	19,877	7,479	33.8	12.3	40.7	11.3	69.5	69.6
1985	20,837	7,753	35.3	12.7	41.2	11.2	69.9	70.3
1986	21,447	8,088	36.1	13.2	41.1	11.3	70.0	70.3
1987	23,132	8,597	38.7	13.9	42.8	11.5	70.3	70.7
1988	24,333	9,055	40.6	14.6	43.7	11.8	70.5	70.9
1989	25,870	9,607	43.0	15.4	45.0	12.0	70.5	71.6
1990	26,872	9,614	44.8	15.4	45.2	11.6	70.6	71.8

[a] Standardized on the age distribution of the model population for the year 1985 in Japan.

TABLE II-12. Cancer Mortality Statistics in Japan (1950–1990)
Cancer of the bone (ICD, 9th revision: 170)

Year	No. of deaths		Crude death rate per 100,000		Age-adjusted death rate per 100,000[a]		Average age at death in years	
	Male	Female	Male	Female	Male	Female	Male	Female
1950	226	186	0.6	0.4	0.9	0.7	51.5	52.3
1951	249	215	0.6	0.5	1.0	0.8	53.9	52.9
1952	386	284	0.9	0.7	1.5	1.0	53.3	52.3
1953	472	396	1.1	0.9	1.9	1.4	55.0	54.7
1954	503	396	1.2	0.9	1.9	1.3	53.3	53.5
1955	470	341	1.1	0.8	1.8	1.1	54.7	53.3
1956	536	369	1.2	0.8	2.0	1.2	53.1	55.0
1957	561	411	1.3	0.9	2.0	1.3	53.5	53.8
1958	554	405	1.2	0.9	1.9	1.2	52.9	54.4
1959	580	426	1.3	0.9	2.0	1.2	53.6	53.7
1960	586	428	1.3	0.9	1.9	1.2	52.5	54.5
1961	617	440	1.3	0.9	2.0	1.2	54.4	53.5
1962	586	489	1.3	1.0	1.8	1.3	52.7	54.1
1963	639	460	1.4	0.9	2.0	1.2	54.4	54.8
1964	583	456	1.2	0.9	1.8	1.2	54.2	55.4
1965	610	434	1.3	0.9	1.8	1.1	54.1	54.1
1966	565	412	1.2	0.8	1.6	1.0	52.9	54.4
1967	538	420	1.1	0.8	1.6	1.0	54.3	53.1
1968	506	414	1.0	0.8	1.4	1.0	52.6	54.0
1969	475	339	1.0	0.7	1.2	0.8	49.5	53.8
1970	537	365	1.1	0.7	1.4	0.8	50.8	53.6
1971	492	338	1.0	0.6	1.3	0.8	51.8	56.1
1972	476	349	0.9	0.7	1.2	0.8	54.9	53.1
1973	479	324	0.9	0.6	1.2	0.7	51.2	53.9
1974	447	344	0.8	0.6	1.1	0.7	54.1	54.1
1975	424	280	0.8	0.5	1.0	0.6	52.6	54.1
1976	398	281	0.7	0.5	0.9	0.5	53.6	54.3
1977	404	280	0.7	0.5	0.9	0.5	52.9	54.5
1978	370	300	0.7	0.5	0.8	0.5	53.9	51.8
1979	334	238	0.6	0.4	0.7	0.4	51.1	52.3
1980	288	221	0.5	0.4	0.6	0.4	51.2	46.4
1981	291	214	0.5	0.4	0.6	0.4	48.4	50.8
1982	275	183	0.5	0.3	0.5	0.3	49.1	54.5
1983	279	203	0.5	0.3	0.5	0.3	49.6	49.9
1984	248	185	0.4	0.3	0.5	0.3	49.4	51.7
1985	278	209	0.5	0.3	0.5	0.3	48.5	52.3
1986	239	201	0.4	0.3	0.4	0.3	46.7	51.4
1987	282	195	0.5	0.3	0.5	0.3	48.7	52.0
1988	262	172	0.4	0.3	0.4	0.2	48.5	51.7
1989	261	197	0.4	0.3	0.4	0.3	44.8	52.0
1990	265	190	0.4	0.3	0.4	0.3	47.8	52.2

[a] Standardized on the age distribution of the model population for the year 1985 in Japan.

TABLE II-13. Cancer Mortality Statistics in Japan (1950–1990)
Cancer of the skin (ICD, 9th revision: 172–173)

Year	No. of deaths		Crude death rate per 100,000		Age-adjusted death rate per 100,000[a]		Average age at death in years	
	Male	Female	Male	Female	Male	Female	Male	Female
1950	292	225	0.7	0.5	1.5	0.9	59.4	59.4
1951	226	239	0.5	0.6	1.2	1.0	60.7	63.0
1952	286	277	0.7	0.6	1.4	1.1	61.1	61.4
1953	279	236	0.7	0.5	1.4	0.9	60.1	63.2
1954	288	272	0.7	0.6	1.4	1.0	61.9	60.7
1955	300	263	0.7	0.6	1.4	1.0	60.5	63.0
1956	308	279	0.7	0.6	1.5	1.0	63.3	63.9
1957	303	310	0.7	0.7	1.4	1.1	62.7	63.7
1958	320	311	0.7	0.7	1.5	1.1	64.8	63.9
1959	344	297	0.8	0.6	1.6	1.0	63.3	64.2
1960	300	310	0.7	0.7	1.3	1.0	64.3	65.6
1961	297	287	0.6	0.6	1.3	0.9	63.2	64.8
1962	328	322	0.7	0.7	1.4	1.0	63.6	65.6
1963	331	319	0.7	0.7	1.3	1.0	62.4	67.9
1964	335	269	0.7	0.5	1.3	0.8	65.2	67.1
1965	325	301	0.7	0.6	1.2	0.9	64.0	68.7
1966	320	306	0.7	0.6	1.2	0.9	64.3	66.7
1967	333	354	0.7	0.7	1.2	1.0	64.7	68.8
1968	352	304	0.7	0.6	1.2	0.8	64.5	67.4
1969	374	301	0.8	0.6	1.3	0.8	65.5	68.2
1970	381	326	0.8	0.6	1.3	0.8	65.1	69.1
1971	362	345	0.7	0.7	1.2	0.9	66.0	69.9
1972	383	324	0.7	0.6	1.2	0.8	64.7	68.2
1973	401	349	0.8	0.6	1.2	0.8	65.6	68.6
1974	378	326	0.7	0.6	1.1	0.7	66.7	68.5
1975	371	333	0.7	0.6	1.0	0.7	66.1	69.0
1976	425	319	0.8	0.6	1.2	0.7	66.0	69.4
1977	409	376	0.7	0.7	1.1	0.7	66.1	68.5
1978	395	353	0.7	0.6	1.0	0.7	67.3	70.8
1979	333	286	0.6	0.5	0.8	0.5	66.0	70.7
1980	327	292	0.6	0.5	0.8	0.5	66.5	71.8
1981	348	293	0.6	0.5	0.8	0.5	67.1	70.6
1982	343	278	0.6	0.5	0.8	0.5	68.2	70.2
1983	324	267	0.6	0.4	0.7	0.4	67.3	70.7
1984	357	289	0.6	0.5	0.7	0.4	67.1	70.8
1985	367	312	0.6	0.5	0.7	0.4	66.5	72.5
1986	335	255	0.6	0.4	0.6	0.4	67.6	72.1
1987	345	338	0.6	0.6	0.6	0.5	67.7	71.4
1988	359	277	0.6	0.5	0.6	0.4	67.4	70.3
1989	343	297	0.6	0.5	0.6	0.4	68.3	71.0
1990	381	304	0.6	0.5	0.6	0.4	69.2	73.5

[a] Standardized on the age distribution of the model population for the year 1985 in Japan.

TABLE II-14. Cancer Mortality Statistics in Japan (1950–1990)
Cancer of the breast (ICD, 9th revision: 174–175)

Year	No. of deaths		Crude death rate per 100,000		Age-adjusted death rate per 100,000[a]		Average age at death in years	
	Male	Female	Male	Female	Male	Female	Male	Female
1950	29	1,419	0.1	3.4	0.2	5.4	59.9	55.8
1951	20	1,402	0.1	3.3	0.1	5.2	58.3	55.6
1952	35	1,446	0.1	3.3	0.2	5.3	61.6	55.5
1953	17	1,452	0.0	3.3	0.1	5.2	57.5	55.7
1954	26	1,526	0.1	3.4	0.1	5.2	61.0	55.1
1955	17	1,572	0.0	3.5	0.1	5.3	69.0	56.2
1956	17	1,544	0.0	3.4	0.1	5.1	62.5	56.7
1957	21	1,458	0.1	3.2	0.1	4.7	64.2	56.4
1958	14	1,692	0.0	3.6	0.1	5.3	65.0	55.8
1959	21	1,652	0.1	3.5	0.1	5.1	62.0	55.8
1960	20	1,683	0.0	3.5	0.1	5.1	61.5	56.4
1961	23	1,741	0.1	3.6	0.1	5.1	67.7	56.3
1962	18	1,740	0.0	3.6	0.1	4.9	65.8	55.8
1963	22	1,857	0.1	3.8	0.1	5.1	66.6	55.5
1964	18	1,853	0.0	3.8	0.1	5.0	68.1	55.9
1965	29	1,966	0.1	3.9	0.1	5.2	64.4	55.4
1966	29	2,100	0.1	4.2	0.1	5.4	64.9	55.6
1967	24	2,107	0.1	4.2	0.1	5.3	66.0	55.9
1968	36	2,248	0.1	4.4	0.1	5.5	66.1	55.9
1969	29	2,208	0.1	4.3	0.1	5.3	62.0	56.1
1970	23	2,486	0.1	4.7	0.1	5.8	64.9	56.3
1971	29	2,689	0.1	5.1	0.1	6.0	65.4	55.6
1972	31	2,762	0.1	5.1	0.1	6.1	65.9	56.0
1973	31	2,995	0.1	5.4	0.1	6.3	67.5	56.1
1974	22	3,059	0.0	5.5	0.1	6.3	67.5	55.8
1975	27	3,262	0.1	5.8	0.1	6.5	65.8	55.9
1976	22	3,347	0.0	5.9	0.1	6.5	71.1	56.2
1977	39	3,570	0.1	6.2	0.1	6.8	68.3	56.6
1978	33	3,755	0.1	6.5	0.1	6.9	71.0	56.8
1979	44	3,878	0.1	6.6	0.1	7.0	67.6	56.6
1980	44	4,141	0.1	7.0	0.1	7.3	66.0	56.9
1981	44	4,364	0.1	7.3	0.1	7.5	70.0	57.1
1982	31	4,311	0.1	7.2	0.1	7.2	68.0	57.5
1983	35	4,417	0.1	7.3	0.1	7.2	68.9	57.5
1984	38	4,825	0.1	7.9	0.1	7.7	68.2	57.5
1985	36	4,922	0.1	8.0	0.1	7.6	70.3	57.9
1986	37	5,127	0.1	8.3	0.1	7.8	69.4	57.9
1987	44	5,231	0.1	8.5	0.1	7.8	68.4	58.3
1988	43	5,602	0.1	9.0	0.1	8.2	68.8	58.2
1989	54	5,746	0.1	9.2	0.1	8.2	72.4	58.3
1990	34	5,848	0.1	9.4	0.1	8.2	70.7	58.5

[a] Standardized on the age distribution of the model population for the year 1985 in Japan.

TABLE II-15. Cancer Mortality Statistics in Japan (1950–1990)
Cancer of the uterus (ICD, 9th revision: 179–182)

Year	No. of deaths	Crude death rate per 100,000	Age-adjusted death rate per 100,000[a]	Average age at death in years
1950	8,356	19.7	31.0	54.1
1951	8,197	19.0	29.9	54.3
1952	8,061	18.4	28.8	54.8
1953	7,638	17.3	26.8	55.4
1954	7,703	17.2	26.4	55.6
1955	7,289	16.1	24.6	56.4
1956	7,343	16.0	24.1	56.3
1957	7,144	15.4	23.0	56.4
1958	7,105	15.2	22.4	57.0
1959	6,999	14.8	21.5	57.1
1960	7,068	14.9	21.3	57.4
1961	6,964	14.5	20.4	57.7
1962	6,940	14.3	19.9	57.8
1963	6,940	14.2	19.5	58.0
1964	6,736	13.6	18.4	58.2
1965	6,689	13.4	18.0	58.9
1966	6,667	13.2	17.5	58.8
1967	6,668	13.1	17.1	59.1
1968	6,610	12.9	16.5	59.4
1969	6,534	12.6	15.9	59.8
1970	6,373	12.1	15.1	60.1
1971	6,194	11.7	14.3	60.5
1972	6,332	11.8	14.2	61.0
1973	6,056	11.0	13.1	61.2
1974	6,149	11.0	12.9	61.7
1975	6,075	10.8	12.4	62.3
1976	5,879	10.3	11.6	62.6
1977	5,694	9.9	10.9	63.2
1978	5,710	9.8	10.6	63.5
1979	5,644	9.6	10.2	64.0
1980	5,465	9.2	9.6	64.5
1981	5,354	9.0	9.1	64.7
1982	5,179	8.6	8.5	65.1
1983	5,133	8.5	8.1	65.4
1984	4,975	8.2	7.6	65.9
1985	4,912	8.0	7.3	65.8
1986	4,744	7.7	6.8	66.0
1987	4,614	7.5	6.4	66.1
1988	4,724	7.6	6.4	66.8
1989	4,632	7.4	6.1	66.9
1990	4,600	7.4	5.9	67.2

[a] Standardized on the age distribution of the model population for the year 1985 in Japan.

TABLE II-16. Cancer Mortality Statistics in Japan (1950–1990)
Cancer of the ovary (ICD, 9th revision: 183.0)

Year	No. of deaths	Crude death rate per 100,000	Age-adjusted death rate per 100,000[a]	Average age at death in years
1950	346	0.8	1.2	47.7
1951	326	0.8	1.1	48.7
1952	329	0.8	1.0	46.0
1953	400	0.9	1.3	47.1
1954	449	1.0	1.4	48.0
1955	473	1.0	1.4	48.3
1956	533	1.2	1.6	47.8
1957	553	1.2	1.6	47.8
1958	557	1.2	1.6	48.5
1959	641	1.4	1.8	48.5
1960	647	1.4	1.8	48.3
1961	731	1.5	2.0	49.7
1962	743	1.5	1.9	49.0
1963	829	1.7	2.1	48.6
1964	842	1.7	2.1	49.6
1965	840	1.7	2.1	50.1
1966	935	1.9	2.3	50.3
1967	964	1.9	2.3	51.2
1968	1,052	2.1	2.4	50.8
1969	1,090	2.1	2.5	50.6
1970	1,129	2.2	2.5	51.7
1971	1,244	2.3	2.7	52.3
1972	1,299	2.4	2.8	53.1
1973	1,392	2.5	2.9	53.5
1974	1,428	2.6	2.9	53.7
1975	1,516	2.7	3.0	54.0
1976	1,730	3.0	3.3	53.9
1977	1,788	3.1	3.4	55.4
1978	1,963	3.4	3.6	56.0
1979	2,070	3.5	3.7	56.4
1980	2,098	3.6	3.7	57.1
1981	2,305	3.9	3.9	57.2
1982	2,349	3.9	3.9	57.5
1983	2,434	4.0	3.9	58.5
1984	2,561	4.2	4.1	58.7
1985	2,675	4.4	4.1	59.1
1986	2,686	4.4	4.0	60.5
1987	3,052	4.9	4.4	61.1
1988	3,118	5.0	4.4	61.3
1989	3,251	5.2	4.5	61.9
1990	3,279	5.3	4.4	61.7

[a] Standardized on the age distribution of the model population for the year 1985 in Japan.

TABLE II-17. Cancer Mortality Statistics in Japan (1950–1990)
Cancer of the prostate (ICD, 9th revision: 185)

Year	No. of deaths	Crude death rate per 100,000	Age-adjusted death rate per 100,000[a]	Average age at death in years
1950	83	0.2	0.5	66.5
1951	128	0.3	0.6	64.5
1952	147	0.4	0.8	67.5
1953	196	0.5	1.0	67.6
1954	235	0.5	1.2	65.8
1955	273	0.6	1.3	68.1
1956	305	0.7	1.5	69.3
1957	358	0.8	1.8	69.6
1958	431	1.0	2.1	70.6
1959	453	1.0	2.2	70.9
1960	480	1.1	2.2	71.0
1961	487	1.1	2.3	71.8
1962	578	1.2	2.5	70.5
1963	599	1.3	2.6	71.1
1964	703	1.5	3.0	72.4
1965	683	1.4	2.8	71.1
1966	717	1.5	2.9	72.2
1967	730	1.5	2.9	72.0
1968	825	1.7	3.1	72.2
1969	937	1.9	3.4	72.3
1970	883	1.8	3.2	72.6
1971	886	1.7	3.0	72.6
1972	975	1.9	3.3	72.8
1973	1,107	2.1	3.6	73.5
1974	1,179	2.2	3.7	73.3
1975	1,267	2.3	3.8	73.7
1976	1,296	2.3	3.8	73.7
1977	1,448	2.6	4.1	74.5
1978	1,499	2.7	4.0	74.5
1979	1,666	2.9	4.4	74.9
1980	1,736	3.0	4.4	75.0
1981	1,866	3.2	4.6	75.4
1982	2,053	3.5	4.8	75.7
1983	2,168	3.7	4.9	76.1
1984	2,315	3.9	5.1	76.3
1985	2,640	4.5	5.6	76.8
1986	2,756	4.6	5.6	76.4
1987	2,969	5.0	5.8	76.9
1988	3,035	5.1	5.7	77.0
1989	3,420	5.7	6.1	76.6
1990	3,460	5.8	6.0	77.2

[a] Standardized on the age distribution of the model population for the year 1985 in Japan.

TABLE II-18. Cancer Mortality Statistics in Japan (1950–1990)
Cancer of the urinary bladder (ICD, 9th revision: 188)

Year	No. of deaths		Crude death rate per 100,000		Age-adjusted death rate per 100,000[a]		Average age at death in years	
	Male	Female	Male	Female	Male	Female	Male	Female
1950	311	203	0.8	0.5	1.7	0.8	64.9	62.5
1951	357	218	0.9	0.5	1.8	0.9	65.1	62.6
1952	348	263	0.8	0.6	1.7	1.0	65.5	64.0
1953	401	267	0.9	0.6	2.0	1.0	66.5	63.4
1954	509	292	1.2	0.7	2.5	1.1	65.9	63.5
1955	528	309	1.2	0.7	2.6	1.1	66.9	65.2
1956	554	352	1.3	0.8	2.6	1.3	67.2	64.7
1957	538	384	1.2	0.8	2.5	1.4	68.0	65.5
1958	612	331	1.4	0.7	2.7	1.1	67.1	66.7
1959	646	379	1.4	0.8	2.9	1.3	68.0	65.8
1960	673	435	1.5	0.9	2.9	1.4	68.7	67.4
1961	736	407	1.6	0.9	3.1	1.3	67.8	67.5
1962	794	466	1.7	1.0	3.3	1.5	68.7	67.4
1963	770	448	1.6	0.9	3.1	1.4	68.6	68.0
1964	810	440	1.7	0.9	3.2	1.3	68.3	68.8
1965	837	454	1.7	0.9	3.2	1.3	68.3	67.2
1966	929	506	1.9	1.0	3.4	1.5	68.4	69.0
1967	951	534	1.9	1.1	3.5	1.5	69.4	68.9
1968	1,005	524	2.0	1.0	3.5	1.4	69.0	68.2
1969	1,019	577	2.0	1.1	3.6	1.5	69.5	69.4
1970	1,030	540	2.0	1.0	3.4	1.4	68.8	69.8
1971	1,000	595	2.0	1.1	3.3	1.5	69.6	70.4
1972	1,177	621	2.3	1.2	3.8	1.5	69.6	70.7
1973	1,198	621	2.3	1.1	3.7	1.4	70.5	70.8
1974	1,267	603	2.4	1.1	3.8	1.3	70.6	71.2
1975	1,174	656	2.2	1.2	3.4	1.4	70.6	72.2
1976	1,304	662	2.4	1.2	3.7	1.4	70.8	72.4
1977	1,373	640	2.5	1.1	3.7	1.3	70.9	72.3
1978	1,440	638	2.6	1.1	3.7	1.2	70.9	73.0
1979	1,515	676	2.7	1.2	3.8	1.2	71.8	73.4
1980	1,606	755	2.8	1.3	3.9	1.3	72.1	73.9
1981	1,615	732	2.8	1.2	3.8	1.2	72.5	74.4
1982	1,671	750	2.9	1.3	3.8	1.2	72.1	74.8
1983	1,670	826	2.9	1.4	3.7	1.3	72.6	75.4
1984	1,669	772	2.8	1.3	3.6	1.1	72.9	74.8
1985	1,705	872	2.9	1.4	3.5	1.2	73.2	75.1
1986	1,807	795	3.0	1.3	3.6	1.1	73.4	76.0
1987	1,815	806	3.0	1.3	3.4	1.0	73.6	77.0
1988	1,851	874	3.1	1.4	3.4	1.1	73.9	76.8
1989	1,999	939	3.3	1.5	3.6	1.1	74.5	77.8
1990	2,110	938	3.5	1.5	3.6	1.0	74.6	77.9

[a] Standardized on the age distribution of the model population for the year 1985 in Japan.

Table II-19. Cancer Mortality Statistics in Japan (1950–1990)
Cancer of the kidney (ICD, 9th revision: 189.0, 189.1)

Year	No. of deaths		Crude death rate per 100,000		Age-adjusted death rate per 100,000[a]		Average age at death in years	
	Male	Female	Male	Female	Male	Female	Male	Female
1950	114	91	0.3	0.2	0.4	0.3	44.3	49.4
1951	110	73	0.3	0.2	0.4	0.3	48.9	53.3
1952	116	86	0.3	0.2	0.4	0.3	47.9	50.2
1953	134	94	0.3	0.2	0.5	0.3	53.9	42.2
1954	165	114	0.4	0.3	0.6	0.4	50.8	48.3
1955	150	112	0.3	0.3	0.5	0.4	52.1	51.7
1956	179	145	0.4	0.3	0.6	0.4	51.0	50.9
1957	205	147	0.5	0.3	0.7	0.4	50.2	50.7
1958	220	162	0.5	0.4	0.8	0.5	53.6	49.4
1959	236	157	0.5	0.3	0.8	0.5	52.8	51.1
1960	277	175	0.6	0.4	0.9	0.5	54.7	50.8
1961	251	204	0.5	0.4	0.8	0.6	54.1	51.9
1962	306	202	0.7	0.4	1.0	0.6	55.8	53.2
1963	307	217	0.7	0.4	1.0	0.6	56.3	54.4
1964	333	191	0.7	0.4	1.0	0.5	56.6	53.5
1965	342	210	0.7	0.4	1.0	0.6	55.4	53.5
1966	361	221	0.7	0.4	1.1	0.6	57.9	54.6
1967	392	227	0.8	0.5	1.1	0.6	57.0	54.6
1968	404	229	0.8	0.5	1.2	0.6	56.0	57.2
1969	417	233	0.8	0.5	1.2	0.6	58.5	57.7
1970	436	248	0.9	0.5	1.2	0.6	59.5	56.9
1971	472	251	0.9	0.5	1.3	0.6	59.9	58.6
1972	509	280	1.0	0.5	1.4	0.6	58.7	55.6
1973	556	311	1.1	0.6	1.5	0.7	61.1	57.0
1974	556	307	1.0	0.6	1.4	0.6	60.4	58.5
1975	618	322	1.1	0.6	1.6	0.7	62.1	64.0
1976	643	307	1.2	0.5	1.6	0.6	60.9	62.1
1977	674	309	1.2	0.5	1.6	0.6	61.9	62.0
1978	754	401	1.3	0.7	1.7	0.7	62.2	62.7
1979	812	414	1.4	0.7	1.8	0.7	63.2	64.1
1980	944	422	1.7	0.7	2.1	0.7	63.9	63.6
1981	932	460	1.6	0.8	2.0	0.8	64.5	64.2
1982	1,079	491	1.9	0.8	2.3	0.8	64.3	63.8
1983	1,151	530	2.0	0.9	2.3	0.8	65.4	66.6
1984	1,275	566	2.2	0.9	2.5	0.9	65.5	67.2
1985	1,338	629	2.3	1.0	2.6	0.9	65.1	67.2
1986	1,384	682	2.3	1.1	2.6	1.0	66.0	69.0
1987	1,477	713	2.5	1.2	2.7	1.0	66.1	68.9
1988	1,580	731	2.6	1.2	2.8	1.0	67.2	70.0
1989	1,608	755	2.7	1.2	2.7	1.0	67.5	70.6
1990	1,763	850	2.9	1.4	2.9	1.0	67.4	70.2

[a] Standardized on the age distribution of the model population for the year 1985 in Japan.

TABLE II-20. Cancer Mortality Statistics in Japan (1950–1990)
Cancer of the lymphatic and hematopoietic systems other than leukemia (ICD, 9th revision: 200–203)

Year	No. of deaths		Crude death rate per 100,000		Age-adjusted death rate per 100,000[a]		Average age at death in years	
	Male	Female	Male	Female	Male	Female	Male	Female
1950	472	307	1.2	0.7	1.7	1.0	46.0	47.5
1951	512	316	1.2	0.7	1.8	1.1	46.0	48.1
1952	591	346	1.4	0.8	2.0	1.1	45.2	47.2
1953	633	366	1.5	0.8	2.2	1.1	46.9	46.6
1954	619	436	1.4	1.0	2.1	1.4	47.5	48.4
1955	718	430	1.6	1.0	2.4	1.3	48.2	47.4
1956	723	446	1.6	1.0	2.3	1.3	46.6	49.5
1957	756	447	1.7	1.0	2.4	1.3	48.3	48.3
1958	816	495	1.8	1.1	2.6	1.4	47.6	49.4
1959	919	563	2.0	1.2	2.9	1.6	48.9	51.4
1960	961	560	2.1	1.2	3.0	1.6	49.5	53.1
1961	1,009	619	2.2	1.3	3.2	1.7	50.6	52.6
1962	1,025	632	2.2	1.3	3.1	1.7	50.5	51.8
1963	1,158	697	2.5	1.4	3.3	1.9	49.3	53.5
1964	1,245	726	2.6	1.5	3.6	1.9	51.0	53.3
1965	1,283	763	2.7	1.5	3.7	1.9	51.7	52.1
1966	1,398	822	2.9	1.6	4.0	2.1	53.3	53.8
1967	1,518	848	3.1	1.7	4.2	2.1	52.4	53.3
1968	1,601	1,027	3.2	2.0	4.5	2.5	54.8	54.9
1969	1,652	1,075	3.3	2.1	4.4	2.5	53.3	56.1
1970	1,649	1,034	3.3	2.0	4.4	2.4	55.1	56.9
1971	1,711	1,057	3.3	2.0	4.5	2.4	55.8	57.5
1972	1,974	1,196	3.8	2.2	5.1	2.6	55.5	57.6
1973	1,933	1,279	3.7	2.3	4.9	2.7	56.0	57.8
1974	2,112	1,323	3.9	2.4	5.2	2.7	57.4	59.5
1975	2,272	1,450	4.2	2.6	5.5	2.9	57.2	59.6
1976	2,364	1,513	4.3	2.7	5.6	2.9	57.6	59.6
1977	2,528	1,599	4.5	2.8	5.8	3.0	58.4	61.4
1978	2,605	1,674	4.6	2.9	5.9	3.1	59.3	61.3
1979	2,731	1,844	4.8	3.2	6.0	3.3	59.7	61.7
1980	2,939	1,953	5.1	3.3	6.3	3.4	60.0	62.8
1981	3,001	2,133	5.2	3.6	6.3	3.6	60.7	64.0
1982	3,096	2,183	5.3	3.6	6.4	3.6	61.6	64.1
1983	3,387	2,264	5.8	3.8	6.8	3.6	61.6	64.0
1984	3,337	2,432	5.7	4.0	6.5	3.7	62.1	65.2
1985	3,552	2,450	6.0	4.0	6.8	3.6	63.7	66.5
1986	3,683	2,682	6.2	4.4	6.8	3.8	63.7	66.8
1987	3,816	2,792	6.4	4.5	6.9	3.8	64.2	67.5
1988	3,823	2,854	6.4	4.6	6.7	3.8	64.9	68.0
1989	3,936	2,932	6.5	4.7	6.7	3.8	65.7	68.5
1990	4,259	3,100	7.1	5.0	7.1	3.9	65.7	68.7

[a] Standardized on the age distribution of the model population for the year 1985 in Japan.

TABLE II-21. Cancer Mortality Statistics in Japan (1950–1990)
Leukemia (ICD, 9th revision: 204–208)

Year	No. of deaths		Crude death rate per 100,000		Age-adjusted death rate per 100,000[a]		Average age at death in years	
	Male	Female	Male	Female	Male	Female	Male	Female
1950	718	508	1.8	1.2	1.8	1.2	26.2	25.2
1951	787	548	1.9	1.3	1.9	1.2	26.3	25.6
1952	796	634	1.9	1.5	1.8	1.4	24.6	26.7
1953	936	723	2.2	1.6	2.2	1.6	27.4	27.4
1954	1,122	747	2.6	1.7	2.6	1.7	26.5	28.0
1955	1,214	824	2.8	1.8	2.8	1.8	26.4	26.7
1956	1,273	900	2.9	2.0	2.9	2.0	28.0	28.5
1957	1,251	971	2.8	2.1	2.9	2.1	29.7	28.6
1958	1,363	1,075	3.0	2.3	3.1	2.4	28.8	30.1
1959	1,380	1,106	3.0	2.3	3.1	2.5	29.6	31.3
1960	1,473	1,155	3.2	2.4	3.4	2.5	30.7	29.9
1961	1,504	1,218	3.3	2.5	3.4	2.7	30.7	32.7
1962	1,606	1,306	3.4	2.7	3.5	2.8	30.5	31.6
1963	1,640	1,316	3.5	2.7	3.7	2.8	31.4	32.2
1964	1,696	1,404	3.6	2.8	3.8	3.0	33.1	33.8
1965	1,765	1,394	3.7	2.8	3.9	2.9	32.8	33.1
1966	1,801	1,465	3.7	2.9	4.0	3.0	33.9	33.8
1967	1,804	1,498	3.7	3.0	4.0	3.1	34.7	35.4
1968	1,848	1,486	3.7	2.9	4.0	3.0	35.4	35.1
1969	1,865	1,561	3.7	3.0	4.1	3.2	36.7	36.3
1970	2,005	1,554	4.0	3.0	4.3	3.1	36.7	36.6
1971	1,957	1,592	3.8	3.0	4.2	3.1	37.7	37.3
1972	2,073	1,735	4.0	3.2	4.4	3.4	38.2	38.3
1973	2,185	1,694	4.1	3.1	4.5	3.2	38.6	39.9
1974	2,223	1,739	4.1	3.1	4.6	3.2	40.2	39.5
1975	2,321	1,843	4.2	3.3	4.7	3.4	40.2	40.9
1976	2,458	1,844	4.4	3.2	5.0	3.3	41.6	42.0
1977	2,527	1,884	4.5	3.3	5.0	3.4	42.5	42.5
1978	2,505	1,849	4.4	3.2	5.0	3.3	44.5	44.1
1979	2,568	1,976	4.5	3.4	5.0	3.5	44.9	46.2
1980	2,624	1,943	4.6	3.3	5.1	3.3	46.0	46.0
1981	2,713	1,978	4.7	3.3	5.2	3.3	47.1	48.0
1982	2,789	2,074	4.8	3.5	5.3	3.4	49.5	49.9
1983	2,783	2,110	4.8	3.5	5.2	3.4	49.6	50.7
1984	2,943	2,269	5.0	3.7	5.4	3.6	51.3	52.0
1985	2,983	2,196	5.1	3.6	5.4	3.4	51.6	52.4
1986	3,116	2,290	5.2	3.7	5.6	3.5	53.1	54.3
1987	3,334	2,308	5.6	3.7	5.8	3.4	53.6	55.4
1988	3,223	2,358	5.4	3.8	5.5	3.4	55.4	54.9
1989	3,397	2,379	5.7	3.8	5.7	3.4	54.8	56.0
1990	3,225	2,408	5.4	3.9	5.3	3.4	55.5	56.9

[a] Standardized on the age distribution of the model population for the year 1985 in Japan.

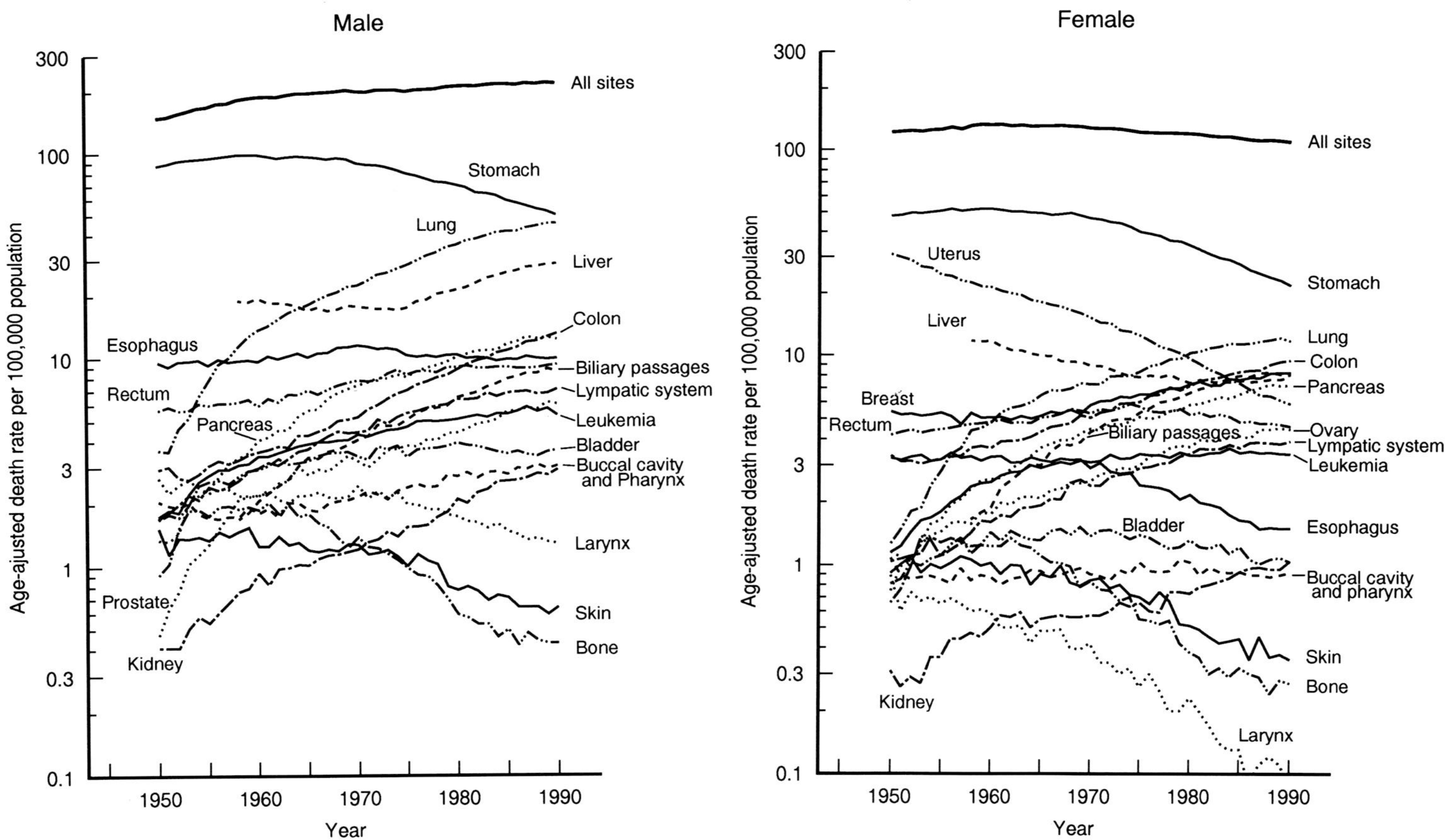

FIG. 2-1. Trends in the age-adjusted death rate* from cancer for selected sites in Japan (1950–1990)
* Standardized on the age distribution of the 'model' population for the year 1985 in Japan.

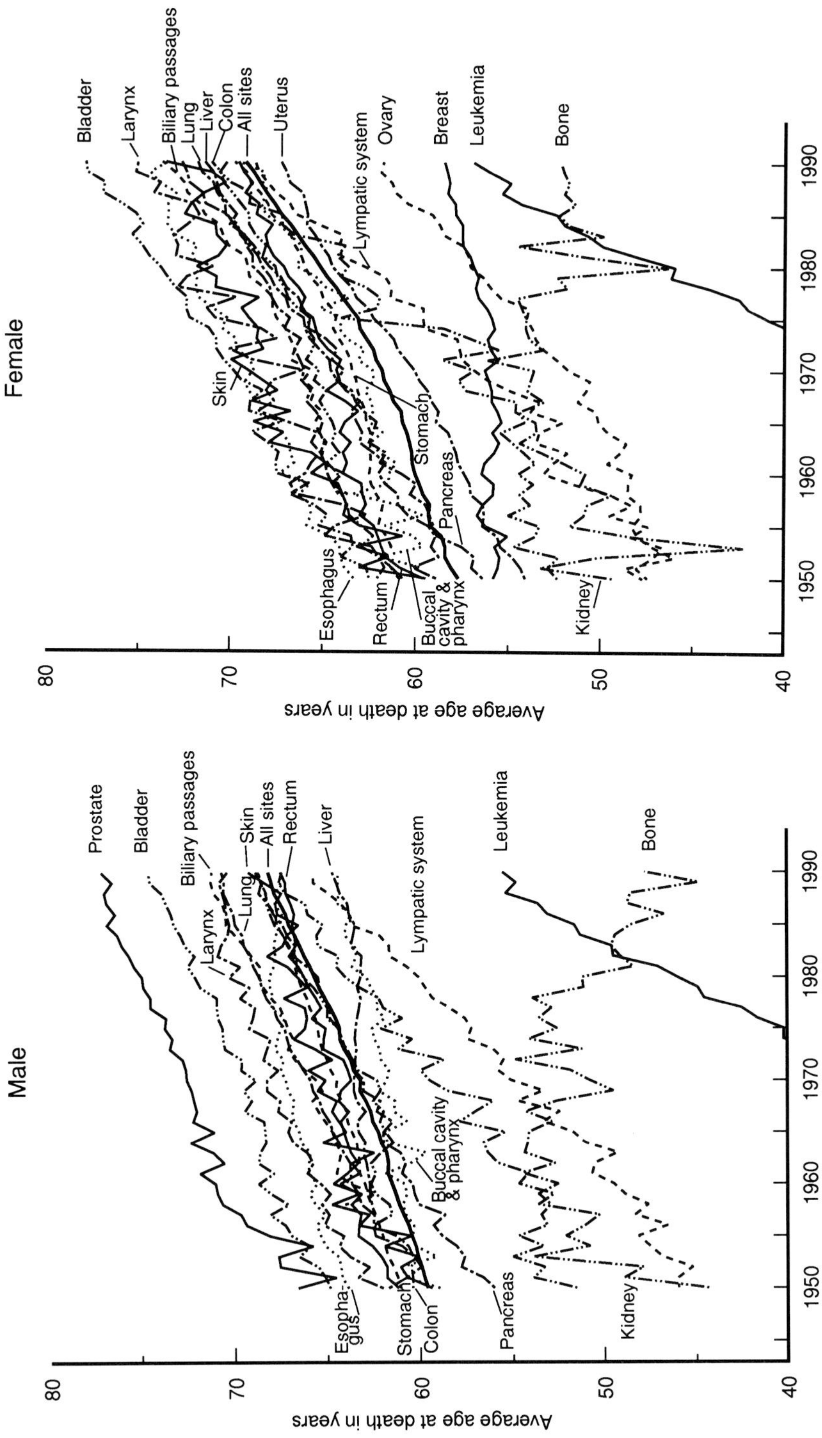

FIG. 2-2. Trends in the average age at death in years for selected sites in Japan (1950–1990)

TABLE III-1. Age- and Sex-Specific Cancer Mortality Rates in Japan (1950–1990)
Cancer of all sites (ICD,9th revision: 140–208)

	1950	1955	1960	1965	1970	1975	1980	1985	1990
Male									
0–4	5.7	6.9	8.7	8.5	8.5	7.8	6.0	4.2	3.8
5–9	2.7	4.4	4.8	6.1	5.6	5.5	5.7	4.7	3.3
10–14	2.9	4.0	4.8	5.3	4.7	4.7	4.8	4.2	3.8
15–19	4.1	5.3	6.2	7.2	7.3	6.5	6.4	6.2	5.4
20–24	4.6	5.7	6.9	8.7	8.8	8.5	6.5	5.9	6.2
25–29	7.7	9.0	10.0	12.5	12.7	11.3	10.9	9.0	8.2
30–34	15.0	17.3	18.7	19.8	20.7	19.3	17.3	15.1	12.4
35–39	29.1	33.5	33.4	35.4	36.0	33.4	32.7	29.1	26.5
40–44	63.4	65.2	65.0	60.3	63.0	60.7	55.9	53.8	49.4
45–49	116.4	126.5	124.2	119.7	114.2	112.6	118.4	102.7	98.7
50–54	211.8	218.7	230.4	219.6	205.2	187.6	214.3	212.8	182.6
55–59	354.0	351.7	386.9	366.3	357.3	345.8	333.7	363.4	373.9
60–64	523.1	570.2	592.2	606.8	579.5	541.2	558.8	543.0	598.8
65–69	713.1	787.8	858.2	884.8	902.0	853.9	850.5	837.3	831.3
70–74	775.1	974.1	1106.7	1128.7	1176.9	1207.6	1247.3	1216.1	1204.1
75–79	713.5	910.7	1166.7	1317.0	1393.5	1468.8	1634.1	1701.8	1645.8
80–84	519.9	721.5	996.2	1234.1	1359.4	1535.6	1850.9	2070.3	2156.2
85–	445.1	501.5	726.3	869.3	1078.6	1285.0	1677.2	2104.8	2451.2
Female									
0–4	4.2	5.4	6.7	6.6	6.7	6.1	5.0	3.8	3.2
5–9	1.9	3.0	3.5	4.3	4.2	4.1	3.8	3.3	2.8
10–14	2.0	3.3	4.0	4.0	4.0	3.8	4.0	3.6	2.8
15–19	3.3	3.5	5.0	5.2	5.5	4.7	4.7	3.8	3.0
20–24	4.9	5.3	7.4	7.8	7.3	6.8	6.0	4.5	4.5
25–29	11.6	11.8	12.7	13.6	13.9	12.6	11.8	9.8	7.2
30–34	26.4	23.6	26.3	27.0	24.5	24.8	20.8	18.9	16.4
35–39	56.0	49.9	49.6	45.5	41.9	38.8	36.7	31.6	32.1
40–44	104.8	91.6	84.2	74.0	71.0	63.4	57.3	55.3	49.8
45–49	152.4	138.1	138.3	120.6	111.9	101.7	89.8	83.8	80.6
50–54	215.5	201.8	189.5	188.6	163.2	156.4	141.5	128.2	118.7
55–59	283.7	273.3	270.6	262.3	243.1	221.2	204.2	185.6	176.0
60–64	375.4	367.1	369.4	358.1	347.7	308.6	296.4	275.4	248.9
65–69	470.6	485.3	495.0	488.7	471.1	446.1	421.8	388.2	363.5
70–74	484.3	578.6	636.5	642.7	639.7	615.4	612.1	563.5	528.0
75–79	463.4	600.0	714.2	756.0	788.3	773.8	814.4	788.6	742.3
80–84	379.6	524.1	667.7	739.2	793.5	850.4	961.8	1004.7	1020.3
85–	295.6	375.9	567.9	557.2	624.2	738.2	893.3	1117.7	1270.2

Mortality rates per 100,000 population.

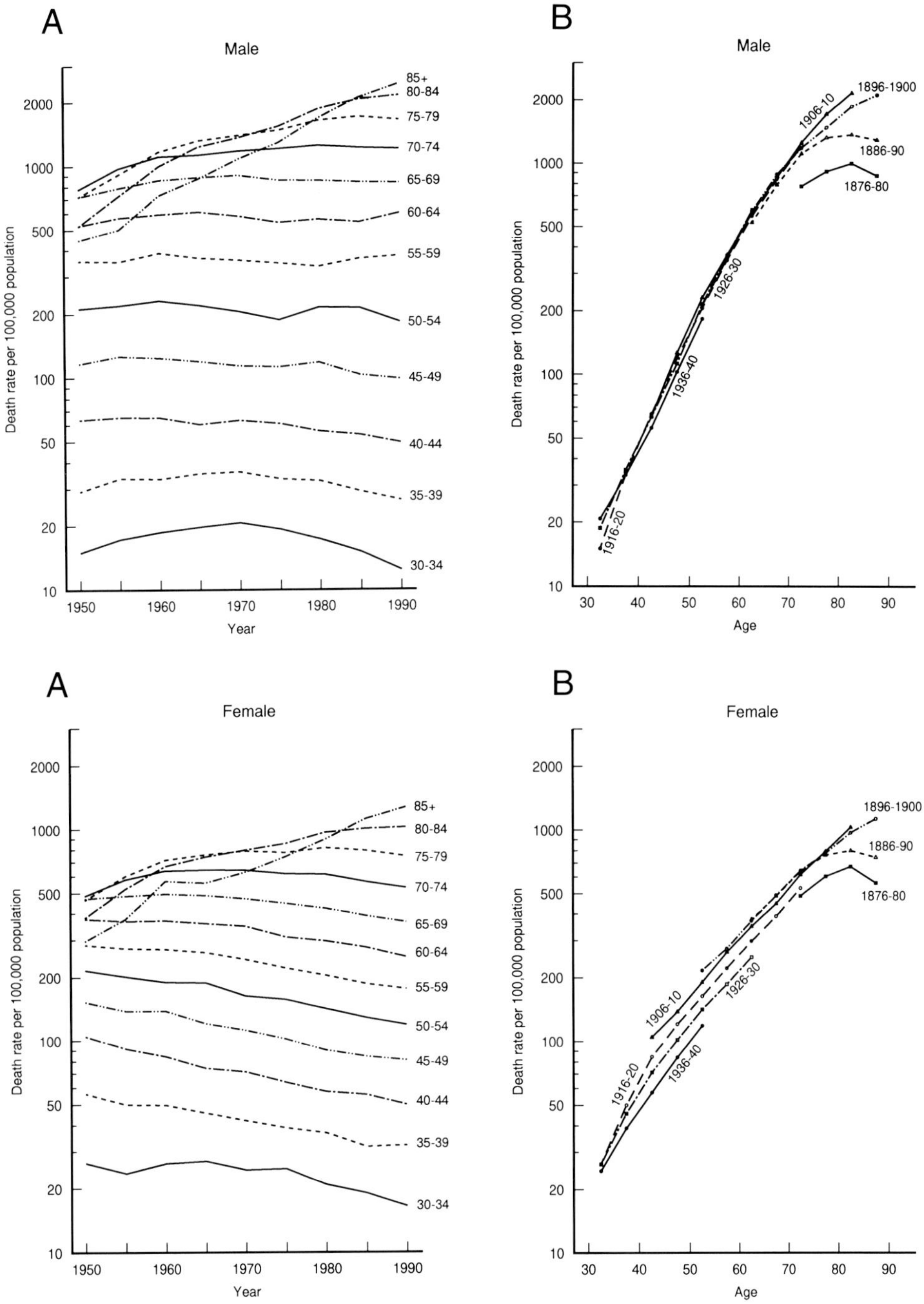

FIG. 3-1. Trends in the age- and sex-specific cancer mortality rate by age group (A) and by birth-year cohort (B) (1950–1990)

Cancer of all sites (ICD, 9th revision, 140–208).

TABLE III-2. Age- and Sex-Specific Cancer Mortality Rates in Japan (1950–1990)
Cancer of the buccal cavity and pharynx (ICD,9th revision: 140–149)

	1950	1955	1960	1965	1970	1975	1980	1985	1990
Male									
0–4	0.1	0.0	0.0	0.0	0.0	0.0	0.0	0.0	0.0
5–9	0.0	0.1	0.0	0.0	0.0	0.0	0.0	0.0	0.0
10–14	0.0	0.1	0.0	0.1	0.0	0.1	0.0	0.0	0.0
15–19	0.1	0.1	0.0	0.1	0.1	0.0	0.0	0.0	0.1
20–24	0.1	0.1	0.1	0.0	0.1	0.1	0.2	0.1	0.1
25–29	0.1	0.1	0.1	0.1	0.1	0.2	0.2	0.1	0.2
30–34	0.3	0.3	0.3	0.2	0.4	0.3	0.4	0.3	0.3
35–39	0.4	0.5	0.4	0.4	0.5	0.7	0.7	0.6	0.5
40–44	0.8	0.7	0.7	0.7	1.2	1.0	1.1	1.2	1.2
45–49	1.8	0.9	1.9	1.5	1.7	1.9	2.5	2.5	2.7
50–54	3.2	2.4	2.5	2.4	2.9	3.2	4.3	4.0	4.2
55–59	4.7	3.4	3.8	3.3	4.8	4.9	5.3	5.8	6.9
60–64	6.2	4.9	5.4	5.5	6.4	7.1	7.7	7.8	9.5
65–69	7.9	7.7	5.4	8.7	9.1	8.9	11.2	11.4	12.5
70–74	8.5	8.1	8.9	8.6	9.9	12.2	11.3	13.0	15.5
75–79	10.5	12.9	13.8	12.2	12.1	16.5	16.4	16.7	15.1
80–84	10.5	9.8	11.2	10.7	11.6	13.0	16.8	18.5	19.5
85–	24.3	7.6	8.9	14.9	19.1	16.3	22.7	20.0	21.1
Female									
0–4	0.0	0.0	0.0	0.1	0.0	0.0	0.0	0.0	0.0
5–9	0.0	0.0	0.0	0.0	0.1	0.0	0.0	0.0	0.0
10–14	0.0	0.0	0.0	0.0	0.0	0.0	0.0	0.0	0.0
15–19	0.0	0.1	0.0	0.0	0.1	0.0	0.1	0.1	0.1
20–24	0.1	0.1	0.2	0.2	0.1	0.0	0.1	0.0	0.1
25–29	0.2	0.0	0.1	0.1	0.1	0.2	0.2	0.1	0.1
30–34	0.2	0.1	0.2	0.2	0.2	0.2	0.2	0.1	0.1
35–39	0.3	0.3	0.2	0.3	0.4	0.3	0.4	0.2	0.3
40–44	0.6	0.5	0.5	0.3	0.5	0.5	0.4	0.6	0.5
45–49	1.1	0.6	1.1	0.6	0.6	0.8	0.8	0.8	0.7
50–54	1.8	1.6	0.7	1.0	1.1	1.3	1.1	0.9	1.0
55–59	1.5	1.6	1.7	2.2	1.6	1.8	1.9	1.9	1.3
60–64	2.7	2.1	1.3	2.2	2.6	3.3	2.2	1.8	2.3
65–69	5.0	2.9	2.9	2.8	2.9	3.3	3.5	3.3	3.1
70–74	4.5	3.8	3.0	4.7	4.6	4.1	4.3	3.8	4.1
75–79	5.3	4.3	5.0	5.7	6.1	7.2	7.1	6.5	5.1
80–84	9.4	7.4	10.2	8.8	5.4	6.8	9.3	8.2	9.5
85–	6.0	7.4	10.6	8.0	8.3	11.2	14.9	13.1	13.2

Mortality rates per 100,000 population.

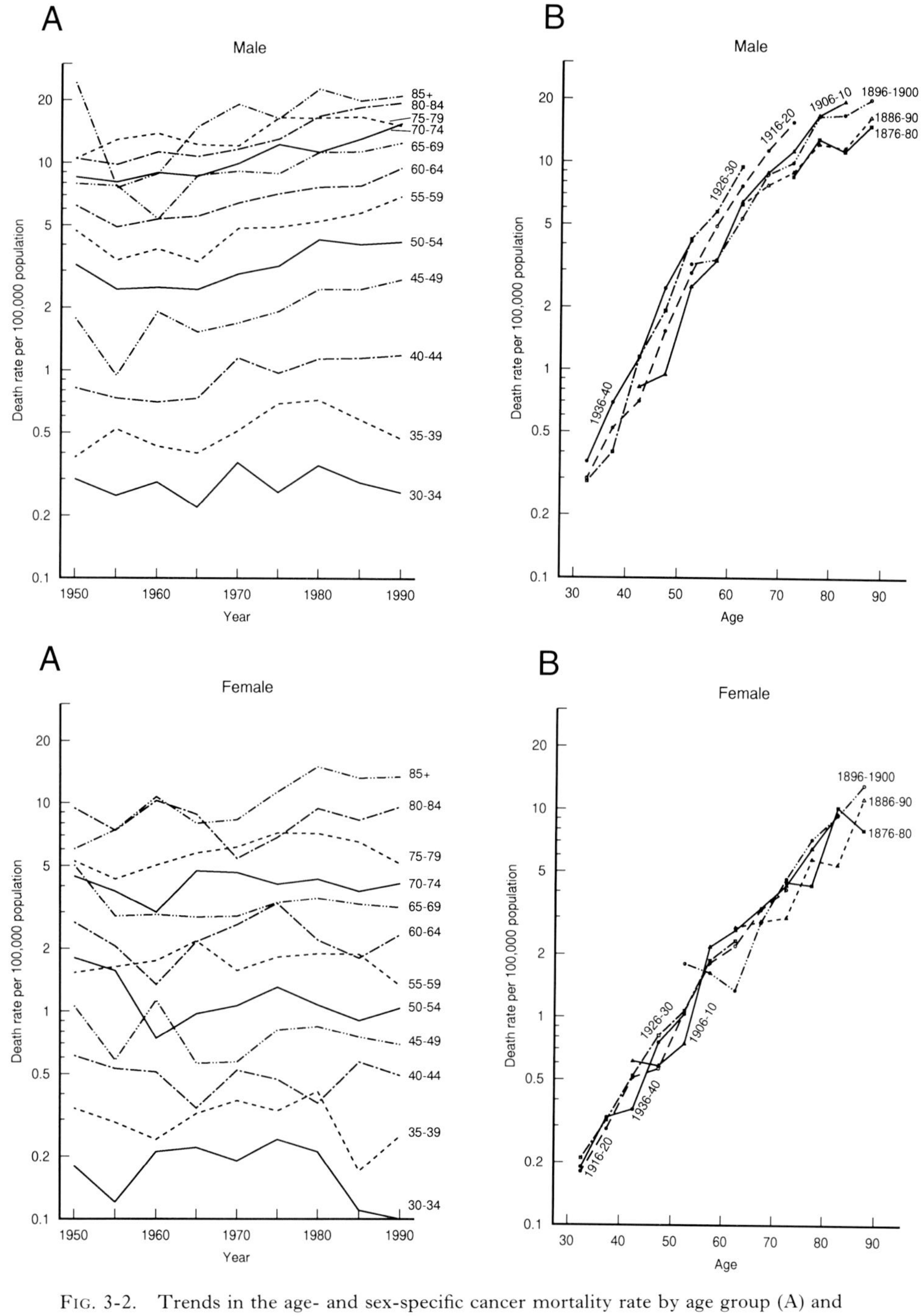

FIG. 3-2. Trends in the age- and sex-specific cancer mortality rate by age group (A) and by birth-year cohort (B) (1950–1990)
Cancer of the buccal cavity and pharynx (ICD, 9th revision, 140–149).

TABLE III-3. Age- and Sex-Specific Cancer Mortality Rates in Japan (1950–1990)
Cancer of the esophagus (ICD, 9th revision: 150)

	1950	1955	1960	1965	1970	1975	1980	1985	1990
Male									
0–4	0.0	0.0	0.0	0.0	0.0	0.0	0.0	0.0	0.0
5–9	0.0	0.0	0.0	0.0	0.0	0.0	0.0	0.0	0.0
10–14	0.0	0.0	0.0	0.0	0.0	0.0	0.0	0.0	0.0
15–19	0.0	0.0	0.0	0.0	0.0	0.0	0.0	0.0	0.0
20–24	0.0	0.1	0.0	0.0	0.0	0.0	0.0	0.0	0.0
25–29	0.1	0.2	0.2	0.0	0.0	0.0	0.0	0.0	0.0
30–34	0.3	0.1	0.2	0.3	0.1	0.1	0.1	0.1	0.1
35–39	0.6	0.5	0.6	0.5	0.6	0.3	0.2	0.4	0.4
40–44	2.1	1.1	1.5	1.5	1.5	1.5	0.9	1.4	1.2
45–49	4.5	3.0	3.5	3.4	4.1	3.9	4.3	4.2	4.5
50–54	10.2	8.4	9.0	7.7	7.9	9.1	10.3	11.0	10.7
55–59	21.3	16.9	18.7	17.7	19.8	17.2	18.3	20.8	21.4
60–64	32.0	31.9	31.2	31.9	36.4	32.0	29.2	29.6	32.3
65–69	52.9	52.9	51.0	51.9	55.9	50.3	48.1	41.9	44.6
70–74	67.6	64.5	63.6	69.2	77.8	65.4	63.3	53.9	57.9
75–79	54.2	59.9	70.1	72.4	82.3	83.5	81.3	74.6	67.2
80–84	38.7	54.1	70.4	73.8	100.9	80.1	90.5	80.8	76.9
85–	27.8	42.8	23.0	70.4	76.5	67.8	91.5	80.6	70.5
Female									
0–4	0.0	0.0	0.0	0.0	0.0	0.0	0.0	0.0	0.0
5–9	0.0	0.0	0.0	0.0	0.0	0.0	0.0	0.0	0.0
10–14	0.0	0.0	0.0	0.0	0.0	0.0	0.0	0.0	0.0
15–19	0.0	0.0	0.0	0.0	0.0	0.0	0.0	0.0	0.0
20–24	0.0	0.0	0.1	0.0	0.0	0.0	0.0	0.0	0.0
25–29	0.1	0.0	0.2	0.1	0.0	0.0	0.0	0.0	0.0
30–34	0.3	0.2	0.0	0.1	0.1	0.0	0.0	0.0	0.1
35–39	0.6	0.5	0.4	0.3	0.3	0.1	0.0	0.0	0.2
40–44	1.4	1.3	0.9	0.4	0.5	0.5	0.4	0.1	0.2
45–49	2.4	1.8	1.5	1.2	1.2	0.7	0.4	0.5	0.6
50–54	4.4	2.9	3.0	2.8	2.1	1.9	1.3	1.0	1.3
55–59	6.4	6.0	5.2	5.6	4.4	3.4	2.6	1.9	2.3
60–64	11.2	9.5	8.4	7.8	6.5	5.7	5.2	3.4	2.9
65–69	15.8	14.4	14.7	13.6	13.0	9.4	8.7	6.7	4.8
70–74	18.2	18.9	19.9	22.4	19.4	14.8	14.5	9.6	8.5
75–79	17.9	25.5	26.1	27.3	25.9	20.5	19.5	15.5	13.8
80–84	14.4	21.3	29.0	26.1	31.7	27.8	26.5	21.0	15.4
85–	13.5	16.9	30.4	21.6	18.0	29.9	28.0	26.9	29.1

Mortality rates per 100,000 population.

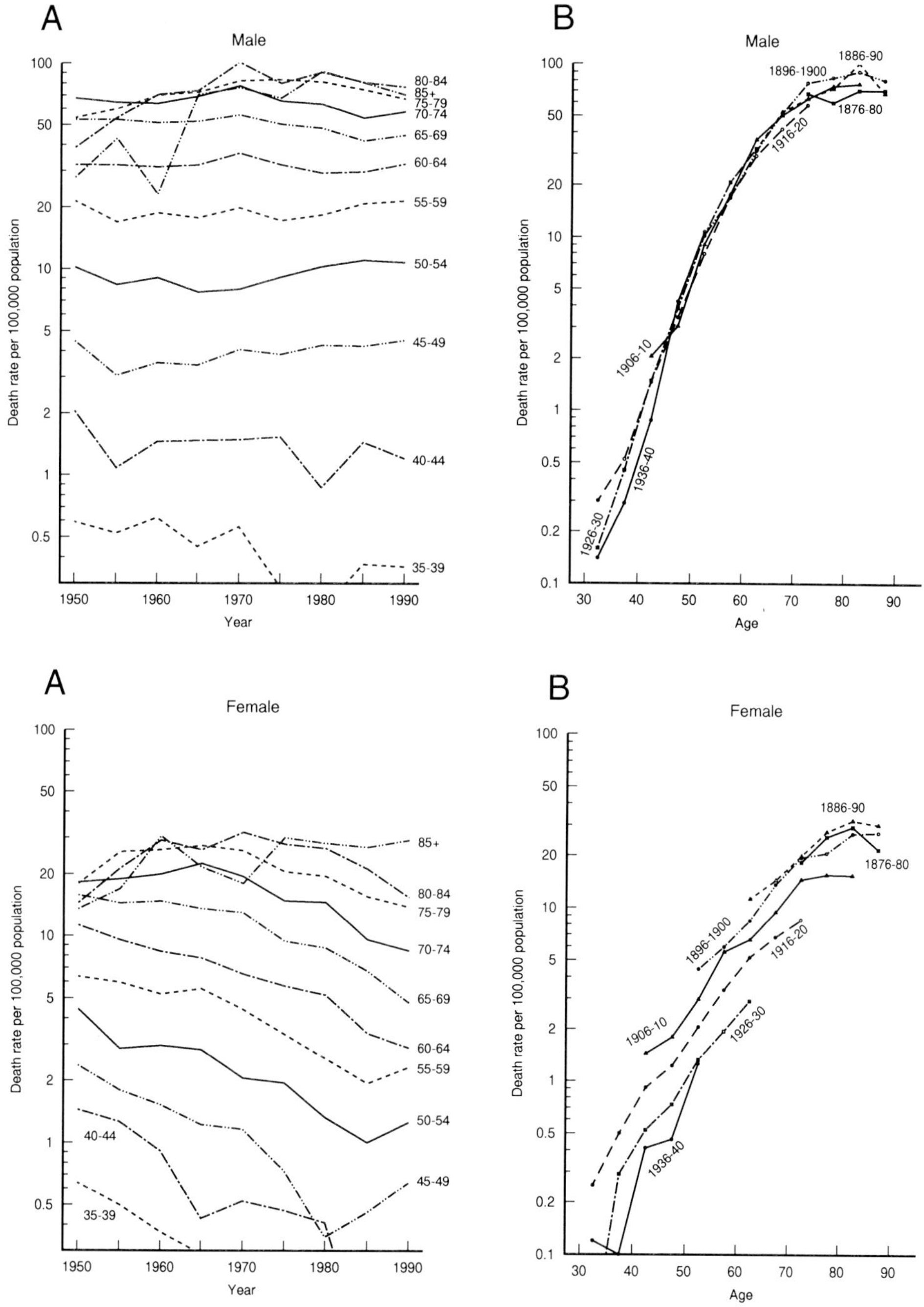

FIG. 3-3. Trends in the age- and sex-specific cancer mortality rate by age group (A) and by birth-year cohort (B) (1950–1990)

Cancer of the esophagus (ICD, 9th revision, 150).

TABLE III-4. Age- and Sex-Specific Cancer Mortality Rates in Japan (1950–1990)
Cancer of the stomach (ICD, 9th revision: 151)

	1950	1955	1960	1965	1970	1975	1980	1985	1990
Male									
0–4	0.1	0.0	0.0	0.0	0.0	0.0	0.0	0.0	0.0
5–9	0.1	0.0	0.0	0.0	0.0	0.0	0.0	0.0	0.0
10–14	0.2	0.0	0.0	0.0	0.0	0.0	0.0	0.0	0.0
15–19	0.2	0.2	0.3	0.3	0.4	0.2	0.1	0.1	0.2
20–24	0.7	0.7	1.1	1.6	1.5	1.3	0.7	0.5	0.4
25–29	2.3	2.8	3.1	3.8	3.6	3.0	2.3	2.2	1.2
30–34	7.0	7.0	8.0	8.5	8.3	6.7	5.7	4.3	2.6
35–39	15.1	17.0	17.0	16.4	15.3	13.4	11.5	8.4	7.1
40–44	35.8	36.7	34.7	28.6	27.5	24.4	19.3	15.9	12.1
45–49	69.6	73.4	67.2	58.8	52.2	45.0	39.4	29.3	24.7
50–54	128.3	128.0	121.9	110.5	93.0	74.0	69.8	56.3	44.5
55–59	219.3	211.3	206.3	189.9	158.4	139.5	105.5	95.8	79.4
60–64	324.6	336.2	317.8	307.2	265.6	218.3	186.4	146.6	132.2
65–69	435.4	456.5	467.2	449.8	409.0	341.1	289.0	230.6	187.0
70–74	463.6	546.2	597.8	568.1	545.5	489.1	417.0	330.8	274.4
75–79	397.1	509.3	607.6	666.1	651.7	602.0	560.7	463.8	386.8
80–84	273.0	359.6	490.1	553.1	604.4	650.8	632.4	605.3	519.2
85–	219.1	234.4	329.5	362.9	391.4	499.2	545.9	607.5	613.7
Female									
0–4	0.0	0.0	0.0	0.0	0.0	0.0	0.0	0.0	0.0
5–9	0.1	0.0	0.0	0.0	0.0	0.0	0.0	0.0	0.0
10–14	0.1	0.0	0.0	0.0	0.0	0.0	0.0	0.0	0.0
15–19	0.2	0.2	0.2	0.2	0.5	0.2	0.1	0.1	0.0
20–24	1.0	1.0	1.3	1.4	1.6	1.4	1.1	0.5	0.6
25–29	3.4	3.1	3.7	4.7	5.1	4.6	4.0	3.2	1.9
30–34	8.5	8.7	10.3	10.5	9.1	10.1	8.1	6.6	4.7
35–39	15.5	17.7	18.2	17.9	16.0	15.0	13.5	10.6	8.7
40–44	29.7	29.9	31.2	26.5	25.6	21.4	17.9	15.2	12.8
45–49	45.4	44.0	45.0	42.2	37.5	31.2	24.8	21.1	15.9
50–54	69.8	69.3	64.7	63.9	54.2	45.1	35.6	28.0	23.0
55–59	108.7	104.8	96.7	88.6	82.4	64.0	52.9	39.7	30.0
60–64	158.3	153.6	142.1	128.9	119.1	97.2	80.9	63.1	45.3
65–69	219.4	223.0	208.7	192.9	175.0	145.6	116.5	88.1	68.7
70–74	235.0	264.2	282.8	275.0	254.4	211.3	173.0	131.8	98.3
75–79	229.5	284.1	321.3	316.1	321.2	279.0	250.9	194.6	150.2
80–84	169.8	253.9	307.2	315.1	332.0	319.1	307.7	268.6	226.2
85–	133.5	162.0	237.2	230.0	239.6	258.1	293.5	316.7	298.2

Mortality rates per 100,000 population.

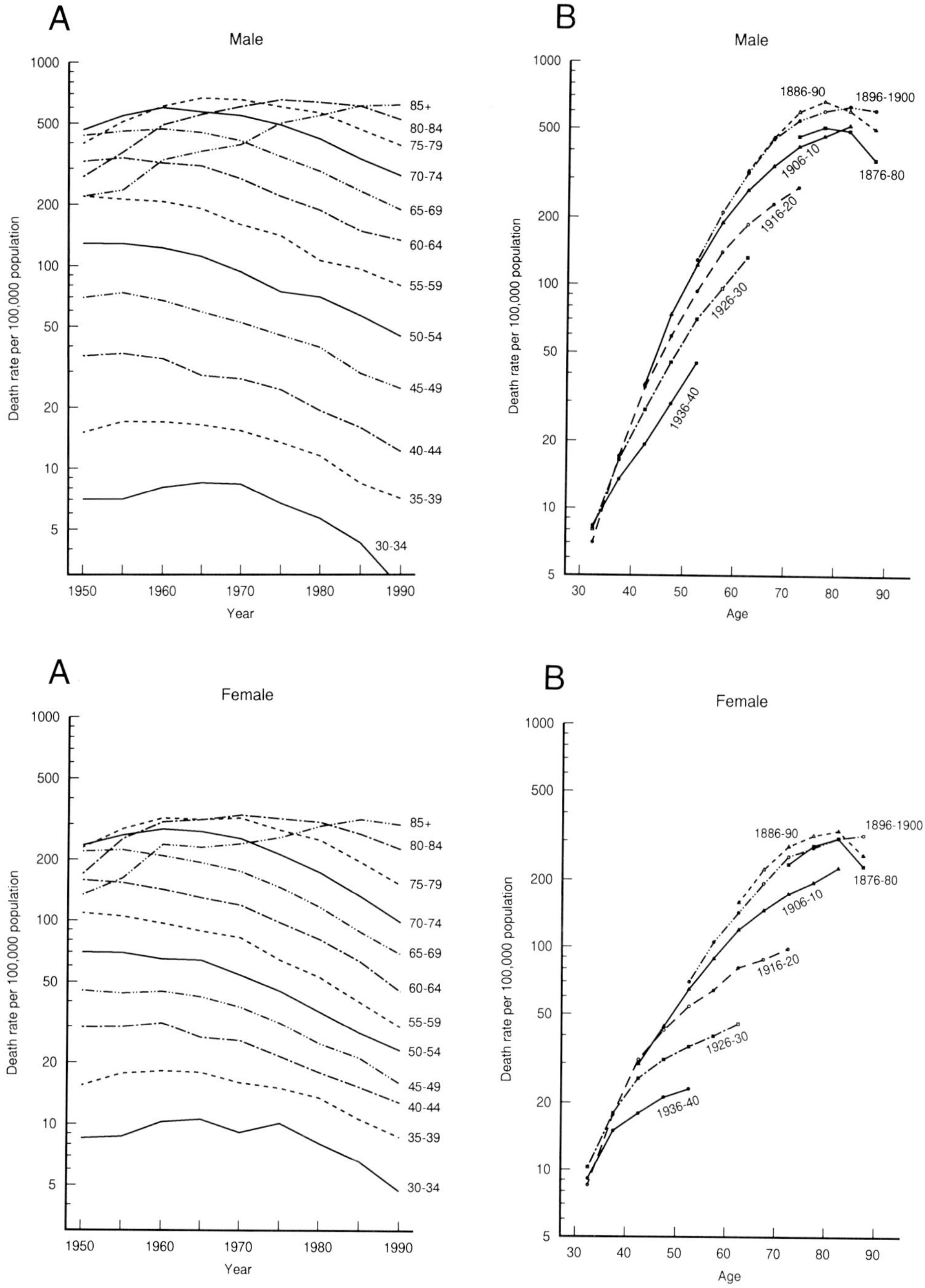

FIG. 3-4. Trends in the age- and sex-specific cancer mortality rate by age group (A) and by birth-year cohort (B) (1950–1990)

Cancer of the stomach (ICD, 9th revision, 151).

TABLE III-5. Age- and Sex-Specific Cancer Mortality Rates in Japan (1950–1990)
Cancer of the colon (ICD, 9th revision: 153)

	1950	1955	1960	1965	1970	1975	1980	1985	1990
Male									
0–4	0.1	0.0	0.1	0.0	0.0	0.0	0.0	0.0	0.0
5–9	0.0	0.0	0.0	0.0	0.0	0.0	0.0	0.0	0.0
10–14	0.1	0.0	0.0	0.1	0.0	0.0	0.0	0.0	0.1
15–19	0.1	0.1	0.1	0.2	0.1	0.1	0.1	0.0	0.1
20–24	0.1	0.1	0.2	0.2	0.5	0.3	0.1	0.3	0.3
25–29	0.2	0.3	0.4	0.6	0.8	0.6	0.6	0.5	0.4
30–34	0.3	0.4	0.5	0.8	1.1	0.9	1.2	1.1	0.8
35–39	0.8	0.9	0.8	1.1	1.5	1.9	2.2	1.3	1.6
40–44	1.4	1.2	1.2	1.9	2.3	3.1	2.7	3.0	3.2
45–49	1.9	2.7	2.2	2.8	3.5	4.0	5.0	5.4	6.2
50–54	3.6	3.0	3.4	4.8	5.1	6.7	7.4	10.0	11.2
55–59	5.9	5.0	6.0	7.2	9.2	11.9	13.4	18.2	21.7
60–64	10.0	10.1	9.4	11.1	11.8	16.5	20.6	26.4	35.2
65–69	13.1	13.0	14.3	16.7	22.7	26.8	33.0	36.0	47.7
70–74	15.0	19.5	21.1	25.7	27.4	36.5	50.6	59.9	66.2
75–79	17.9	16.4	24.4	28.6	40.7	53.0	67.9	86.6	91.0
80–84	15.7	16.5	24.8	30.0	40.3	64.5	93.4	117.1	146.3
85–	13.9	20.2	39.0	29.8	27.0	67.0	79.8	130.0	188.1
Female									
0–4	0.0	0.0	0.1	0.0	0.0	0.0	0.0	0.0	0.0
5–9	0.0	0.0	0.0	0.1	0.0	0.0	0.0	0.0	0.0
10–14	0.0	0.0	0.0	0.0	0.0	0.0	0.0	0.0	0.0
15–19	0.0	0.0	0.1	0.0	0.0	0.1	0.1	0.1	0.0
20–24	0.1	0.2	0.1	0.4	0.2	0.1	0.3	0.2	0.3
25–29	0.3	0.2	0.3	0.3	0.6	0.5	0.5	0.6	0.3
30–34	0.5	0.5	0.5	0.8	0.8	1.1	0.9	0.8	0.9
35–39	0.9	0.9	1.3	0.9	1.4	1.8	1.7	1.7	1.6
40–44	1.9	1.7	1.5	1.7	2.2	2.8	2.6	3.4	3.2
45–49	2.2	2.2	2.3	3.1	3.3	4.0	4.5	5.4	5.9
50–54	4.0	3.8	3.4	5.3	5.2	6.8	7.9	9.6	9.1
55–59	7.4	5.6	6.4	6.5	7.6	9.8	11.4	13.3	15.5
60–64	11.6	9.1	9.4	10.7	11.7	13.3	17.1	19.5	22.1
65–69	15.6	14.7	14.2	15.1	18.3	20.8	24.8	28.0	32.1
70–74	18.1	19.5	22.1	26.7	29.3	34.1	37.5	42.0	47.8
75–79	16.3	19.7	24.7	34.9	42.4	44.9	56.1	61.8	68.0
80–84	16.7	16.8	28.4	32.0	44.9	56.8	68.7	89.0	100.5
85–	10.5	15.9	23.6	30.7	30.6	45.2	71.5	92.2	131.3

Mortality rates per 100,000 population.

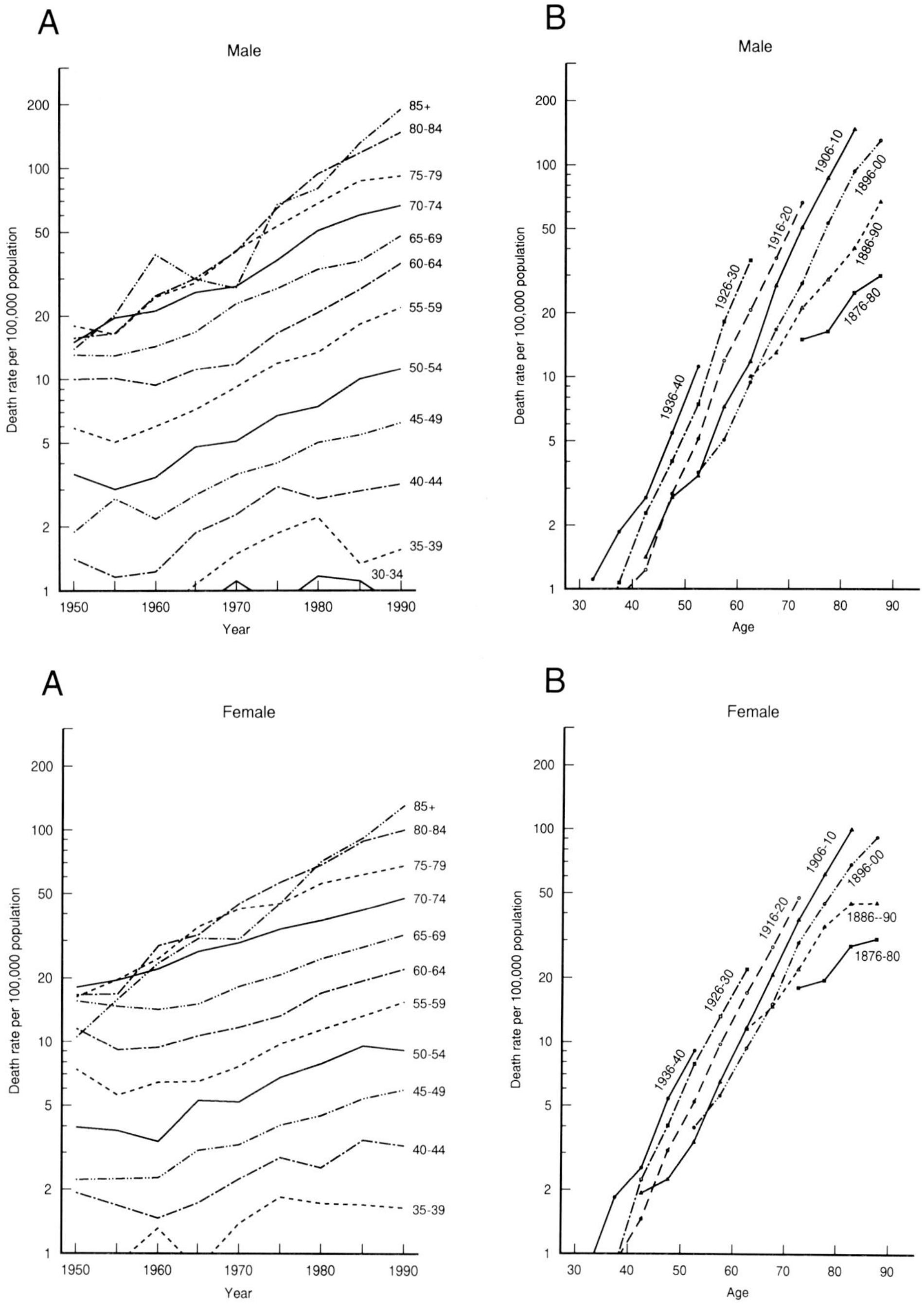

FIG. 3-5. Trends in the age- and sex-specific cancer mortality rate by age group (A) and by birth-year cohort (B) (1950–1990)

Cancer of the colon (ICD, 9th revision, 153).

TABLE III-6. Age- and Sex-Specific Cancer Mortality Rates in Japan (1950–1990)
Cancer of the rectum (ICD, 9th revision: 154)

	1950	1955	1960	1965	1970	1975	1980	1985	1990
Male									
0–4	0.0	0.0	0.0	0.0	0.0	0.0	0.0	0.0	0.0
5–9	0.0	0.0	0.0	0.0	0.0	0.0	0.0	0.0	0.0
10–14	0.0	0.0	0.0	0.0	0.0	0.0	0.0	0.0	0.0
15–19	0.1	0.1	0.1	0.1	0.1	0.1	0.0	0.0	0.0
20–24	0.1	0.1	0.2	0.6	0.4	0.2	0.1	0.1	0.0
25–29	0.6	0.3	0.2	0.5	1.1	0.6	0.4	0.3	0.2
30–34	0.9	0.6	0.7	0.9	1.2	1.5	1.0	0.6	0.6
35–39	1.3	1.2	0.6	1.0	2.1	2.2	2.1	1.6	1.4
40–44	1.9	2.3	2.0	1.9	2.8	3.2	3.6	3.3	2.9
45–49	4.8	3.8	2.8	4.2	4.4	4.9	6.0	5.5	6.0
50–54	7.0	4.9	4.9	6.4	7.1	6.4	9.1	10.3	10.4
55–59	11.5	9.6	8.9	10.7	12.0	12.3	12.0	16.1	17.4
60–64	17.8	17.2	17.4	17.7	19.2	19.9	20.0	20.9	25.2
65–69	25.0	25.8	23.6	29.3	30.5	32.2	32.1	31.8	33.6
70–74	34.4	39.2	41.1	39.5	44.1	47.2	51.4	46.6	44.6
75–79	38.5	46.2	44.6	52.9	59.5	65.6	69.3	67.4	60.4
80–84	20.9	38.3	46.7	71.7	70.6	84.0	90.2	93.2	93.3
85–	13.9	32.8	46.1	56.9	66.4	69.4	102.0	97.1	111.2
Female									
0–4	0.0	0.0	0.0	0.0	0.0	0.0	0.0	0.0	0.0
5–9	0.0	0.0	0.0	0.0	0.0	0.0	0.0	0.0	0.0
10–14	0.0	0.0	0.0	0.0	0.0	0.0	0.0	0.0	0.0
15–19	0.0	0.1	0.1	0.0	0.0	0.0	0.0	0.0	0.0
20–24	0.1	0.2	0.1	0.4	0.1	0.1	0.1	0.1	0.1
25–29	0.4	0.3	0.3	0.6	0.9	0.5	0.3	0.2	0.1
30–34	1.0	0.3	0.5	0.9	1.3	1.4	0.8	0.5	0.5
35–39	1.7	1.1	1.1	1.2	1.6	2.0	1.7	0.9	1.0
40–44	3.0	2.9	2.0	2.3	2.3	2.6	2.8	2.4	1.6
45–49	4.5	3.5	4.0	3.9	3.3	4.3	3.9	4.0	4.3
50–54	6.9	6.7	6.0	5.6	7.0	6.1	6.0	5.8	6.5
55–59	10.2	10.1	9.6	9.2	8.3	9.6	7.9	8.1	8.3
60–64	12.6	13.5	13.3	11.6	11.9	12.3	11.4	11.3	11.3
65–69	18.2	17.1	18.5	20.0	19.4	18.8	15.7	15.6	14.7
70–74	18.6	21.8	29.0	28.5	27.1	30.8	26.2	23.7	20.2
75–79	15.3	27.2	33.7	36.5	41.8	41.0	40.4	32.3	29.5
80–84	16.1	25.4	29.6	41.6	44.4	54.6	53.5	45.7	42.1
85–	15.0	16.9	24.3	28.4	38.3	50.8	53.8	62.5	61.2

Mortality rates per 100,000 population.

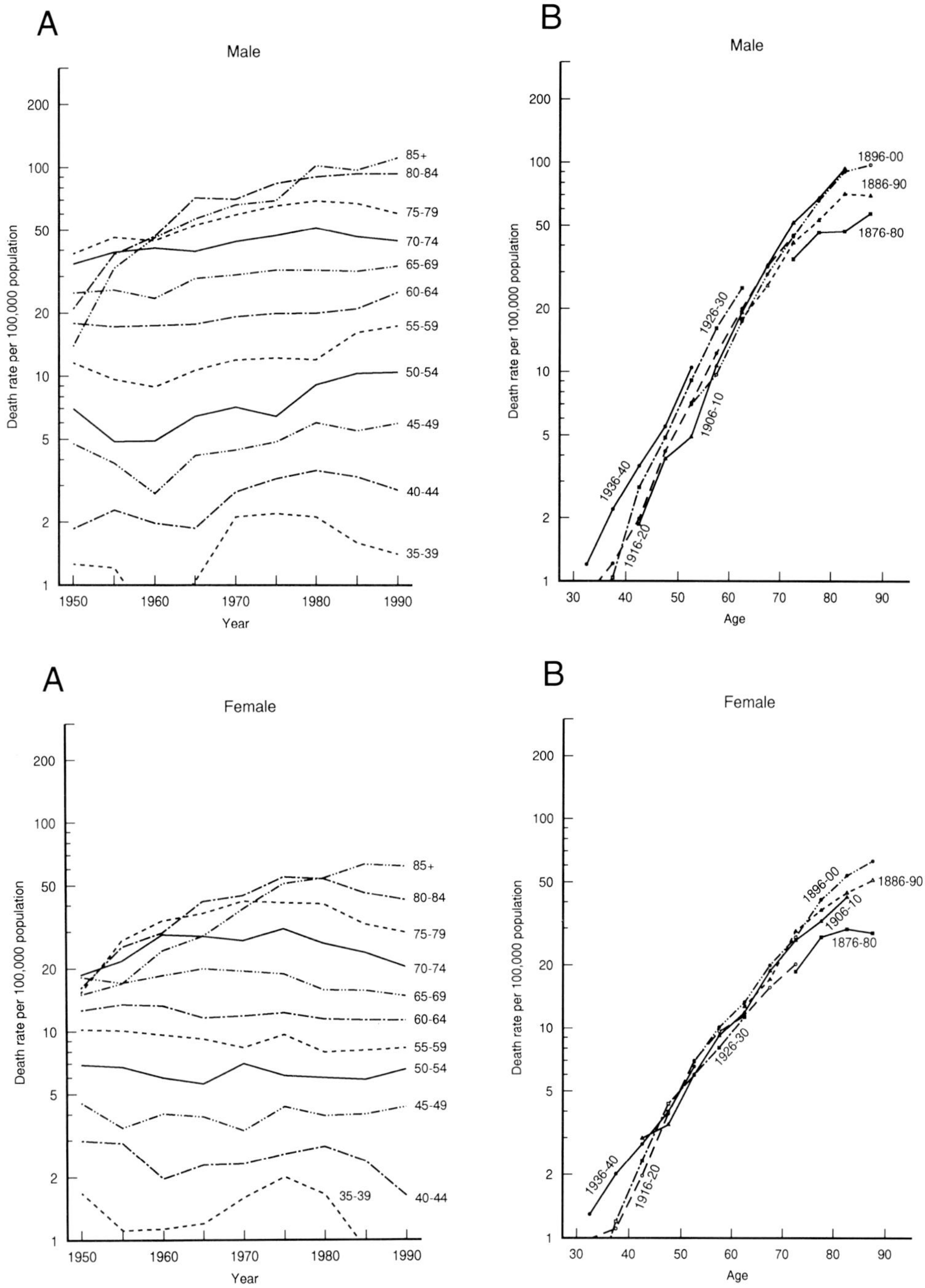

FIG. 3-6. Trends in the age- and sex-specific cancer mortality rate by age group (A) and by birth-year cohort (B) (1950–1990)

Cancer of the rectum (ICD, 9th revision, 154).

TABLE III-7. Age- and Sex-Specific Cancer Mortality Rates in Japan (1950–1990)
Cancer of the liver (ICD, 9th revision: 155)

	1950	1955	1960	1965	1970	1975	1980	1985	1990
Male									
0–4			0.2	0.3	0.4	0.5	0.3	0.4	0.2
5–9			0.1	0.1	0.2	0.1	0.1	0.1	0.0
10–14			0.1	0.1	0.1	0.0	0.1	0.1	0.0
15–19			0.2	0.1	0.0	0.1	0.1	0.1	0.1
20–24			0.4	0.2	0.3	0.3	0.2	0.1	0.1
25–29			0.5	0.5	0.4	0.4	0.4	0.3	0.2
30–34			1.1	0.9	0.9	1.4	1.3	1.0	0.7
35–39			2.4	2.8	3.1	2.7	2.9	3.6	2.7
40–44			6.3	6.3	6.4	6.9	6.3	7.3	7.2
45–49			12.5	13.1	12.4	13.6	20.7	17.5	15.5
50–54			28.6	20.5	23.7	23.5	37.3	50.9	35.1
55–59			42.6	33.1	37.2	38.9	50.0	72.8	95.0
60–64			64.1	53.3	50.6	51.0	69.6	87.1	115.3
65–69			83.9	71.7	76.7	74.1	79.6	98.4	118.8
70–74			115.4	90.0	94.5	92.3	107.2	114.7	128.1
75–79			127.2	114.9	117.6	101.0	113.6	133.1	137.9
80–84			87.5	125.2	115.8	113.6	132.0	146.3	157.9
85–			76.2	81.2	106.9	107.0	107.2	130.0	155.0
Female									
0–4			0.3	0.4	0.3	0.3	0.2	0.3	0.2
5–9			0.0	0.0	0.1	0.1	0.0	0.1	0.0
10–14			0.0	0.1	0.0	0.1	0.1	0.1	0.1
15–19			0.1	0.1	0.1	0.0	0.0	0.1	0.0
20–24			0.3	0.2	0.2	0.2	0.0	0.0	0.1
25–29			0.3	0.3	0.3	0.3	0.1	0.2	0.2
30–34			0.7	1.0	0.7	0.4	0.3	0.4	0.3
35–39			2.1	1.5	1.3	1.2	1.1	0.7	0.5
40–44			4.3	3.0	2.7	2.4	1.9	1.4	0.9
45–49			7.9	6.5	5.3	4.5	3.2	3.3	2.1
50–54			13.1	11.0	9.4	7.8	6.0	6.4	4.9
55–59			20.8	18.0	15.7	13.1	12.1	13.0	12.8
60–64			36.8	28.3	23.9	20.9	19.0	22.2	24.2
65–69			49.7	45.4	37.1	32.9	30.5	30.7	37.1
70–74			70.0	57.5	54.3	47.5	45.3	43.8	49.0
75–79			80.3	74.8	72.5	59.7	60.9	59.3	58.0
80–84			71.4	65.1	61.8	65.8	69.8	70.2	71.0
85–			64.6	51.7	60.1	56.0	62.5	72.5	86.2

Mortality rates per 100,000 population.

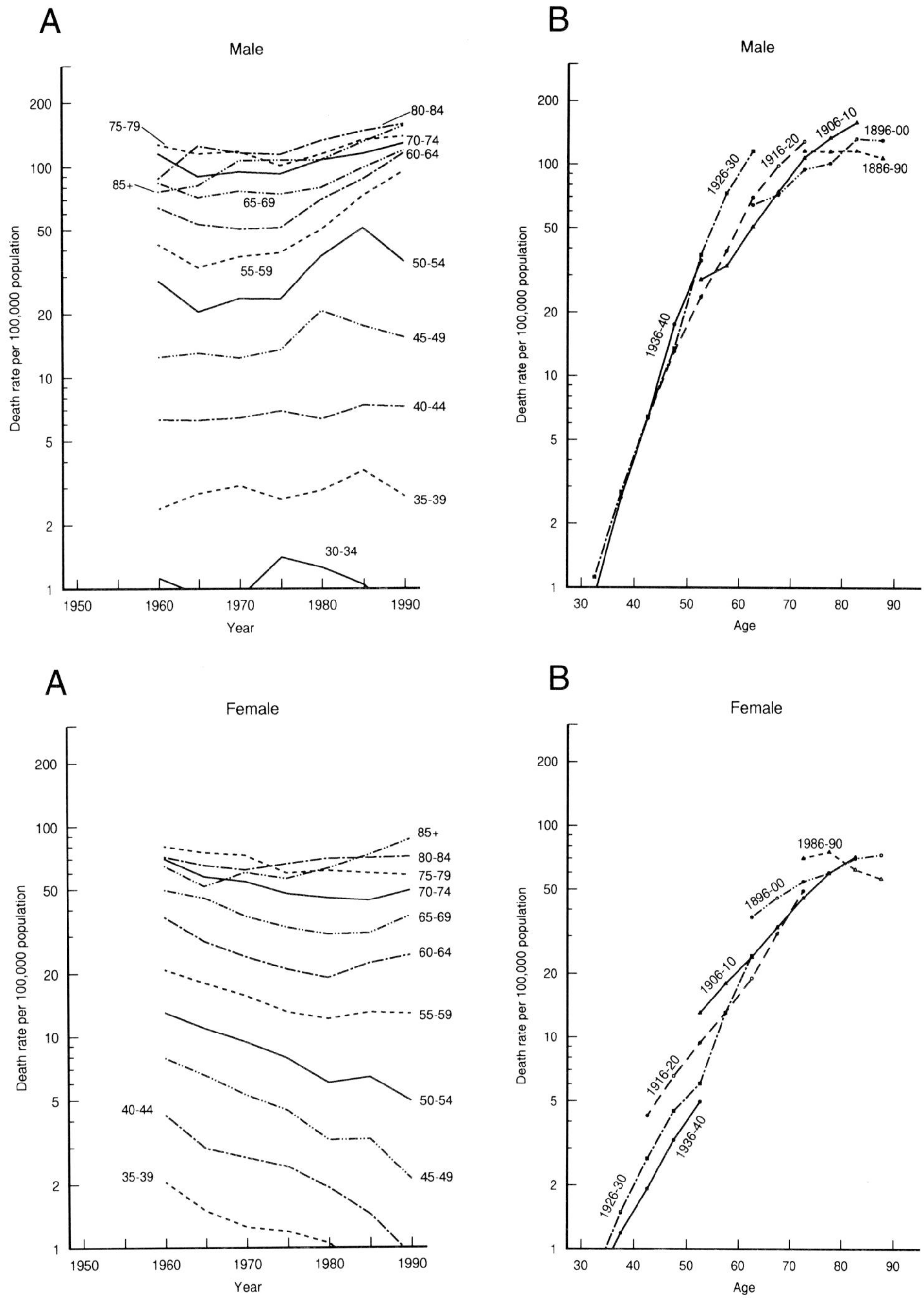

FIG. 3-7. Trends in the age- and sex-specific cancer mortality rate by age group (A) and by birth-year cohort (B) (1950–1990)

Cancer of the liver (ICD, 9th revision, 155).

Table III-8. Age- and Sex-specific Cancer Mortality Rates in Japan (1950–1990)
Cancer of the biliary passages (ICD, 9th revision: 156)

	1950	1955	1960	1965	1970	1975	1980	1985	1990
Male									
0–4			0.0	0.0	0.0	0.0	0.0	0.0	0.0
5–9			0.0	0.0	0.0	0.0	0.0	0.0	0.0
10–14			0.0	0.0	0.0	0.0	0.0	0.0	0.0
15–19			0.0	0.0	0.0	0.0	0.0	0.0	0.0
20–24			0.0	0.0	0.1	0.0	0.1	0.0	0.1
25–29			0.0	0.1	0.0	0.1	0.1	0.1	0.1
30–34			0.0	0.1	0.1	0.2	0.1	0.2	0.2
35–39			0.3	0.4	0.4	0.5	0.4	0.5	0.6
40–44			0.5	0.7	0.8	0.8	0.8	1.3	1.1
45–49			1.0	1.8	2.1	2.6	2.5	2.6	2.7
50–54			2.6	4.1	4.4	4.3	4.9	4.1	4.9
55–59			4.9	6.2	7.9	8.9	9.7	9.0	10.4
60–64			7.4	10.8	12.0	12.6	15.9	17.9	19.2
65–69			9.6	16.3	19.9	23.3	29.5	34.6	31.5
70–74			15.0	21.8	24.8	34.0	42.5	49.7	56.8
75–79			11.7	23.2	31.1	42.0	54.5	75.8	80.3
80–84			7.1	23.0	29.9	41.0	64.3	90.3	102.5
85–			8.9	8.1	14.6	36.0	60.0	95.5	120.2
Female									
0–4			0.0	0.0	0.0	0.0	0.0	0.0	0.0
5–9			0.0	0.0	0.0	0.0	0.0	0.0	0.0
10–14			0.0	0.0	0.0	0.0	0.0	0.0	0.0
15–19			0.0	0.0	0.1	0.0	0.0	0.0	0.0
20–24			0.1	0.0	0.0	0.1	0.1	0.0	0.1
25–29			0.0	0.0	0.1	0.1	0.1	0.1	0.1
30–34			0.1	0.2	0.2	0.2	0.2	0.3	0.2
35–39			0.1	0.3	0.4	0.5	0.4	0.6	0.5
40–44			0.7	0.8	1.1	1.2	1.4	1.5	1.0
45–49			1.3	1.3	2.2	2.4	2.6	3.1	2.8
50–54			2.6	3.7	4.4	4.6	5.9	5.8	5.3
55–59			4.3	6.8	8.3	10.4	10.7	10.9	9.3
60–64			6.3	10.7	16.7	15.1	18.5	17.7	16.6
65–69			10.1	13.5	21.6	25.1	29.3	31.2	29.1
70–74			9.7	16.3	27.2	35.4	43.4	51.1	49.3
75–79			9.9	21.3	26.3	43.7	56.5	73.7	73.2
80–84			7.7	18.8	24.5	35.0	59.3	89.5	109.2
85–			9.9	9.1	13.1	27.6	41.5	84.1	117.1

Mortality rates per 100,000 population.

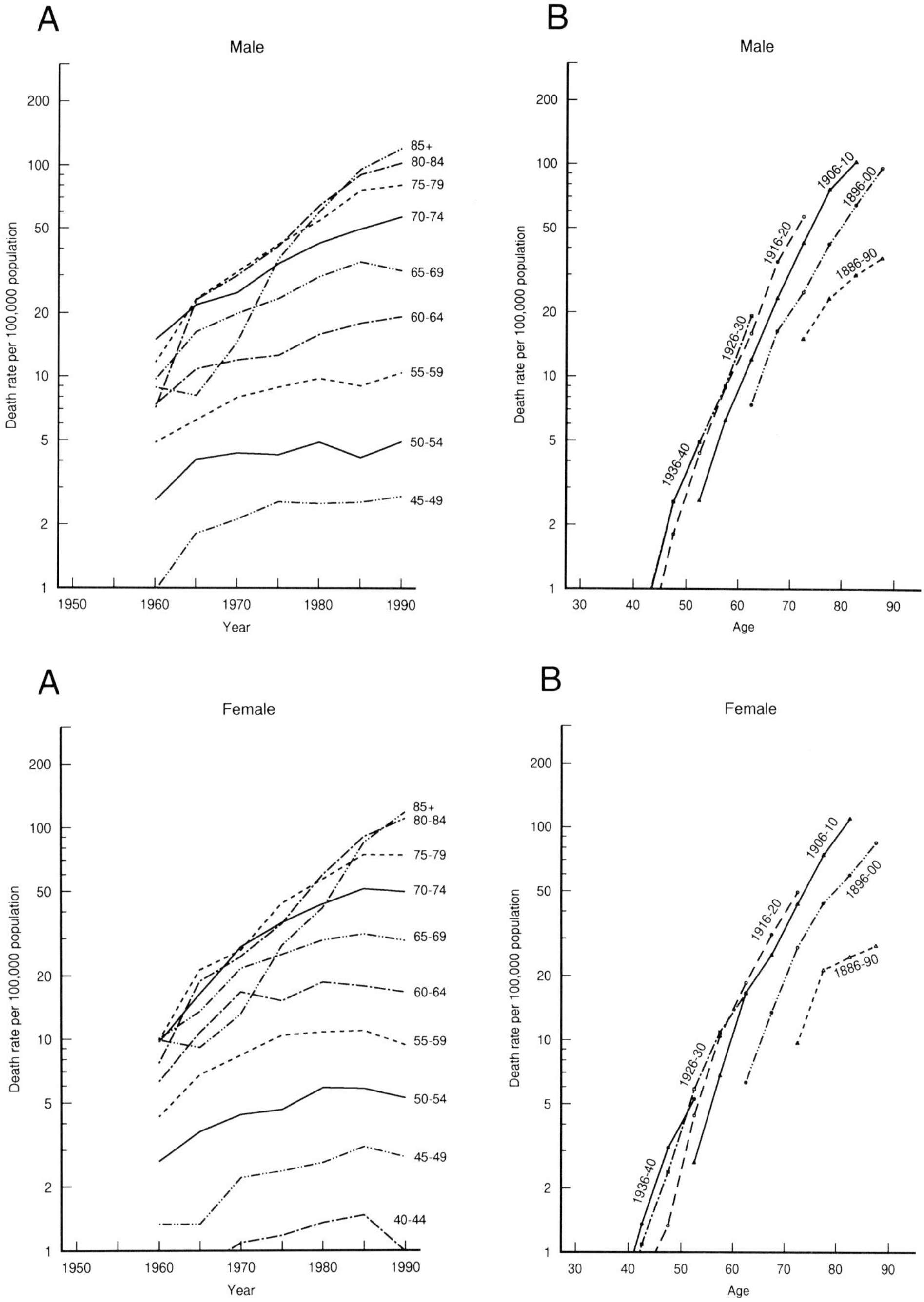

FIG. 3-8. Trends in the age- and sex-specific cancer mortality rate by age group (A) and by birth-year cohort (B) (1950–1990)

Cancer of the biliary passages (ICD, 9th revision, 156).

TABLE III-9. Age- and Sex-Specific Cancer Mortality Rates in Japan (1950–1990)
Cancer of the pancreas (ICD, 9th revision: 157)

	1950	1955	1960	1965	1970	1975	1980	1985	1990
Male									
0–4	0.0	0.0	0.0	0.0	0.0	0.0	0.0	0.0	0.0
5–9	0.0	0.0	0.0	0.0	0.0	0.0	0.0	0.0	0.0
10–14	0.0	0.0	0.0	0.0	0.1	0.0	0.0	0.0	0.0
15–19	0.0	0.0	0.0	0.1	0.0	0.1	0.0	0.0	0.0
20–24	0.1	0.0	0.1	0.1	0.2	0.1	0.1	0.0	0.0
25–29	0.0	0.1	0.2	0.2	0.2	0.3	0.3	0.0	0.0
30–34	0.3	0.3	0.4	0.6	0.6	0.4	0.4	0.4	0.3
35–39	0.6	0.6	0.9	0.9	1.4	1.1	1.4	0.9	1.3
40–44	1.4	1.5	1.9	1.9	2.4	2.2	3.1	2.8	2.8
45–49	1.7	2.3	4.4	4.5	4.1	5.2	6.1	6.3	6.3
50–54	2.7	5.0	6.6	9.1	10.1	9.7	10.9	11.5	11.1
55–59	4.7	7.0	11.1	13.4	18.1	17.0	19.1	20.8	18.6
60–64	6.2	9.3	13.9	20.6	25.5	26.6	32.3	31.9	33.1
65–69	4.0	11.8	20.5	25.5	36.7	38.8	45.2	51.4	49.2
70–74	3.7	9.9	17.3	30.2	42.7	47.6	57.6	69.6	71.7
75–79	1.5	5.6	19.6	28.6	35.8	52.0	71.2	89.5	99.8
80–84	2.1	2.3	10.1	23.0	34.0	41.7	67.9	92.7	115.5
85–	3.5	2.5	5.3	13.5	28.1	31.9	54.8	92.4	126.9
Female									
0–4	0.0	0.0	0.0	0.0	0.0	0.0	0.0	0.0	0.0
5–9	0.0	0.0	0.0	0.0	0.0	0.0	0.0	0.0	0.0
10–14	0.1	0.0	0.0	0.0	0.0	0.0	0.0	0.0	0.0
15–19	0.0	0.0	0.0	0.0	0.0	0.0	0.1	0.0	0.0
20–24	0.1	0.0	0.0	0.0	0.1	0.1	0.0	0.1	0.1
25–29	0.1	0.1	0.1	0.2	0.2	0.1	0.2	0.2	0.1
30–34	0.3	0.2	0.4	0.3	0.5	0.3	0.3	0.3	0.4
35–39	0.3	0.7	0.4	0.5	0.8	0.6	0.6	0.6	1.0
40–44	0.6	1.5	1.3	1.7	1.5	1.4	1.3	1.7	1.2
45–49	1.0	1.8	2.6	3.0	2.9	3.5	3.0	3.0	2.8
50–54	1.1	2.6	5.0	5.3	6.0	6.6	5.9	4.9	5.0
55–59	3.0	5.0	7.4	10.3	9.4	10.0	9.3	9.4	9.7
60–64	3.4	5.4	8.2	14.0	15.5	15.5	17.7	17.2	16.2
65–69	2.4	8.1	12.7	17.2	21.0	23.2	26.7	26.0	27.5
70–74	1.6	5.8	11.6	15.9	27.4	31.0	40.3	43.5	42.2
75–79	1.4	5.1	9.5	18.5	27.2	36.6	42.1	54.4	63.4
80–84	0.6	2.9	7.3	11.4	17.7	29.0	43.6	62.5	82.9
85–	3.0	3.2	0.8	5.7	10.2	16.4	32.0	58.3	97.6

Mortality rates per 100,000 population.

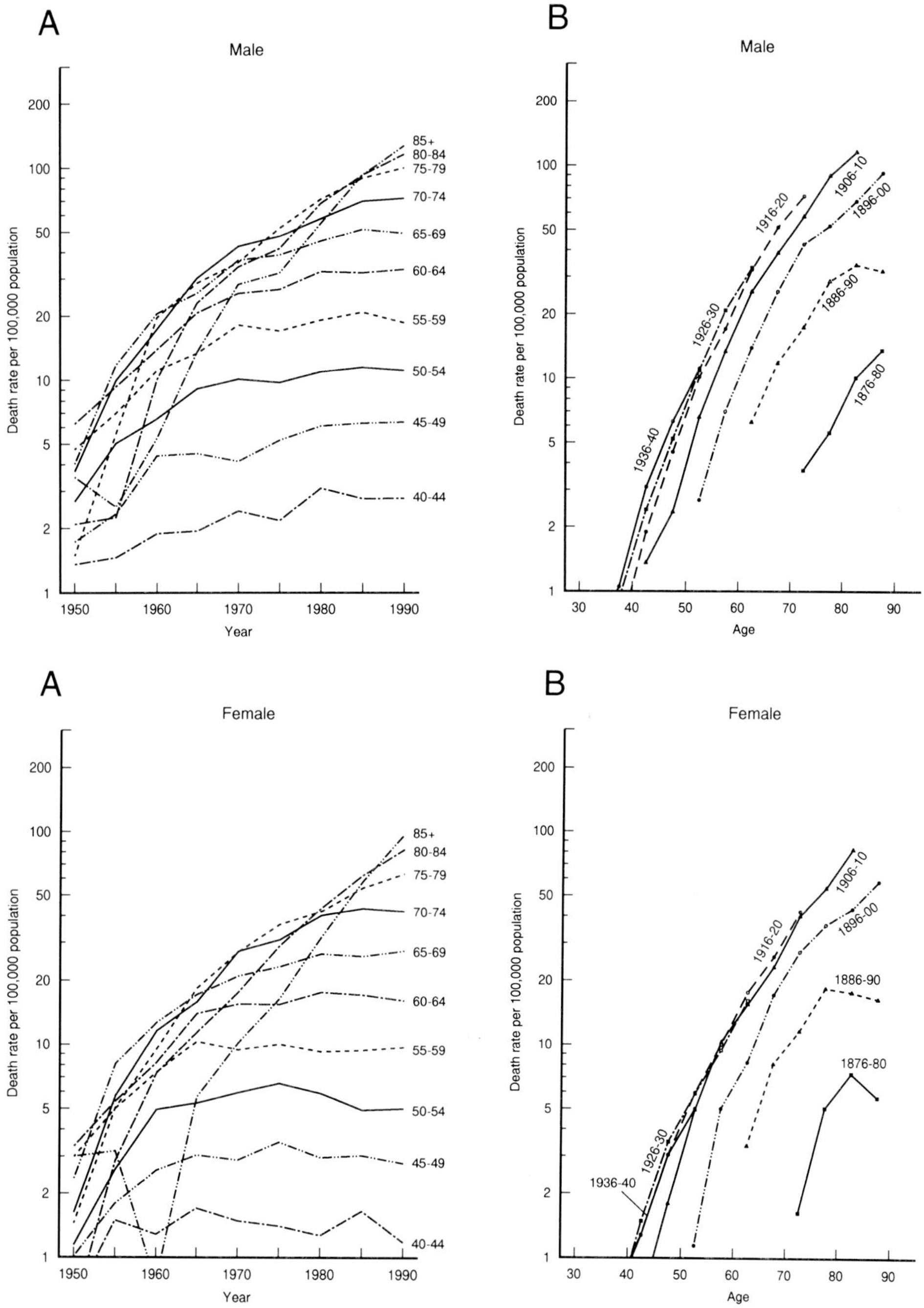

FIG. 3-9. Trends in the age- and sex-specific cancer mortality rate by age group (A) and by birth-year cohort (B) (1950–1990)

Cancer of the pancreas (ICD, 9th revision, 157).

TABLE III-10. Age- and Sex-Specific Cancer Mortality Rates in Japan (1950–1990)
Cancer of the larynx (ICD, 9th revision: 161)

	1950	1955	1960	1965	1970	1975	1980	1985	1990
Male									
0–4	0.0	0.0	0.0	0.0	0.0	0.0	0.0	0.0	0.0
5–9	0.0	0.0	0.0	0.0	0.0	0.0	0.0	0.0	0.0
10–14	0.0	0.0	0.0	0.0	0.0	0.0	0.0	0.0	0.0
15–19	0.0	0.0	0.0	0.0	0.0	0.0	0.0	0.0	0.0
20–24	0.0	0.0	0.0	0.0	0.0	0.0	0.0	0.0	0.0
25–29	0.0	0.0	0.0	0.0	0.0	0.0	0.0	0.0	0.0
30–34	0.1	0.0	0.0	0.0	0.1	0.0	0.0	0.0	0.0
35–39	0.5	0.0	0.2	0.0	0.1	0.0	0.0	0.0	0.0
40–44	0.7	0.4	0.3	0.4	0.3	0.1	0.1	0.2	0.1
45–49	1.9	1.1	0.8	0.5	0.6	0.6	0.6	0.3	0.3
50–54	3.7	2.7	2.0	1.6	1.3	1.0	1.0	0.7	0.8
55–59	7.8	5.4	4.4	3.3	3.1	2.6	2.6	2.5	2.3
60–64	8.2	8.8	8.0	7.6	7.8	5.4	3.8	3.6	3.3
65–69	13.7	10.7	10.8	12.0	12.6	9.9	7.0	6.1	5.6
70–74	17.4	17.5	12.0	15.3	16.2	12.8	11.7	10.0	8.3
75–79	11.6	12.0	15.1	16.4	21.3	20.7	16.1	13.2	9.5
80–84	8.4	7.5	18.9	18.2	20.8	21.8	21.6	16.5	15.2
85–	7.0	5.0	10.6	9.5	22.5	9.8	19.2	16.4	16.6
Female									
0–4	0.0	0.0	0.0	0.0	0.0	0.0	0.0	0.0	0.0
5–9	0.0	0.0	0.0	0.0	0.0	0.0	0.0	0.0	0.0
10–14	0.0	0.0	0.0	0.0	0.0	0.0	0.0	0.0	0.0
15–19	0.0	0.0	0.0	0.0	0.0	0.0	0.0	0.0	0.0
20–24	0.0	0.0	0.0	0.0	0.0	0.0	0.0	0.0	0.0
25–29	0.1	0.0	0.0	0.0	0.0	0.0	0.0	0.0	0.0
30–34	0.0	0.1	0.0	0.0	0.1	0.0	0.0	0.0	0.0
35–39	0.1	0.1	0.1	0.0	0.1	0.0	0.0	0.0	0.0
40–44	0.5	0.3	0.3	0.1	0.2	0.0	0.0	0.0	0.0
45–49	0.8	0.5	0.4	0.2	0.1	0.1	0.0	0.1	0.0
50–54	1.4	0.7	0.5	0.5	0.2	0.3	0.2	0.1	0.1
55–59	2.2	1.0	1.4	1.0	1.0	0.4	0.3	0.1	0.1
60–64	3.5	2.1	1.7	1.7	1.4	0.6	0.7	0.3	0.1
65–69	4.2	3.2	2.3	2.2	1.8	0.9	0.9	0.5	0.2
70–74	4.6	4.3	2.8	2.9	2.4	1.5	1.7	0.7	0.7
75–79	2.2	4.1	5.2	3.6	3.5	2.0	1.4	0.9	1.1
80–84	2.8	3.3	4.8	3.8	2.5	4.2	2.8	2.3	1.0
85–	4.5	2.1	3.0	2.3	2.4	3.7	3.4	1.3	1.4

Mortality rates per 100,000 population.

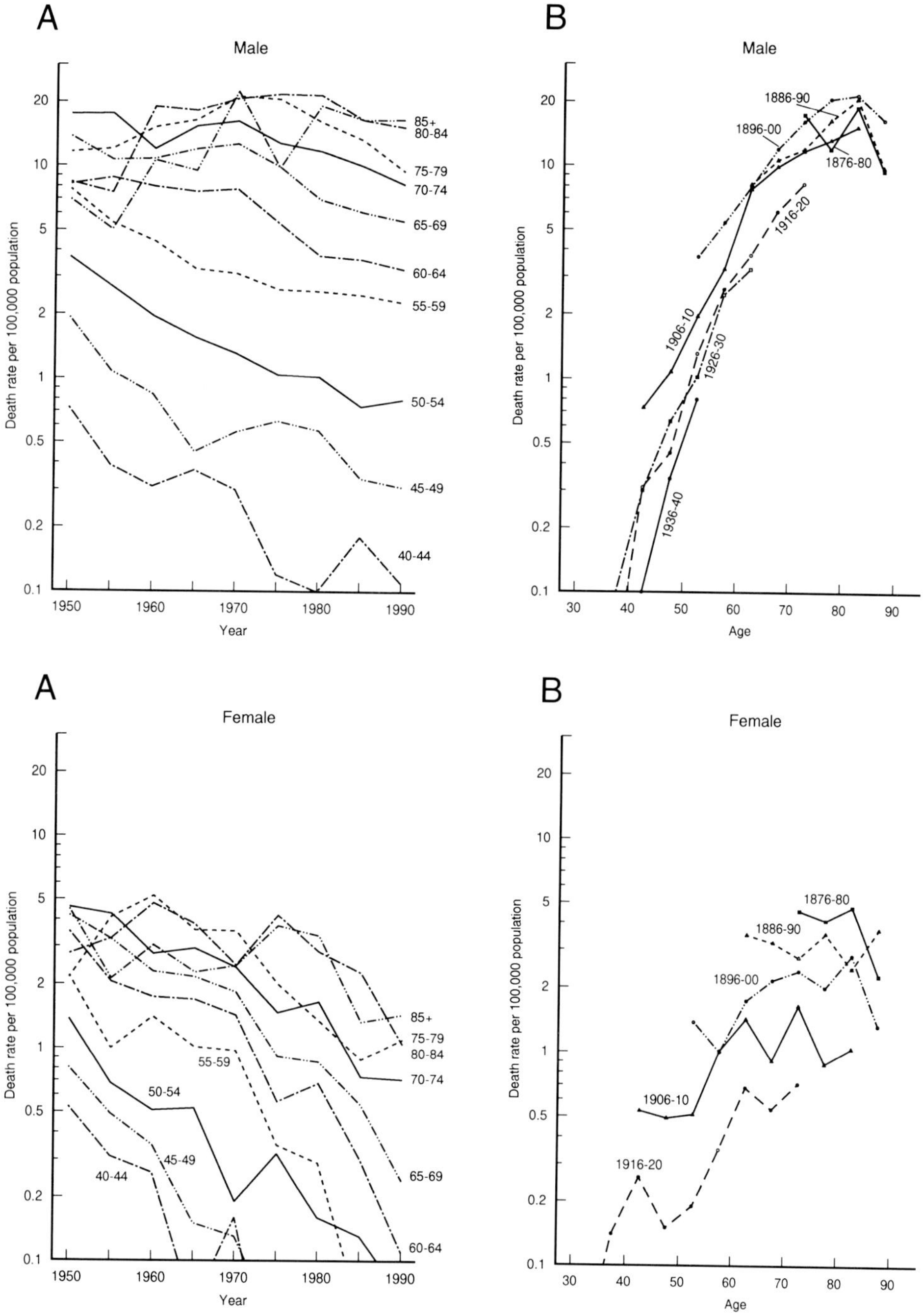

FIG. 3-10. Trends in the age- and sex-specific cancer mortality rate by age group (A) and by birth-year cohort (B) (1950–1990)

Cancer of the larynx (ICD, 9th revision, 161).

Table III-11. Age- and Sex-Specific Cancer Mortality Rates in Japan (1950–1990)
Cancer of the trachea, bronchus, and lung (ICD, 9th revision: 162)

	1950	1955	1960	1965	1970	1975	1980	1985	1990
Male									
0–4	0.0	0.0	0.1	0.0	0.0	0.0	0.1	0.0	0.0
5–9	0.0	0.0	0.0	0.0	0.0	0.0	0.0	0.0	0.0
10–14	0.1	0.1	0.0	0.1	0.0	0.0	0.0	0.0	0.0
15–19	0.2	0.1	0.2	0.1	0.1	0.1	0.1	0.0	0.0
20–24	0.1	0.2	0.2	0.4	0.2	0.2	0.1	0.2	0.1
25–29	0.3	0.3	0.4	0.5	0.5	0.4	0.5	0.3	0.4
30–34	0.1	0.5	0.7	0.8	0.8	0.9	0.9	1.0	1.0
35–39	0.4	0.8	1.1	1.8	1.6	1.9	2.5	2.9	3.3
40–44	0.9	2.0	2.7	3.6	4.6	4.9	5.0	6.1	6.8
45–49	2.1	4.9	7.7	8.5	8.5	11.4	11.2	11.1	13.0
50–54	4.9	10.1	15.8	18.7	20.1	20.8	26.4	25.2	23.1
55–59	7.7	15.5	30.5	32.0	40.7	43.9	48.8	53.6	53.6
60–64	13.7	29.5	46.5	66.3	71.5	79.7	96.0	98.2	113.4
65–69	21.9	43.2	71.4	93.1	125.0	139.4	157.2	179.1	190.9
70–74	20.4	51.5	86.9	118.5	156.6	210.5	252.7	282.5	301.3
75–79	21.3	36.3	81.8	126.1	160.9	238.3	329.1	396.4	421.1
80–84	8.4	27.0	62.1	105.9	127.0	191.7	321.4	435.4	516.7
85–	3.5	15.1	37.2	39.3	77.6	127.4	242.3	391.5	499.4
Female									
0–4	0.0	0.0	0.0	0.0	0.0	0.0	0.0	0.0	0.0
5–9	0.0	0.1	0.0	0.0	0.0	0.0	0.0	0.0	0.0
10–14	0.1	0.0	0.0	0.0	0.0	0.0	0.0	0.0	0.0
15–19	0.1	0.1	0.1	0.1	0.1	0.0	0.0	0.1	0.0
20–24	0.0	0.1	0.2	0.2	0.1	0.0	0.1	0.1	0.0
25–29	0.1	0.2	0.2	0.3	0.2	0.3	0.3	0.2	0.2
30–34	0.2	0.6	0.9	0.9	0.8	0.7	0.8	0.4	0.7
35–39	0.4	1.1	1.3	1.8	1.2	1.7	1.7	1.8	2.0
40–44	0.8	1.9	1.8	2.7	2.9	2.5	2.9	3.3	3.1
45–49	1.1	3.0	4.9	3.9	5.2	5.4	5.1	5.3	5.7
50–54	2.7	4.4	6.4	9.3	8.0	9.4	9.6	9.4	10.4
55–59	3.6	6.6	10.5	14.1	14.2	15.9	15.9	16.4	15.7
60–64	4.1	9.4	16.7	20.7	24.5	23.3	27.4	28.0	25.3
65–69	5.0	13.2	22.1	27.8	32.0	35.9	42.1	43.4	42.8
70–74	5.9	14.1	23.3	35.9	41.3	51.1	63.7	65.9	69.4
75–79	4.6	9.4	25.4	41.8	46.7	58.5	84.4	94.6	99.8
80–84	3.3	6.5	19.8	31.7	47.6	55.2	90.4	119.3	120.0
85–	1.5	4.2	16.0	17.0	25.7	51.2	67.8	114.2	150.5

Mortality rates per 100,000 population.

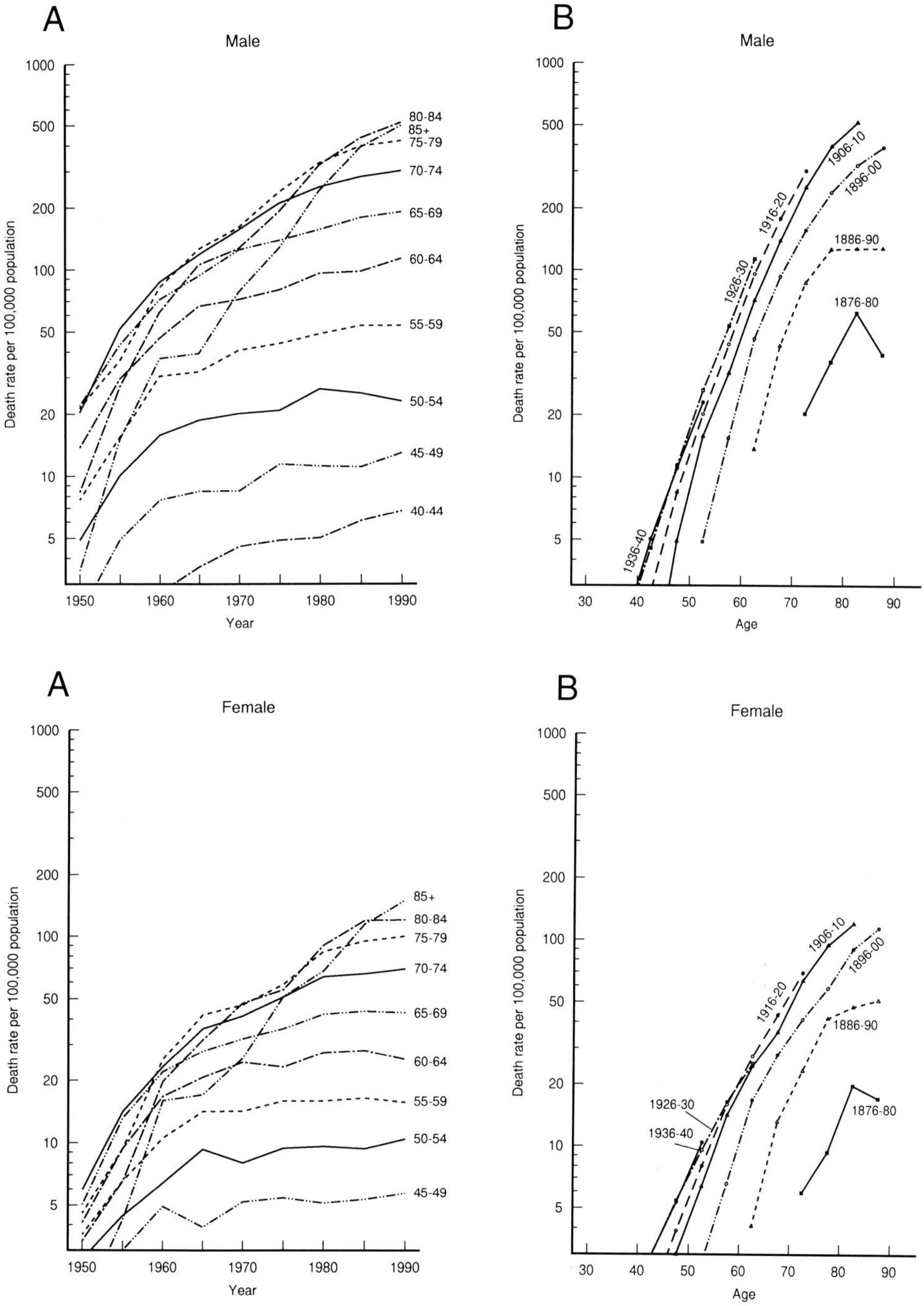

FIG. 3-11. Trends in the age- and sex-specific cancer mortality rate by age group (A) and by birth-year cohort (B) (1950–1990)

Cancer of the trachea, bronchus, and lung (ICD, 9th revision, 162).

TABLE III-12. Age- and Sex-Specific Cancer Mortality Rates in Japan (1950–1990)
Cancer of the bone (ICD, 9th revision: 170)

	1950	1955	1960	1965	1970	1975	1980	1985	1990
Male									
0–4	0.1	0.1	0.1	0.2	0.1	0.0	0.1	0.0	0.1
5–9	0.0	0.1	0.1	0.2	0.2	0.1	0.1	0.1	0.1
10–14	0.2	0.3	0.4	0.5	0.6	0.6	0.4	0.4	0.3
15–19	0.4	0.4	0.9	0.8	1.2	0.7	0.6	1.0	0.9
20–24	0.1	0.3	0.3	0.4	0.7	0.7	0.4	0.3	0.4
25–29	0.1	0.2	0.2	0.3	0.4	0.3	0.2	0.2	0.2
30–34	0.1	0.5	0.3	0.3	0.2	0.4	0.2	0.1	0.1
35–39	0.4	0.6	1.0	0.4	0.4	0.1	0.2	0.2	0.2
40–44	0.6	0.7	1.5	0.8	0.4	0.2	0.2	0.2	0.2
45–49	0.7	1.6	1.5	1.0	1.3	0.4	0.4	0.3	0.3
50–54	1.5	2.5	2.8	2.1	1.4	1.0	0.5	0.4	0.3
55–59	2.0	3.2	4.0	3.4	2.1	1.5	0.8	0.5	0.6
60–64	2.9	6.0	6.5	4.9	3.6	2.2	1.4	0.6	0.7
65–69	3.4	6.9	7.1	8.0	4.9	3.3	1.4	1.2	0.9
70–74	3.2	9.1	7.2	9.1	6.6	5.4	3.5	1.7	1.1
75–79	4.5	8.2	7.7	10.8	5.5	5.4	3.1	2.8	1.4
80–84	4.2	8.3	6.5	7.0	9.1	3.9	1.9	4.3	2.7
85–	0.0	2.5	1.8	5.4	5.6	8.2	3.5	1.6	2.5
Female									
0–4	0.1	0.1	0.0	0.2	0.1	0.0	0.1	0.1	0.0
5–9	0.0	0.1	0.0	0.1	0.2	0.2	0.1	0.2	0.1
10–14	0.1	0.2	0.4	0.4	0.5	0.4	0.5	0.5	0.4
15–19	0.2	0.3	0.4	0.5	0.6	0.3	0.6	0.4	0.3
20–24	0.1	0.1	0.2	0.3	0.2	0.3	0.4	0.2	0.2
25–29	0.1	0.4	0.1	0.2	0.2	0.2	0.3	0.1	0.2
30–34	0.1	0.2	0.4	0.3	0.2	0.1	0.2	0.1	0.2
35–39	0.4	0.5	0.5	0.3	0.3	0.1	0.1	0.1	0.1
40–44	0.5	0.8	0.8	0.7	0.4	0.4	0.1	0.1	0.1
45–49	0.7	1.3	1.8	0.7	0.7	0.4	0.3	0.1	0.2
50–54	1.0	1.8	1.5	1.7	0.9	0.5	0.3	0.4	0.2
55–59	2.0	2.0	3.2	1.7	1.7	1.1	0.4	0.2	0.2
60–64	1.5	3.0	3.4	3.8	1.8	1.0	0.7	0.5	0.5
65–69	1.7	2.5	3.4	3.2	2.3	1.8	1.1	0.7	0.6
70–74	2.3	4.9	4.7	5.1	3.3	1.8	1.1	0.9	0.7
75–79	3.8	4.9	6.2	5.1	4.1	3.0	0.8	2.1	1.1
80–84	3.3	5.3	4.5	7.3	5.6	4.2	1.5	2.0	1.3
85–	0.0	5.3	3.8	2.3	4.4	2.6	2.0	1.9	1.3

Mortality rates per 100,000 population.

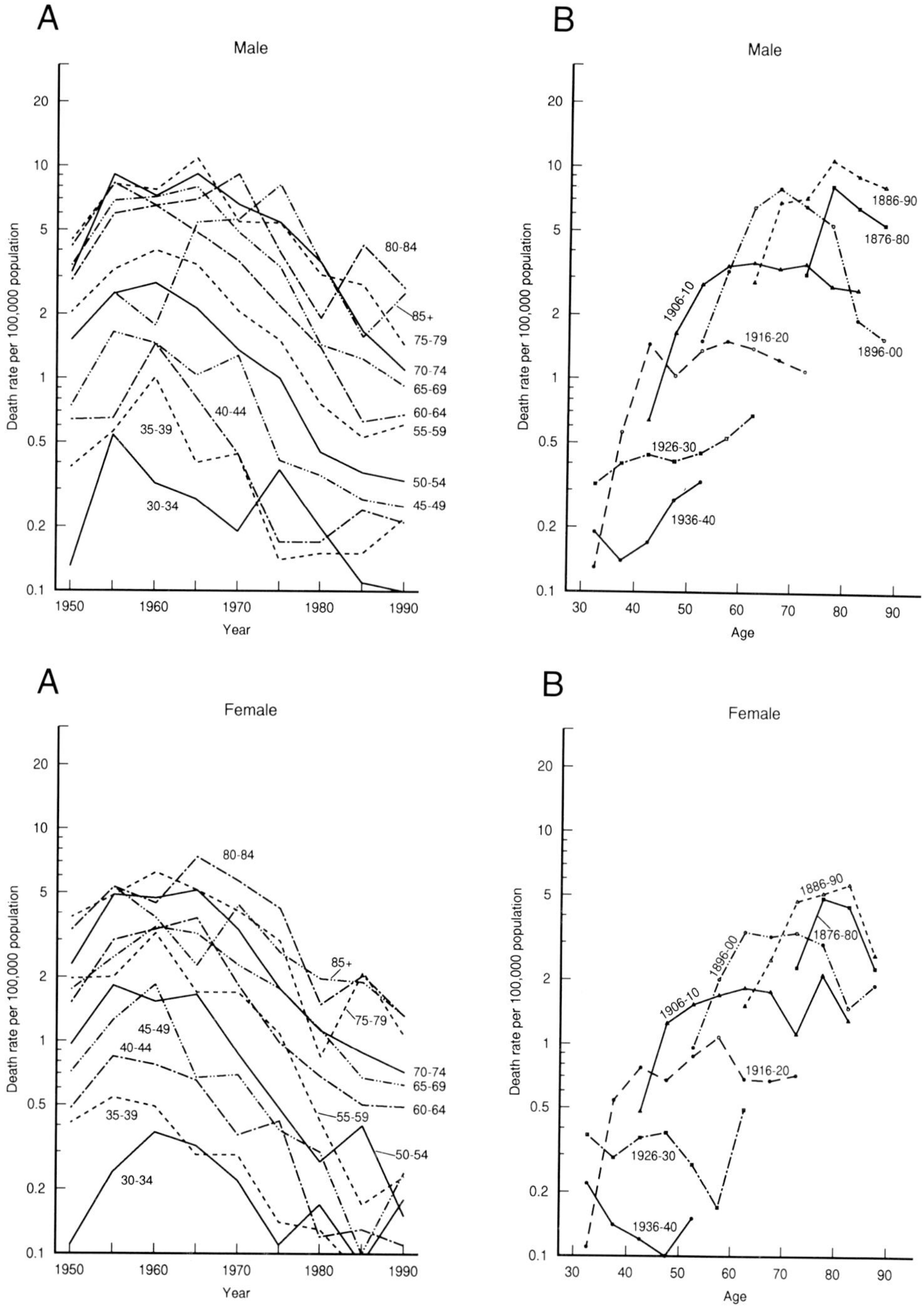

FIG. 3-12. Trends in the age- and sex-specific cancer mortality rate by age group (A) and by birth-year cohort (B) (1950–1990)

Cancer of the bone (ICD, 9th revision, 170).

Table III-13. Age- and Sex-Specific Cancer Mortality Rates in Japan (1950–1990)
Cancer of the skin (ICD, 9th revision: 172–173)

	1950	1955	1960	1965	1970	1975	1980	1985	1990
Male									
0–4	0.1	0.1	0.1	0.1	0.1	0.0	0.0	0.0	0.0
5–9	0.1	0.1	0.0	0.0	0.1	0.0	0.0	0.0	0.0
10–14	0.1	0.1	0.1	0.0	0.1	0.0	0.0	0.0	0.0
15–19	0.1	0.0	0.0	0.1	0.0	0.0	0.0	0.1	0.0
20–24	0.1	0.1	0.0	0.0	0.1	0.1	0.0	0.0	0.0
25–29	0.1	0.1	0.1	0.1	0.1	0.1	0.1	0.1	0.1
30–34	0.1	0.2	0.1	0.2	0.2	0.0	0.2	0.1	0.1
35–39	0.3	0.3	0.2	0.2	0.2	0.3	0.2	0.2	0.0
40–44	0.5	0.5	0.1	0.6	0.3	0.3	0.3	0.4	0.2
45–49	1.0	0.6	0.8	0.7	0.7	0.6	0.4	0.3	0.3
50–54	1.3	1.5	1.0	1.2	0.9	0.9	0.9	0.8	0.6
55–59	1.8	1.9	1.7	1.1	2.0	1.2	1.0	1.1	1.0
60–64	2.8	3.3	2.5	1.9	2.4	2.3	1.6	1.2	1.3
65–69	7.2	5.1	5.7	4.4	3.5	3.8	1.6	2.3	1.9
70–74	7.4	6.7	4.9	4.8	5.1	5.3	3.8	3.5	2.7
75–79	9.3	9.4	9.0	12.0	10.0	7.3	5.3	4.5	4.5
80–84	17.8	13.5	21.9	16.1	15.4	10.1	8.6	7.4	6.7
85–	24.3	17.6	14.2	17.6	32.6	18.8	18.6	14.1	15.4
Female									
0–4	0.1	0.1	0.1	0.1	0.1	0.0	0.0	0.0	0.0
5–9	0.0	0.1	0.0	0.0	0.0	0.0	0.0	0.0	0.0
10–14	0.0	0.0	0.1	0.0	0.1	0.0	0.0	0.0	0.0
15–19	0.1	0.1	0.0	0.0	0.1	0.1	0.0	0.0	0.0
20–24	0.1	0.0	0.1	0.1	0.0	0.0	0.0	0.0	0.1
25–29	0.1	0.1	0.1	0.0	0.1	0.1	0.0	0.0	0.0
30–34	0.1	0.2	0.1	0.2	0.1	0.1	0.1	0.1	0.1
35–39	0.5	0.3	0.3	0.1	0.1	0.2	0.2	0.1	0.2
40–44	0.6	0.2	0.3	0.2	0.2	0.2	0.2	0.2	0.2
45–49	0.9	0.7	0.6	0.5	0.4	0.4	0.2	0.2	0.3
50–54	1.0	1.4	0.9	0.7	0.6	0.3	0.6	0.5	0.3
55–59	1.5	1.3	1.5	0.8	1.1	0.7	0.7	0.4	0.3
60–64	2.3	1.9	1.9	1.7	1.4	1.4	0.6	0.7	0.6
65–69	3.9	2.9	2.4	2.6	2.1	2.3	1.2	1.3	0.8
70–74	3.8	5.0	4.0	4.9	3.3	3.1	2.1	2.0	1.2
75–79	4.6	6.2	9.9	5.0	7.4	6.2	3.0	3.0	1.8
80–84	3.9	12.3	10.5	13.8	12.0	7.2	6.5	5.0	3.8
85–	15.0	11.7	22.1	22.2	20.9	17.2	18.5	13.1	12.3

Mortality rates per 100,000 population.

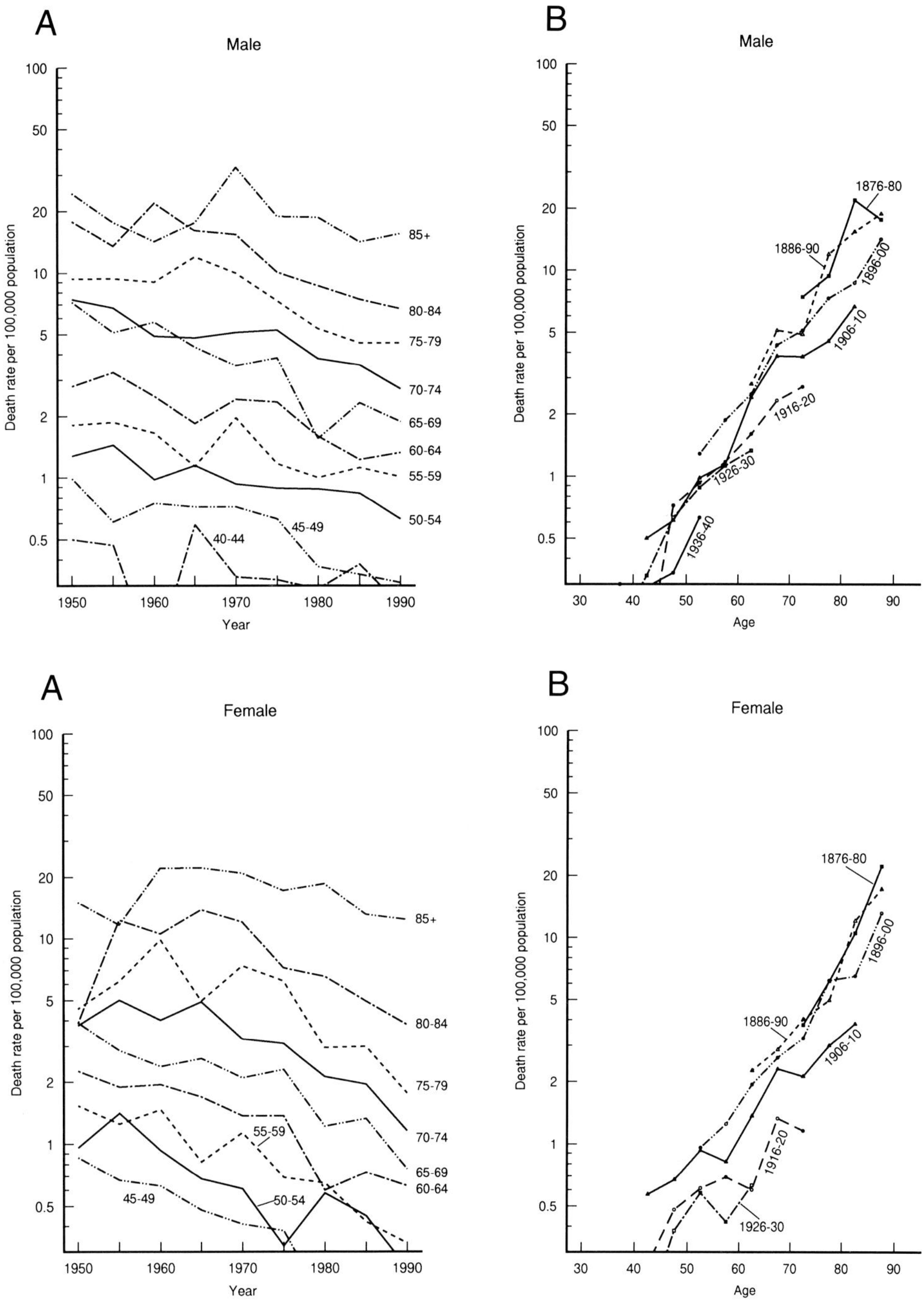

FIG. 3-13. Trends in the age- and sex-specific cancer mortality rate by age group (A) and by birth-year cohort (B) (1950–1990)

Cancer of the skin (ICD, 9th revision, 172, 173).

TABLE III-14. Age- and Sex-Specific Cancer Mortality Rates in Japan (1950–1990)
Cancer of the breast (ICD, 9th revision: 174)

	1950	1955	1960	1965	1970	1975	1980	1985	1990
Female									
0–4	0.0	0.0	0.0	0.0	0.0	0.0	0.0	0.0	0.0
5–9	0.0	0.0	0.0	0.0	0.0	0.0	0.0	0.0	0.0
10–14	0.0	0.0	0.0	0.0	0.0	0.0	0.0	0.0	0.0
15–19	0.0	0.1	0.0	0.0	0.0	0.0	0.0	0.0	0.0
20–24	0.1	0.1	0.1	0.0	0.1	0.2	0.1	0.2	0.1
25–29	0.4	0.5	0.4	0.5	0.6	0.5	1.0	0.8	0.8
30–34	1.8	1.8	1.6	1.7	2.0	2.3	2.5	3.0	2.6
35–39	3.6	4.3	4.1	4.0	4.2	4.6	5.5	5.5	6.4
40–44	7.0	6.4	6.5	6.8	7.2	8.6	8.6	9.5	10.8
45–49	9.0	8.7	9.5	9.4	10.6	12.3	13.3	13.1	15.8
50–54	10.9	10.1	9.6	12.6	13.2	17.1	17.2	17.9	19.3
55–59	13.6	11.6	11.5	12.6	14.2	16.4	19.9	20.7	22.5
60–64	15.2	13.6	10.3	11.9	14.0	15.8	17.2	19.9	20.2
65–69	15.0	14.7	11.9	12.9	12.5	14.6	18.2	19.1	19.6
70–74	14.8	16.9	15.6	12.6	15.3	14.8	18.0	19.7	20.1
75–79	17.0	18.4	17.8	12.7	14.4	15.4	18.2	17.6	18.6
80–84	15.5	18.0	21.7	17.0	23.3	18.2	20.2	19.5	20.9
85–	15.0	23.3	28.1	20.5	30.1	24.3	23.3	26.3	23.3

Mortality rates per 100,000 population.

TABLE III-15. Age- and Sex-Specific Cancer Mortality Rates in Japan (1950–1990)
Cancer of the uterus (ICD, 9th revision: 179–182)

	1950	1955	1960	1965	1970	1975	1980	1985	1990
Female									
0–4	0.0	0.0	0.0	0.0	0.0	0.0	0.0	0.0	0.0
5–9	0.0	0.0	0.0	0.0	0.0	0.0	0.0	0.0	0.0
10–14	0.0	0.1	0.0	0.1	0.0	0.0	0.0	0.0	0.0
15–19	0.1	0.1	0.2	0.1	0.2	0.0	0.0	0.1	0.0
20–24	0.8	0.5	0.8	0.6	0.2	0.3	0.2	0.2	0.3
25–29	3.0	2.3	2.3	1.7	1.2	0.5	0.6	0.5	0.5
30–34	8.8	5.1	4.5	3.8	2.6	1.7	1.1	1.3	1.0
35–39	23.5	12.5	9.9	7.3	5.6	2.9	2.2	1.9	2.4
40–44	43.8	27.0	19.0	13.7	12.0	7.1	4.7	3.9	3.2
45–49	62.8	43.7	34.5	23.5	19.5	14.8	9.5	7.1	5.4
50–54	76.8	58.8	46.9	36.5	26.8	22.1	15.0	10.9	7.9
55–59	80.3	65.6	55.7	46.6	37.1	28.7	21.1	14.2	12.3
60–64	84.2	70.2	64.7	57.0	49.3	36.9	27.8	20.6	14.3
65–69	85.5	71.9	68.0	63.3	52.5	47.5	35.7	26.7	20.1
70–74	72.2	79.9	71.9	65.5	61.9	57.0	43.8	32.6	25.2
75–79	53.6	65.8	71.6	70.2	62.3	59.5	54.2	41.3	34.2
80–84	52.2	50.3	52.0	66.2	59.4	56.6	64.5	56.4	47.2
85–	22.5	39.2	43.3	39.2	48.0	52.3	53.5	52.6	51.9

Mortality rates per 100,000 population.

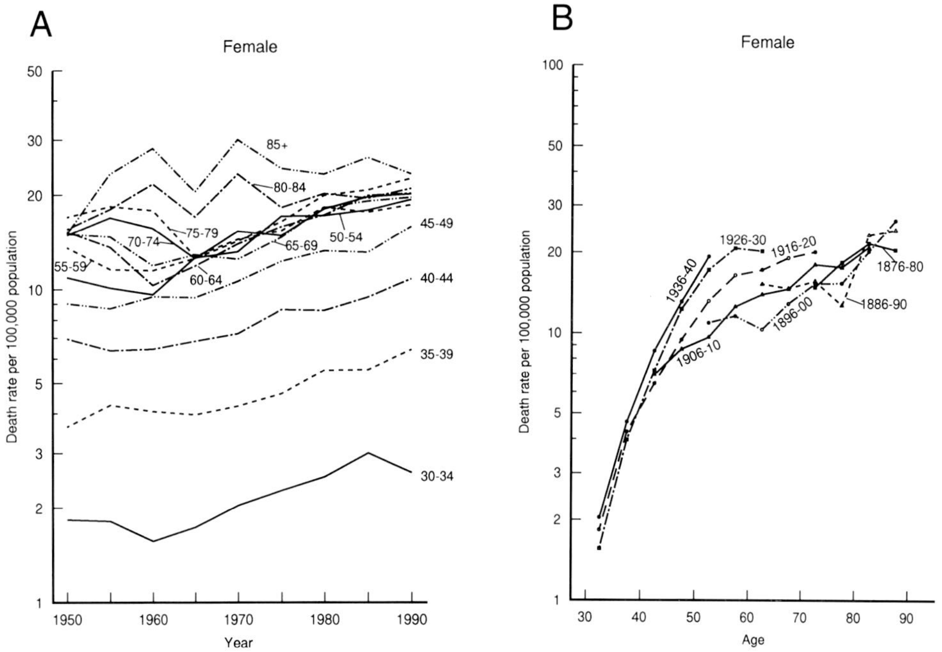

FIG. 3-14. Trends in the age- and sex-specific cancer mortality rate by age group (A) and by birth-year cohort (B) (1950–1990)
Cancer of the breast (ICD, 9th revision, 174).

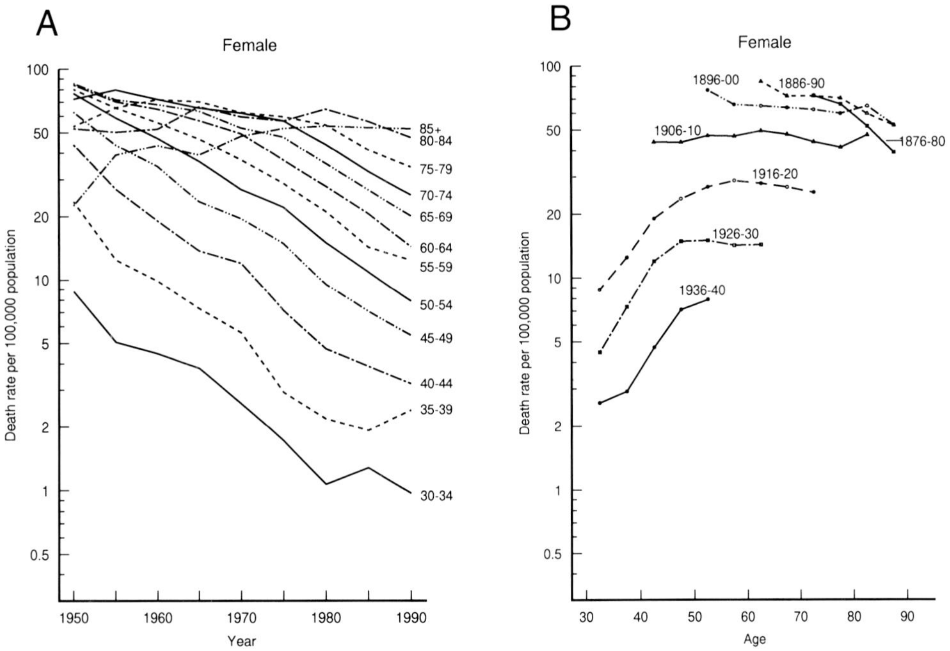

FIG. 3-15. Trends in the age- and sex-specific cancer mortality rate by age group (A) and by birth-year cohort (B) (1950–1990)
Cancer of the uterus (ICD, 9th revision, 179–182).

Table III-16. Age- and Sex-Specific Cancer Mortality Rates in Japan (1950–1990)
Cancer of the ovary (ICD, 9th revision: 183.0)

	1950	1955	1960	1965	1970	1975	1980	1985	1990
Female									
0–4	0.0	0.0	0.0	0.0	0.1	0.1	0.0	0.0	0.0
5–9	0.0	0.0	0.1	0.1	0.1	0.1	0.1	0.0	0.0
10–14	0.1	0.2	0.4	0.3	0.2	0.3	0.3	0.2	0.1
15–19	0.4	0.2	0.6	0.4	0.7	0.5	0.4	0.4	0.1
20–24	0.6	0.5	0.5	0.7	1.0	0.6	0.8	0.5	0.4
25–29	0.7	0.7	0.7	0.8	0.9	0.8	0.8	0.6	0.6
30–34	0.6	0.8	0.7	1.0	1.2	1.0	1.1	1.2	0.9
35–39	1.1	1.5	1.9	1.6	1.4	1.7	1.5	1.9	2.1
40–44	1.2	1.8	1.9	2.4	2.5	3.4	3.4	4.1	3.8
45–49	2.2	3.0	3.1	4.5	4.2	4.7	5.7	5.9	7.4
50–54	2.8	3.4	3.7	4.8	4.9	7.7	9.3	10.4	9.3
55–59	2.2	3.9	4.1	4.5	6.1	7.1	8.8	10.1	11.2
60–64	2.5	2.6	4.4	5.2	6.0	8.2	9.6	10.7	11.9
65–69	2.7	2.5	3.6	4.4	7.0	7.9	10.9	10.9	11.4
70–74	2.3	2.5	3.7	4.4	5.9	7.0	11.2	12.9	15.0
75–79	3.1	3.2	2.9	3.1	7.5	7.2	11.7	14.3	17.1
80–84	1.1	0.8	4.1	3.8	4.4	7.0	9.5	13.8	16.9
85–	0.0	1.1	0.8	2.8	3.4	3.4	5.3	12.1	21.0

Mortality rates per 100,000 population.

Table III-17. Age- and Sex-Specific Cancer Mortality Rates in Japan (1950–1990)
Cancer of the prostate (ICD, 9th revision: 185)

	1950	1955	1960	1965	1970	1975	1980	1985	1990
Male									
0–4	0.0	0.0	0.0	0.0	0.0	0.0	0.0	0.0	0.0
5–9	0.0	0.0	0.0	0.0	0.0	0.0	0.0	0.0	0.0
10–14	0.0	0.0	0.0	0.0	0.0	0.0	0.0	0.0	0.0
15–19	0.0	0.0	0.0	0.0	0.0	0.1	0.0	0.0	0.0
20–24	0.0	0.1	0.0	0.0	0.0	0.0	0.0	0.0	0.0
25–29	0.0	0.0	0.0	0.0	0.0	0.1	0.0	0.0	0.1
30–34	0.0	0.0	0.1	0.1	0.1	0.0	0.0	0.0	0.1
35–39	0.0	0.0	0.1	0.1	0.1	0.0	0.0	0.0	0.0
40–44	0.1	0.0	0.0	0.1	0.1	0.1	0.1	0.0	0.1
45–49	0.2	0.1	0.4	0.1	0.2	0.2	0.2	0.3	0.1
50–54	0.3	0.7	0.5	0.9	0.7	0.6	0.8	0.6	0.6
55–59	0.9	1.5	1.4	2.1	1.9	2.0	2.1	2.3	2.4
60–64	0.8	3.4	4.2	4.0	4.9	5.5	5.8	5.2	7.6
65–69	2.5	6.5	8.5	10.3	11.3	11.0	12.5	13.6	13.4
70–74	2.8	11.1	16.7	20.4	19.8	27.5	27.4	32.3	35.3
75–79	3.7	11.7	26.8	32.5	36.0	45.3	53.1	67.2	65.7
80–84	6.3	14.3	32.5	44.9	49.0	64.5	80.4	109.5	118.5
85–	3.5	2.5	23.0	32.5	77.6	74.3	98.5	158.5	184.2

Mortality rates per 100,000 population.

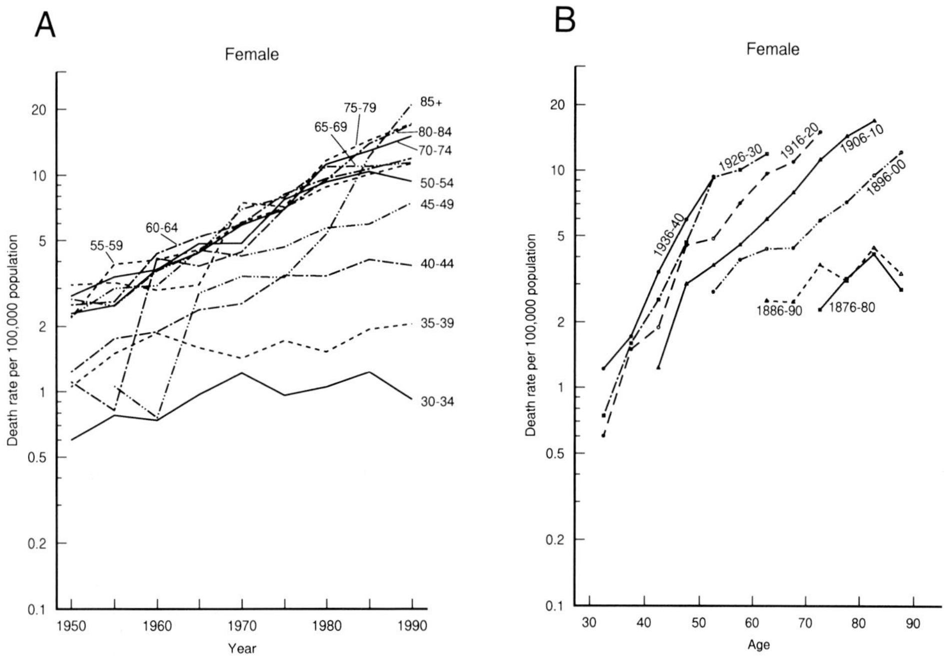

FIG. 3-16. Trends in the age- and sex-specific cancer mortality rate by age group (A) and by birth-year cohort (B) (1950–1990)

Cancer of the ovary (ICD, 9th revision, 183.0).

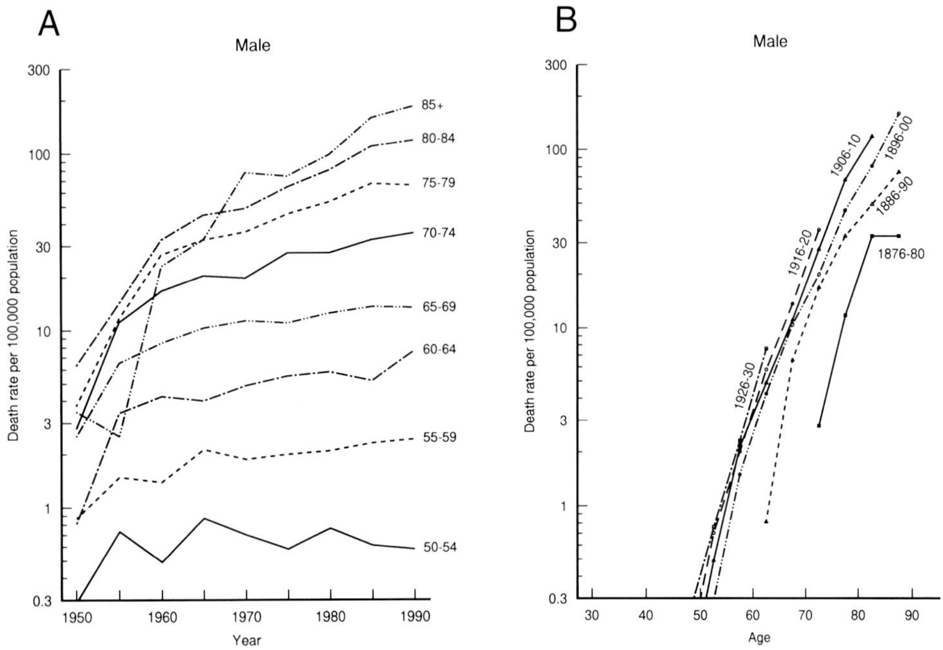

FIG. 3-17. Trends in the age- and sex-specific cancer mortality rate by age group (A) and by birth-year cohort (B) (1950–1990)

Cancer of the prostate (ICD, 9th revision, 185).

TABLE III-18. Age- and Sex-Specific Cancer Mortality Rates in Japan (1950–1990)
Cancer of the urinary bladder (ICD, 9th revision: 188)

	1950	1955	1960	1965	1970	1975	1980	1985	1990
Male									
0–4	0.0	0.0	0.0	0.0	0.0	0.1	0.0	0.0	0.0
5–9	0.0	0.0	0.0	0.0	0.0	0.0	0.0	0.0	0.0
10–14	0.0	0.0	0.0	0.0	0.0	0.0	0.0	0.0	0.0
15–19	0.1	0.0	0.0	0.0	0.0	0.0	0.0	0.0	0.0
20–24	0.0	0.0	0.0	0.0	0.0	0.0	0.0	0.0	0.0
25–29	0.0	0.0	0.0	0.1	0.0	0.0	0.0	0.0	0.0
30–34	0.1	0.2	0.0	0.1	0.1	0.1	0.0	0.1	0.1
35–39	0.1	0.2	0.1	0.2	0.3	0.0	0.0	0.1	0.0
40–44	0.2	0.4	0.2	0.6	0.4	0.4	0.4	0.3	0.3
45–49	0.7	1.0	0.6	1.1	0.8	0.8	0.8	0.6	0.7
50–54	1.2	1.8	1.7	2.0	2.0	1.2	1.8	1.2	1.2
55–59	2.1	3.1	3.7	3.4	4.2	4.3	4.0	3.8	3.1
60–64	4.6	5.0	6.8	6.4	8.2	6.3	6.9	5.7	6.1
65–69	8.7	12.2	12.5	12.6	13.6	12.0	14.4	11.3	10.4
70–74	9.8	18.0	20.8	21.4	22.3	23.4	21.7	20.3	20.7
75–79	12.7	20.2	26.8	31.0	31.5	29.9	40.0	36.5	35.0
80–84	19.9	31.5	34.3	37.4	40.7	50.1	63.1	54.2	55.6
85–	13.9	25.2	35.4	47.4	41.6	51.5	69.9	70.9	100.5
Female									
0–4	0.0	0.0	0.0	0.0	0.0	0.0	0.0	0.0	0.0
5–9	0.0	0.0	0.0	0.0	0.0	0.0	0.0	0.0	0.0
10–14	0.0	0.0	0.0	0.0	0.0	0.0	0.0	0.0	0.0
15–19	0.0	0.0	0.0	0.0	0.0	0.0	0.0	0.0	0.0
20–24	0.0	0.0	0.0	0.0	0.0	0.0	0.0	0.0	0.0
25–29	0.1	0.1	0.0	0.0	0.0	0.1	0.0	0.0	0.0
30–34	0.0	0.0	0.0	0.1	0.0	0.0	0.0	0.0	0.0
35–39	0.0	0.0	0.0	0.2	0.1	0.1	0.1	0.0	0.0
40–44	0.5	0.5	0.3	0.2	0.2	0.0	0.1	0.2	0.1
45–49	0.7	0.7	0.6	0.5	0.8	0.4	0.4	0.3	0.2
50–54	1.4	1.3	1.1	1.5	0.6	0.6	0.5	0.5	0.3
55–59	1.3	1.9	1.7	2.3	1.1	1.4	1.2	1.0	0.5
60–64	3.3	3.4	6.0	3.6	3.2	3.0	2.3	1.9	1.5
65–69	3.8	5.4	7.1	5.0	6.3	5.2	4.0	4.1	2.9
70–74	3.9	7.6	7.9	8.0	8.5	8.8	7.8	7.0	5.3
75–79	4.6	8.3	10.9	12.1	15.8	13.8	13.1	13.9	10.8
80–84	2.8	5.7	10.8	12.9	14.5	21.4	22.1	17.2	18.8
85–	3.0	3.2	11.4	6.8	11.2	18.7	25.5	27.1	29.1

Mortality rates per 100,000 population.

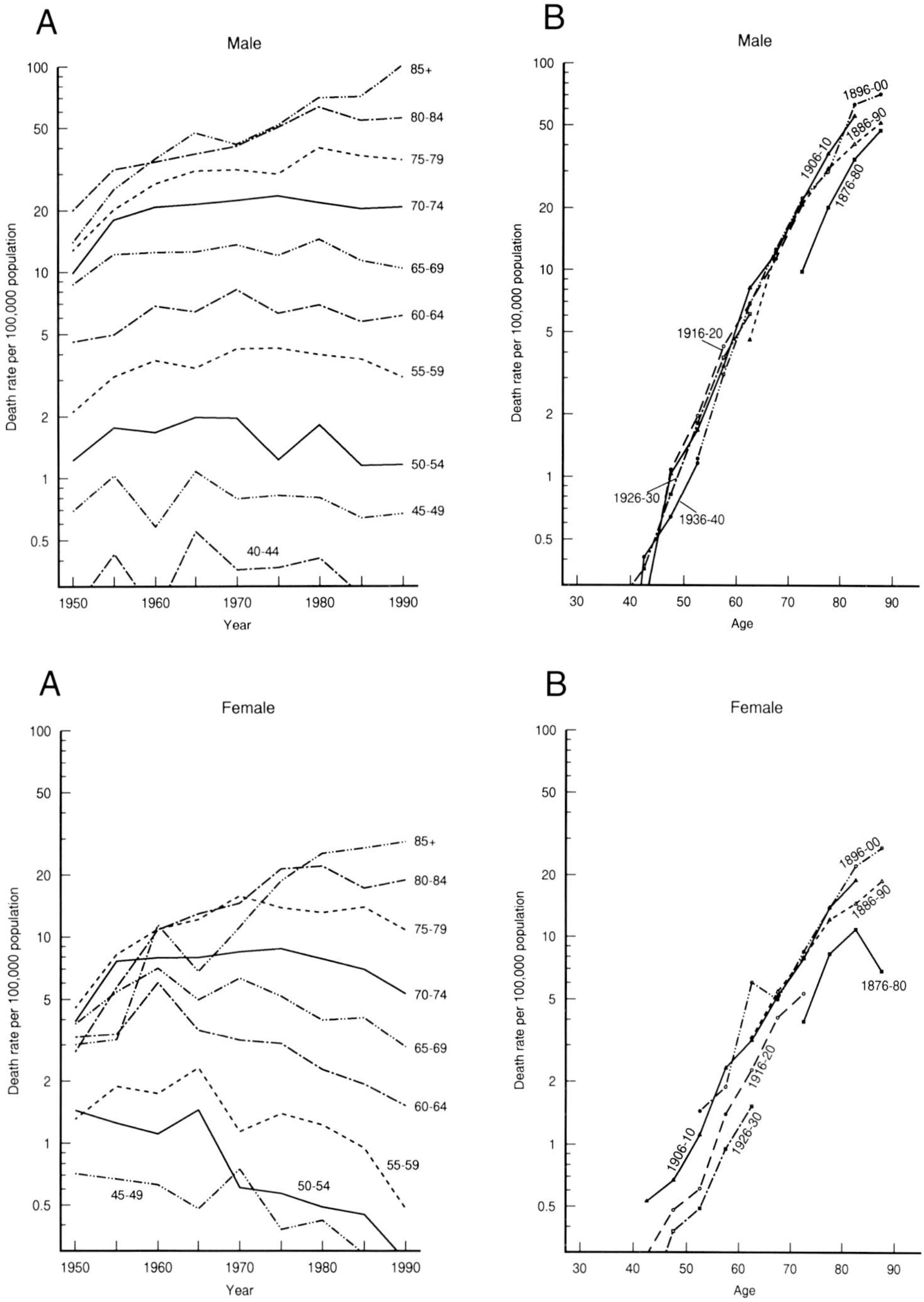

Fig. 3-18. Trends in the age- and sex-specific cancer mortality rate by age group (A) and by birth-year cohort (B) (1950–1990)
Cancer of the urinary bladder (ICD, 9th revision, 188).

Table III-19. Age- and Sex-Specific Cancer Mortality Rates in Japan (1950–1990)
Cancer of the kidney (ICD, 9th revision: 189.0,189.1)

	1950	1955	1960	1965	1970	1975	1980	1985	1990
Male									
0–4	0.4	0.2	0.4	0.5	0.4	0.3	0.3	0.2	0.1
5–9	0.0	0.1	0.1	0.1	0.1	0.1	0.1	0.1	0.0
10–14	0.1	0.0	0.1	0.0	0.0	0.0	0.0	0.0	0.0
15–19	0.0	0.0	0.0	0.0	0.0	0.0	0.1	0.1	0.1
20–24	0.0	0.1	0.1	0.2	0.1	0.1	0.0	0.0	0.1
25–29	0.1	0.0	0.2	0.1	0.0	0.1	0.0	0.2	0.0
30–34	0.0	0.0	0.1	0.1	0.2	0.0	0.0	0.3	0.2
35–39	0.2	0.3	0.1	0.2	0.1	0.2	0.1	0.2	0.3
40–44	0.6	0.2	0.4	0.2	0.4	0.6	0.7	0.5	0.7
45–49	0.5	0.5	0.9	0.9	0.9	0.6	1.5	1.5	1.3
50–54	0.6	0.7	1.2	1.8	1.8	1.9	2.7	3.0	3.0
55–59	0.7	1.1	2.4	2.4	2.3	4.2	4.2	4.9	5.3
60–64	1.4	2.5	3.3	3.7	4.7	5.0	6.8	7.9	8.6
65–69	1.6	1.9	3.9	4.5	6.0	7.7	9.0	12.8	12.0
70–74	1.1	3.2	3.6	4.8	6.5	9.0	10.1	14.0	16.7
75–79	0.8	1.5	4.8	3.8	5.7	7.6	14.3	16.9	22.6
80–84	2.1	0.0	3.0	2.7	4.6	8.1	15.4	16.5	24.3
85–	0.0	2.5	1.8	2.7	3.4	4.1	12.8	16.4	23.6
Female									
0–4	0.2	0.2	0.5	0.6	0.5	0.1	0.3	0.1	0.2
5–9	0.1	0.1	0.2	0.1	0.1	0.1	0.1	0.1	0.0
10–14	0.0	0.0	0.0	0.0	0.0	0.0	0.0	0.1	0.1
15–19	0.1	0.0	0.0	0.0	0.0	0.1	0.1	0.0	0.0
20–24	0.1	0.0	0.1	0.0	0.0	0.0	0.0	0.0	0.0
25–29	0.1	0.1	0.1	0.0	0.1	0.0	0.0	0.2	0.1
30–34	0.0	0.1	0.1	0.1	0.1	0.0	0.0	0.1	0.1
35–39	0.2	0.1	0.2	0.1	0.1	0.2	0.2	0.1	0.1
40–44	0.3	0.4	0.3	0.1	0.2	0.2	0.2	0.3	0.4
45–49	0.2	0.3	0.4	0.5	0.4	0.3	0.3	0.3	0.4
50–54	0.5	0.9	0.7	0.8	0.7	0.6	0.9	0.8	0.9
55–59	0.4	0.5	0.9	0.8	1.0	1.4	1.3	1.4	1.8
60–64	0.5	0.9	1.3	1.6	1.8	2.1	2.4	3.0	2.4
65–69	1.4	1.2	1.3	2.0	2.5	3.7	3.2	3.7	3.7
70–74	1.5	1.3	2.5	2.9	3.8	3.4	4.7	4.6	5.6
75–79	1.4	1.5	2.6	3.1	2.0	4.0	4.7	7.2	8.2
80–84	0.6	1.6	1.3	2.1	1.7	3.0	2.7	8.1	10.9
85–	1.5	1.1	2.3	0.6	1.9	4.1	4.2	6.8	11.8

Mortality rates per 100,000 population.

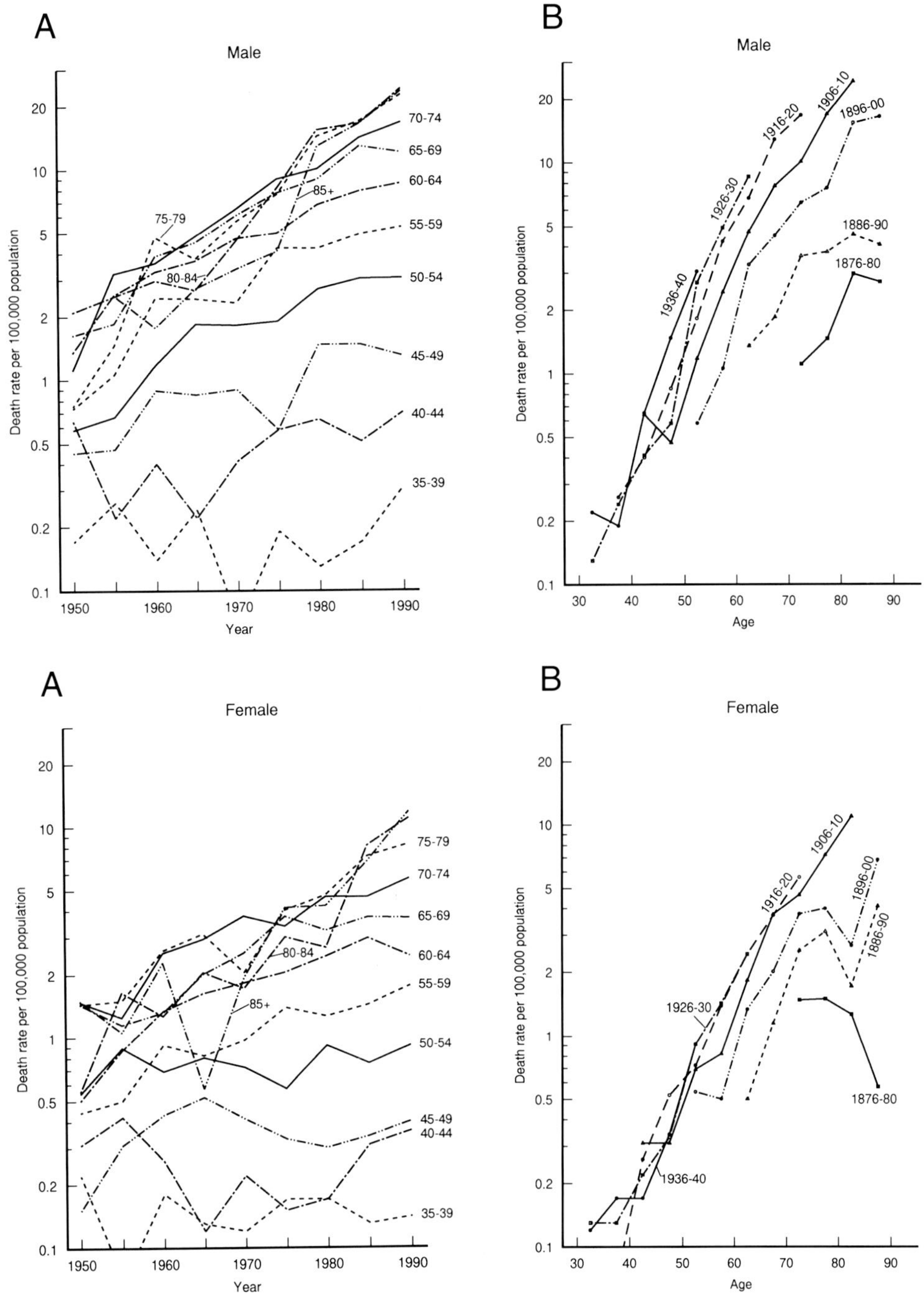

FIG. 3-19. Trends in the age- and sex-specific cancer mortality rate by age group (A) and by birth-year cohort (B) (1950–1990)

Cancer of the kidney (ICD, 9th revision, 189.0, 189.1).

TABLE III-20. Age- and Sex-Specific Cancer Mortality Rates in Japan (1950–1990)
Cancer of the lymphatic and hematopoietic systems other than leukemia (ICD, 9th revision: 200–203)

	1950	1955	1960	1965	1970	1975	1980	1985	1990
Male									
0–4	0.7	0.5	0.7	0.8	0.4	0.6	0.6	0.7	0.3
5–9	0.4	0.4	0.7	0.8	0.5	0.5	0.7	0.5	0.5
10–14	0.3	0.4	0.6	0.6	0.9	0.9	0.7	0.7	0.4
15–19	0.4	0.8	0.6	0.8	0.8	1.2	1.3	1.0	0.7
20–24	0.5	0.3	0.7	0.7	1.0	1.0	0.8	0.6	0.8
25–29	0.5	0.8	0.6	1.0	1.0	1.0	1.0	0.7	1.0
30–34	0.7	1.0	1.2	1.3	1.4	1.0	1.0	0.7	1.1
35–39	1.1	1.4	1.6	1.7	1.6	1.9	1.8	1.8	1.2
40–44	1.1	1.7	2.2	2.7	2.6	3.0	2.7	2.1	2.2
45–49	2.1	3.4	3.2	3.3	3.7	4.9	5.1	4.0	4.1
50–54	2.7	4.0	5.2	5.3	5.4	6.7	8.1	6.6	5.6
55–59	3.8	5.0	7.1	6.9	9.6	11.2	11.2	11.1	12.3
60–64	4.7	7.0	9.0	11.7	13.6	15.2	16.6	16.9	19.2
65–69	6.4	7.1	8.6	14.1	16.8	21.9	23.4	23.9	23.9
70–74	5.4	8.9	10.4	14.1	19.7	24.8	32.2	38.2	38.6
75–79	5.6	7.6	8.8	12.6	19.0	26.7	38.5	49.1	53.4
80–84	4.2	4.5	7.7	10.7	16.6	27.7	38.4	59.4	62.1
85–	0.0	7.6	12.4	14.9	19.1	21.2	40.2	52.1	64.3
Female									
0–4	0.4	0.7	0.3	0.5	0.4	0.4	0.4	0.4	0.3
5–9	0.3	0.4	0.4	0.5	0.2	0.2	0.2	0.2	0.2
10–14	0.1	0.2	0.3	0.3	0.3	0.5	0.2	0.3	0.2
15–19	0.3	0.3	0.3	0.5	0.3	0.4	0.5	0.4	0.4
20–24	0.1	0.3	0.3	0.5	0.5	0.4	0.4	0.3	0.5
25–29	0.3	0.3	0.5	0.5	0.3	0.6	0.7	0.5	0.3
30–34	0.4	0.7	0.6	0.8	0.7	0.8	0.7	0.6	0.7
35–39	0.8	0.6	0.7	0.7	1.2	1.0	0.9	0.9	1.0
40–44	1.2	0.6	0.8	1.2	1.2	1.1	1.5	1.2	1.5
45–49	1.6	1.3	2.0	2.0	2.2	2.3	2.3	2.1	2.2
50–54	1.1	1.9	2.6	2.8	3.5	4.0	4.0	3.4	3.3
55–59	2.8	3.4	3.1	4.6	5.7	6.1	7.0	5.7	6.0
60–64	2.3	3.6	3.8	4.8	8.1	8.2	9.3	8.8	9.5
65–69	3.4	4.1	4.9	7.7	9.1	12.2	12.3	14.5	13.6
70–74	3.0	3.9	7.0	6.2	9.4	12.8	18.1	19.6	21.3
75–79	1.7	3.8	5.7	7.1	11.6	15.7	21.9	27.4	29.0
80–84	3.9	4.5	8.0	5.3	5.4	13.0	19.9	27.0	39.2
85–	3.0	3.2	6.8	5.1	4.9	11.6	15.1	28.4	30.1

Mortality rates per 100,000 population.

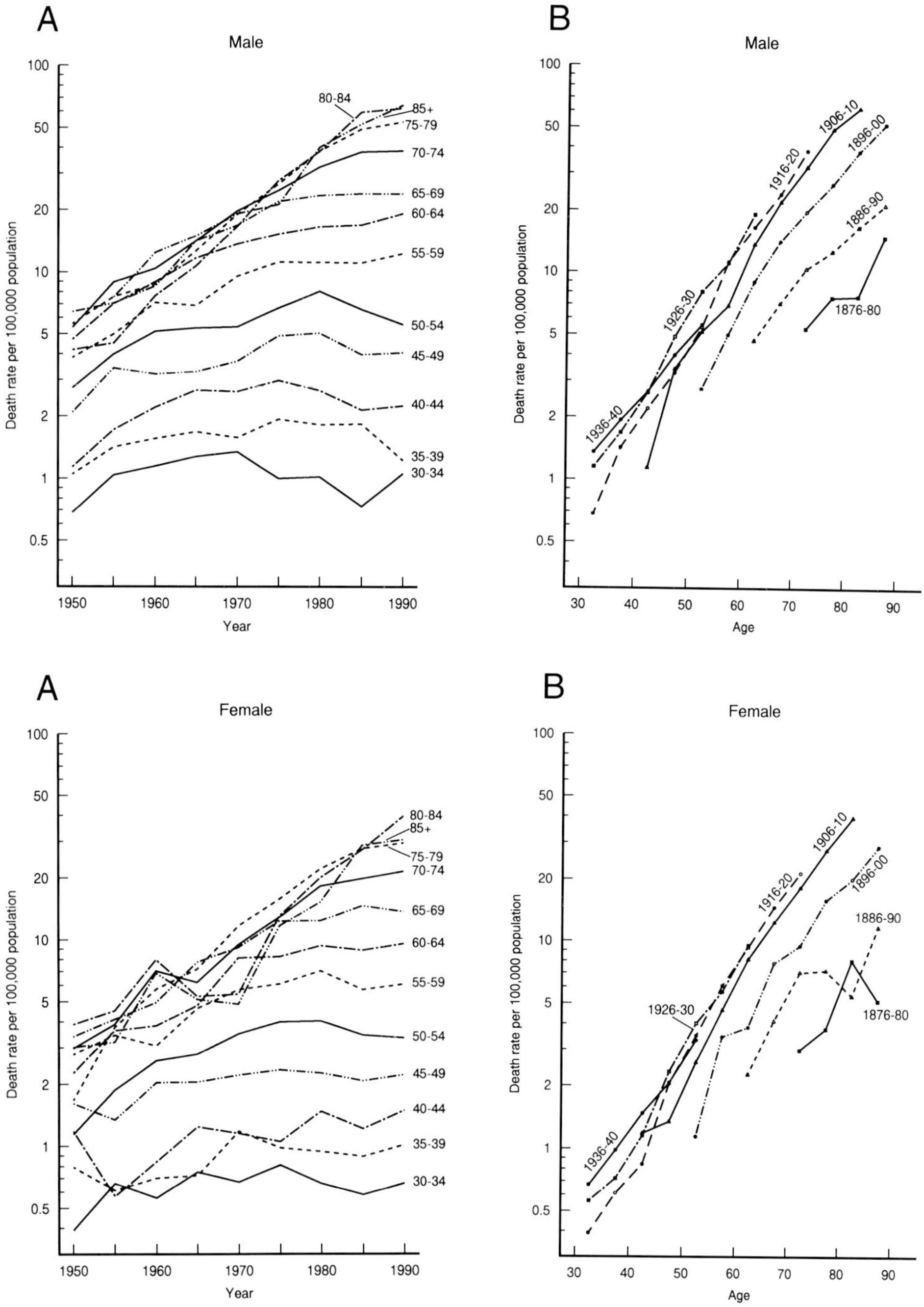

FIG. 3-20. Trends in the age- and sex-specific cancer mortality rate by age group (A) and by birth-year cohort (B) (1950–1990)

Cancer of the lymphatic and hematopoietic systems other than leukemia (ICD, 9th revision, 200–203).

TABLE III-21. Age- and Sex-Specific Cancer Mortality Rates in Japan (1950–1990)
Leukemia (ICD, 9th revision: 204–208)

	1950	1955	1960	1965	1970	1975	1980	1985	1990
Male									
0–4	2.5	4.1	4.5	4.4	4.6	3.9	2.8	1.3	1.4
5–9	1.5	2.8	2.9	3.7	3.5	3.5	3.3	2.6	1.4
10–14	1.5	2.4	2.8	3.0	2.2	2.3	2.6	2.2	2.0
15–19	1.7	2.5	2.8	3.3	3.2	2.8	2.5	2.7	2.2
20–24	1.2	2.1	2.4	2.7	2.5	2.6	2.0	2.2	2.3
25–29	1.4	2.3	2.3	2.6	2.7	2.4	2.8	2.1	2.1
30–34	1.7	2.2	2.4	2.4	2.9	3.4	2.4	2.8	2.2
35–39	1.7	2.6	2.5	3.2	3.5	3.5	3.5	3.4	3.1
40–44	1.9	3.4	3.5	3.0	3.8	4.0	4.0	3.7	3.5
45–49	2.1	3.0	3.7	4.6	5.0	4.9	4.9	4.8	4.3
50–54	2.3	2.8	4.0	4.9	5.1	5.6	5.7	5.8	6.0
55–59	1.9	3.3	5.4	5.2	6.2	6.4	7.1	7.5	8.4
60–64	2.5	3.2	4.6	7.1	7.5	8.5	8.4	10.1	11.9
65–69	2.0	3.1	5.0	7.0	8.9	10.2	12.5	14.6	13.2
70–74	0.7	2.9	5.6	5.2	9.7	11.7	16.8	20.3	18.2
75–79	1.9	1.8	3.2	5.1	8.1	13.1	19.6	25.4	24.6
80–84	1.1	0.8	4.1	2.1	4.2	10.4	21.1	25.9	33.1
85–	0.0	0.0	1.8	2.7	3.4	6.5	17.5	23.1	31.4
Female									
0–4	2.0	2.7	3.7	3.5	3.6	3.1	2.0	1.4	1.4
5–9	1.0	1.9	2.2	2.7	2.8	2.7	2.3	1.7	1.4
10–14	1.1	1.8	2.1	2.4	2.3	1.9	1.9	1.6	1.2
15–19	1.0	1.5	2.0	2.6	2.3	2.2	2.2	1.7	1.2
20–24	1.0	1.4	2.1	1.8	2.0	2.0	1.7	1.3	1.2
25–29	1.1	1.9	1.7	2.0	1.8	2.1	1.5	1.5	1.3
30–34	0.7	1.2	2.6	2.1	1.6	2.5	2.2	2.0	1.7
35–39	1.4	1.7	2.4	2.8	2.7	2.4	2.5	2.3	2.5
40–44	1.0	2.3	2.6	2.9	3.0	3.1	3.4	3.0	2.6
45–49	1.5	2.2	3.3	3.3	4.2	3.5	3.3	3.6	3.7
50–54	1.6	1.9	2.3	3.7	3.0	4.1	4.5	4.6	4.3
55–59	1.2	2.3	2.9	4.1	5.7	5.6	4.3	5.4	5.6
60–64	1.4	1.9	3.0	4.6	5.0	5.4	6.0	6.4	6.5
65–69	1.1	1.7	3.3	3.8	5.2	6.8	7.1	7.5	8.2
70–74	0.8	1.3	1.8	3.4	5.6	6.4	8.4	9.9	10.6
75–79	0.0	0.4	2.3	3.1	2.6	8.6	9.4	12.6	12.0
80–84	0.0	0.0	1.0	1.2	3.4	4.6	8.8	12.6	18.0
85–	0.0	0.0	0.0	0.0	0.0	3.7	5.9	11.9	13.6

Mortality rates per 100,000 population.

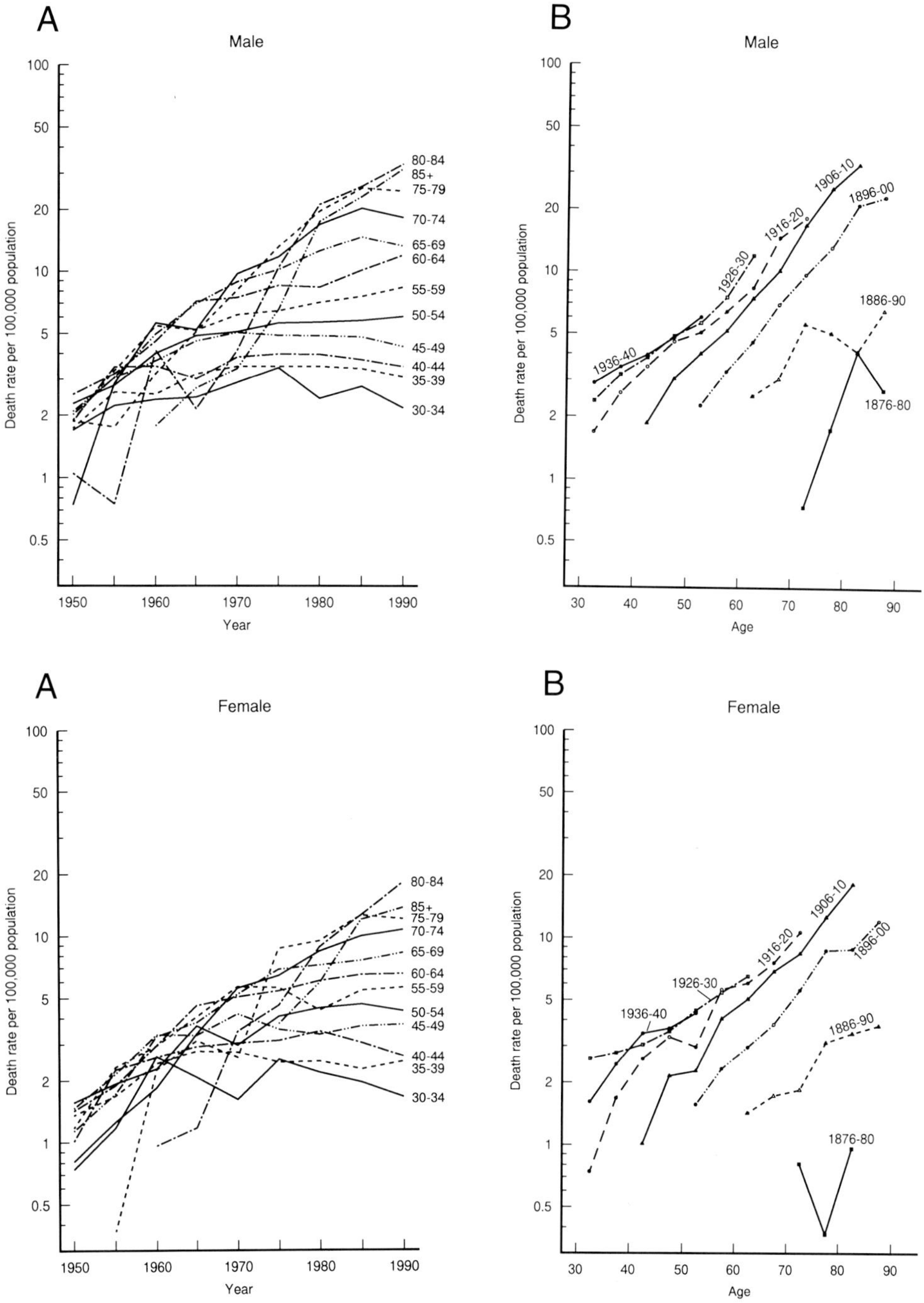

FIG. 3-21. Trends in the age- and sex-specific cancer mortality rate by age group (A) and by birth-year cohort (B) (1950–1990)
Leukemia (ICD, 9th revision, 204–208).

TABLE IV-1. Age-Adjusted Death Rates[a] for Cancer by Site for Cities and Counties in Japan (1970)

ICD (8th revision)	Site	Rate per 100,000 population[b]				
		All Japan	All cities	10 large cities[c]	Other cities	Counties
Male						
140–209	All sites	198.3	204.0	206.6	203.3	189.0
140–149	Buccal cavity and pharynx	2.2	2.4	2.8	2.2	1.8
150	Esophagus	11.4	11.9	12.6	11.7	10.4
151	Stomach	88.5	90.0	86.9	91.2	86.3
153	Colon	5.2	5.6	5.9	5.4	4.5
154	Rectum	7.8	8.1	8.4	8.0	7.1
155, 197.7, 197.8	Liver	17.6	17.7	16.9	18.0	17.6
156	Biliary passages	4.0	4.1	4.7	3.9	4.0
157	Pancreas	7.4	7.5	7.9	7.4	7.0
161	Larynx	2.4	2.7	3.2	2.5	2.0
162	Trachea, bronchus, and lung	22.4	24.0	27.1	22.9	19.5
170	Bone	1.4	1.4	1.2	1.5	1.4
172, 173	Skin	1.3	1.1	1.2	1.1	1.5
185	Prostate	3.2	3.3	3.4	3.3	3.1
188	Urinary bladder	3.4	3.6	4.0	3.4	3.1
189.0, 189.1	Kidney	1.2	1.4	1.7	1.2	0.9
204–207	Leukemia	4.3	4.3	4.1	4.3	4.4
200–203, 208–209	Lymphatic and hematopoietic systems other than leukemia	4.5	4.5	4.1	4.6	4.5
Female						
140–209	All sites	126.5	129.6	131.9	128.8	120.6
140–149	Buccal cavity and pharynx	0.9	1.0	1.1	0.9	0.7
150	Esophagus	2.9	2.9	3.0	2.9	2.8
151	Stomach	46.3	46.9	46.0	47.3	45.3
153	Colon	5.0	5.2	5.9	4.9	4.7
154	Rectum	5.3	5.3	5.6	5.3	5.2
155, 197.7, 197.8	Liver	8.9	8.6	7.8	8.9	9.4
156	Biliary passages	4.3	4.4	4.2	4.5	4.1
157	Pancreas	4.5	4.7	4.4	4.8	4.0
161	Larynx	0.4	0.4	0.6	0.4	0.4
162	Trachea, bronchus, and lung	7.3	7.9	8.5	7.7	6.1
170	Bone	0.8	0.8	0.8	0.8	0.9
172, 173	Skin	0.8	0.9	0.9	0.8	0.8
174	Breast	5.8	6.2	7.4	5.8	4.8
180–182	Uterus	15.1	15.7	16.3	15.5	13.8
183.0	Ovary	2.5	2.7	2.9	2.6	2.1
188	Urinary bladder	1.4	1.4	1.5	1.4	1.3
189.0, 189.1	Kidney	0.6	0.6	0.8	0.5	0.5
204–207	Leukemia	3.1	3.0	3.1	3.0	3.2
200–203, 208–209	Lymphatic and hematopoietic systems other than leukemia	2.4	2.3	2.5	2.3	2.6

[a] Standardized on the age distribution of the 'model' population for the year 1985 in Japan.

[b] Based on the total population (including foreigners).

[c] 10 large cities: Sapporo, Tokyo, Yokohama, Kawasaki, Nagoya, Kyoto, Osaka, Kobe, Kitakyushu, and Fukuoka.

TABLE IV-2. Age-Adjusted Death Rates[a] for Cancer by Site for Cities and Counties in Japan (1980)

ICD (9th revision)	Site	Rate per 100,000 population[b]				
		All Japan	All cities	10 large cities[c]	Other cities	Counties
Male						
140–208	All sites	209.9	215.6	226.8	211.8	197.8
140–149	Buccal cavity and pharynx	2.7	2.9	3.1	2.8	2.2
150	Esophagus	10.3	10.6	12.1	10.1	9.4
151	Stomach	69.6	70.3	71.3	69.9	68.4
153	Colon	8.7	9.6	11.1	9.1	6.7
154	Rectum	8.9	9.0	8.9	9.1	8.7
155	Liver	21.2	22.3	24.6	21.5	18.7
156	Biliary passages	6.4	6.5	6.5	6.5	6.3
157	Pancreas	10.0	10.1	10.0	10.1	9.9
161	Larynx	1.7	1.8	2.2	1.7	1.5
162	Trachea, bronchus, and lung	35.3	36.4	38.7	35.6	33.1
170	Bone	0.6	0.6	0.5	0.6	0.7
172, 173	Skin	0.8	0.7	0.7	0.8	0.8
185	Prostate	4.4	4.5	4.6	4.5	4.1
188	Urinary bladder	3.9	4.2	4.6	4.0	3.3
189.0, 189.1	Kidney	2.1	2.3	2.6	2.1	1.7
204–208	Leukemia	5.1	5.2	5.5	5.0	4.8
200–203	Lymphoid tissue and multiple myeloma	6.3	6.4	6.8	6.2	6.3
Female						
140–208	All sites	118.4	121.3	126.2	119.6	111.8
140–149	Buccal cavity and pharynx	1.0	1.1	1.1	1.1	0.9
150	Esophagus	2.2	2.2	2.4	2.1	2.1
151	Stomach	34.0	34.1	34.2	34.1	33.9
153	Colon	7.1	7.4	8.0	7.3	6.3
154	Rectum	5.2	5.2	5.5	5.1	5.1
155	Liver	7.3	7.2	7.1	7.3	7.6
156	Biliary passages	6.6	6.6	6.7	6.6	6.6
157	Pancreas	5.8	6.0	6.1	6.0	5.4
161	Larynx	0.2	0.2	0.2	0.2	0.2
162	Trachea, bronchus, and lung	10.1	10.8	12.4	10.3	8.7
170	Bone	0.4	0.4	0.3	0.4	0.3
172, 173	Skin	0.5	0.5	0.4	0.5	0.6
174	Breast	7.2	7.9	9.6	7.3	5.5
179–182	Uterus	9.5	10.0	10.8	9.7	8.3
183.0	Ovary	3.7	3.8	4.0	3.8	3.2
188	Urinary bladder	1.3	1.4	1.3	1.4	1.2
189.0, 189.1	Kidney	0.7	0.8	1.0	0.7	0.7
204–208	Leukemia	3.3	3.3	3.2	3.4	3.3
200–203	Lymphoid tissue and multiple myeloma	3.4	3.4	3.5	3.4	3.4

[a] Standardized on the age distribution of the 'model' population for the year 1985 in Japan.
[b] Based on the total population (including foreigners).
[c] 10 large cities: Sapporo, Tokyo, Yokohama, Kawasaki, Nagoya, Kyoto, Osaka, Kobe, Kitakyushu, and Fukuoka.

TABLE IV-3. Age-Adjusted Death Rates[a] for Cancer by Site for Cities and Counties in Japan (1990)

ICD (9th revision)	Site	Rate per 100,000 population[b]				
		All Japan	All cities	10 large cities[c]	Other cities	Counties
Male						
140–208	All sites	215.3	219.6	233.7	214.9	204.9
140–149	Buccal cavity and pharynx	3.0	3.2	3.7	3.0	2.7
150	Esophagus	9.8	10.2	11.6	9.7	8.9
151	Stomach	49.5	49.8	50.8	49.8	48.8
153	Colon	12.9	13.6	15.3	13.1	11.0
154	Rectum	9.1	9.2	9.5	9.1	9.0
155	Liver	28.4	30.0	34.6	28.4	24.2
156	Biliary passages	8.5	8.5	8.6	8.4	8.7
157	Pancreas	12.1	12.1	12.4	12.0	12.2
161	Larynx	1.3	1.3	1.4	1.3	1.3
162	Trachea, bronchus, and lung	45.0	45.9	49.4	44.7	42.8
170	Bone	0.4	0.4	0.4	0.4	0.4
172, 173	Skin	0.6	0.6	0.6	0.6	0.7
185	Prostate	6.0	6.0	6.1	5.9	6.0
188	Urinary bladder	3.6	3.7	3.8	3.7	3.3
189.0, 189.1	Kidney	2.9	3.1	3.4	2.9	2.5
204–208	Leukemia	5.3	5.1	4.8	5.2	5.8
200–203	Lymphoid tissue and multiple myeloma	7.0	7.0	7.2	6.9	7.1
Female						
140–208	All sites	107.4	110.1	118.9	107.3	100.4
140–149	Buccal cavity and pharynx	0.9	1.0	1.1	0.9	0.8
150	Esophagus	1.5	1.6	2.0	1.4	1.2
151	Stomach	21.5	21.5	21.6	21.5	21.5
153	Colon	9.3	9.7	10.7	9.3	8.5
154	Rectum	4.6	4.6	4.7	4.6	4.4
155	Liver	7.8	8.2	9.8	7.7	6.8
156	Biliary passages	8.0	8.0	8.0	8.0	7.8
157	Pancreas	7.1	7.3	7.6	7.2	6.6
161	Larynx	0.1	0.1	0.1	0.1	0.1
162	Trachea, bronchus, and lung	11.5	12.1	14.6	11.3	10.1
170	Bone	0.3	0.3	0.3	0.3	0.2
172, 173	Skin	0.4	0.3	0.4	0.3	0.4
174	Breast	8.2	8.6	10.3	8.1	6.8
179–182	Uterus	5.8	6.1	6.5	6.0	5.1
183.0	Ovary	4.4	4.6	4.8	4.5	3.9
188	Urinary bladder	1.0	1.0	1.1	1.0	1.0
189.0, 189.1	Kidney	1.0	1.1	1.3	1.0	0.9
204–208	Leukemia	3.3	3.2	3.0	3.3	3.7
200–203	Lymphoid tissue and multiple myeloma	3.9	3.9	3.9	3.9	3.8

[a] Standardized on the age distribution of the 'model' population for the year 1985 in Japan.
[b] Based on the total population (including foreigners).
[c] 10 large cities: Sapporo, Tokyo, Yokohama, Kawasaki, Nagoya, Kyoto, Osaka, Kobe, Kitakyushu, and Fukuoka.

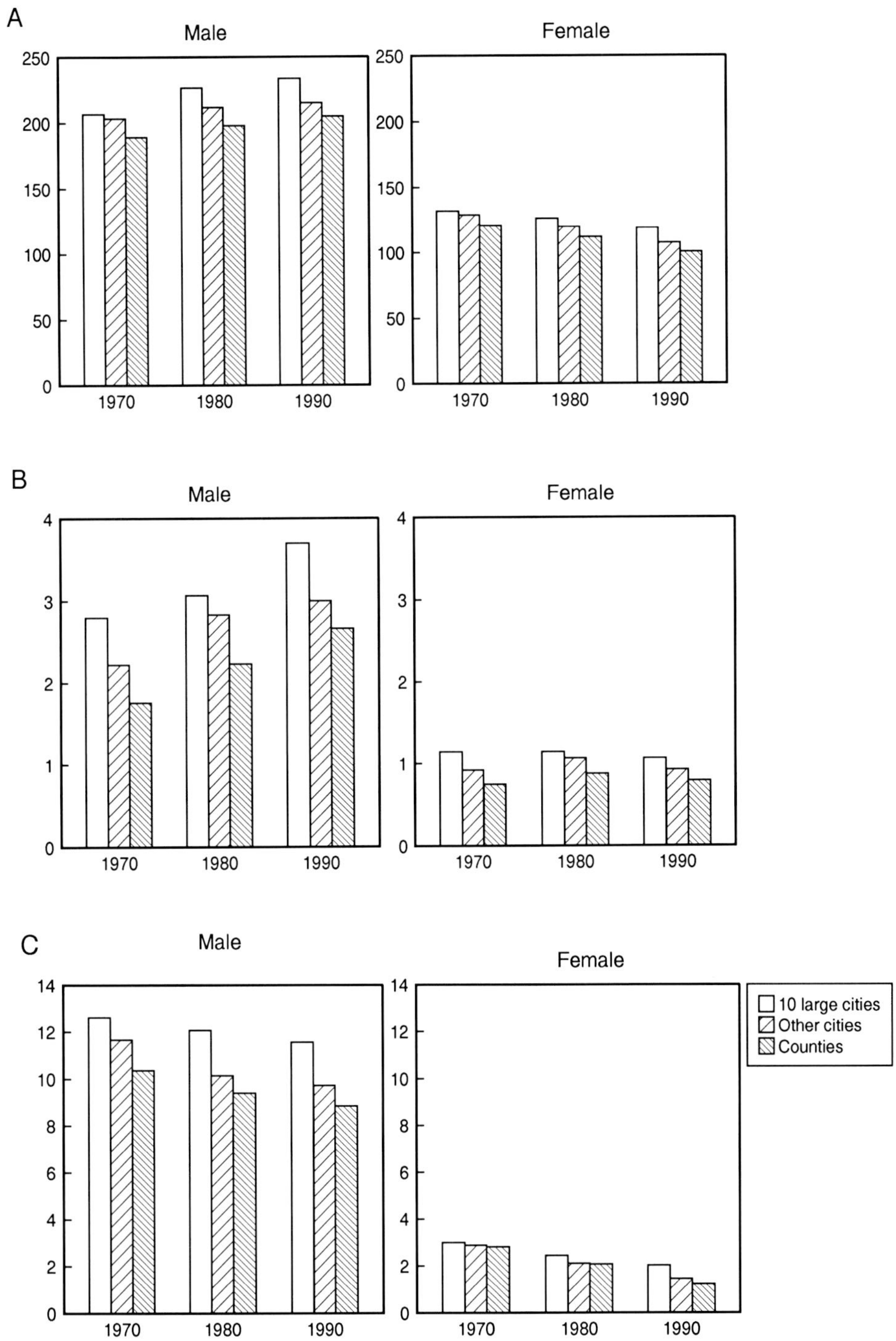

FIG. 4-1. Age-adjusted death rates for cancer for 10 large cities, other cities, and counties (1970, 1980, 1990)

A: cancer of all sites (ICD, 9th revision, 140–208). B: cancer of the buccal cavity and pharynx (ICD, 9th revision, 140–149). C: cancer of the esophagus (ICD, 9th revision, 150).

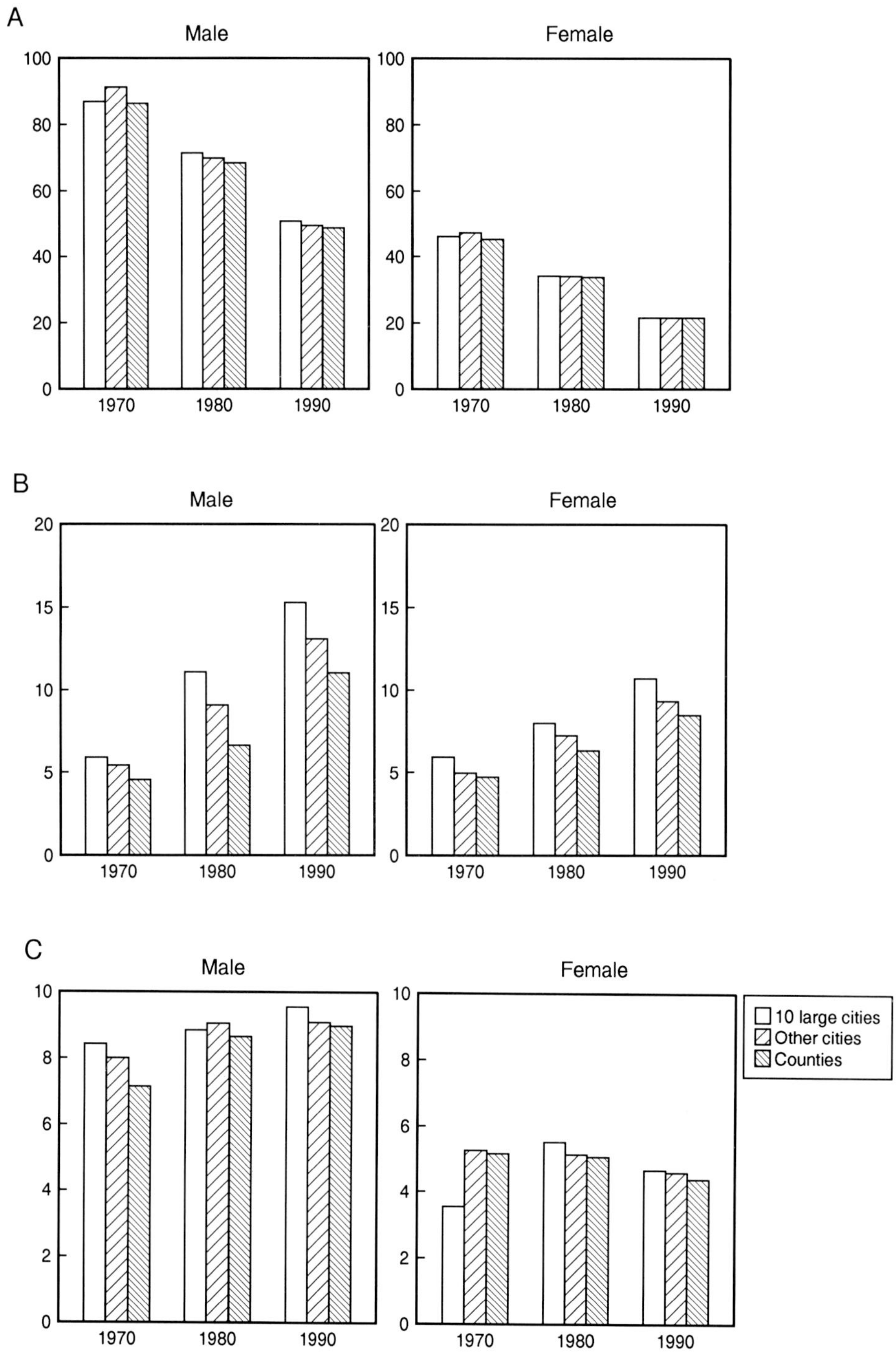

FIG. 4-2. Age-adjusted death rates for cancer for 10 large cities, other cities, and counties (1970, 1980, 1990)

A: cancer of the stomach (ICD, 9th revision, 151). B: cancer of the colon (ICD, 9th revision, 153). C: cancer of the rectum (ICD, 9th revision, 154).

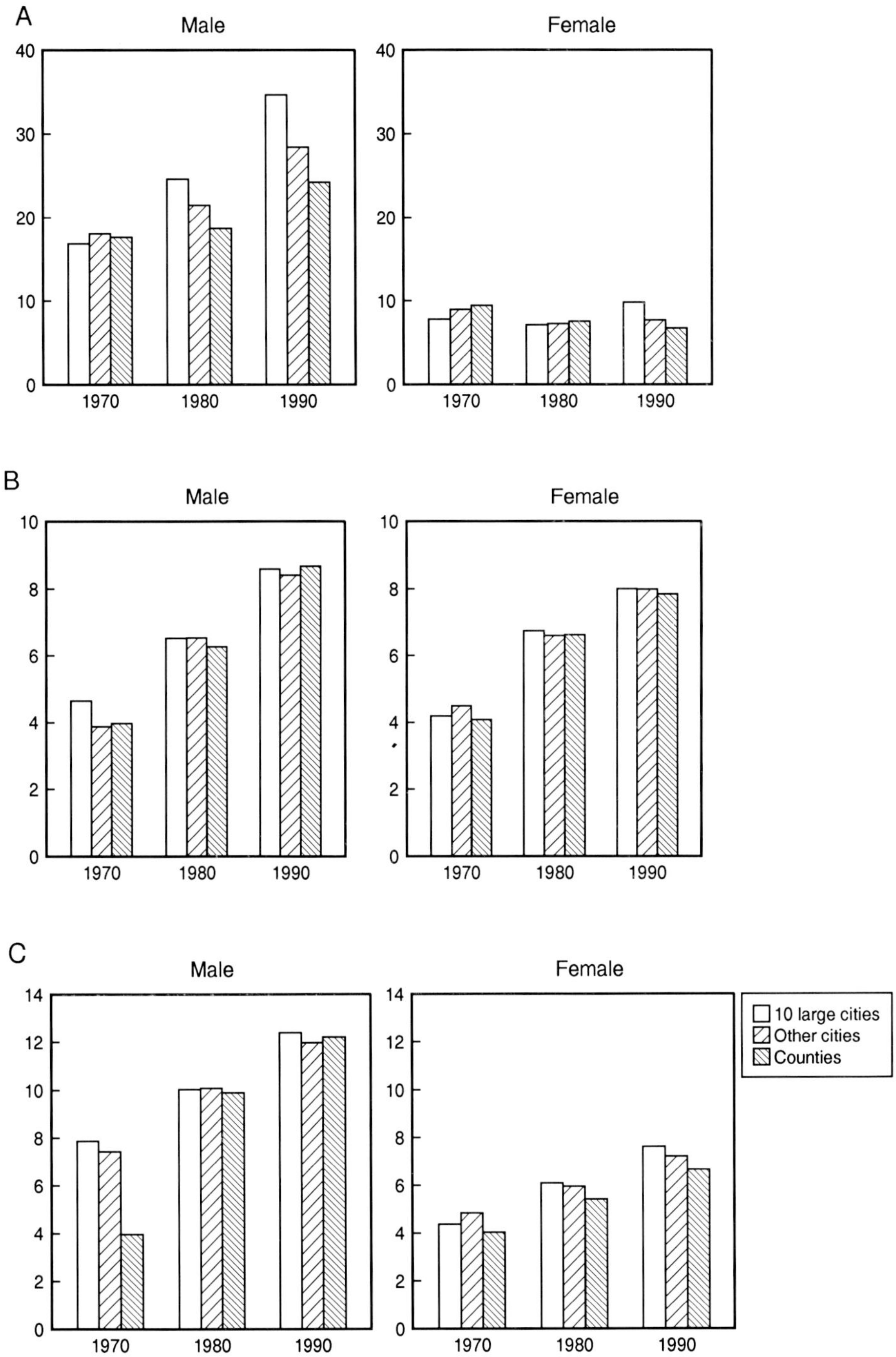

FIG. 4-3. Age-adjusted death rates for cancer for 10 large cities, other cities, and counties (1970, 1980, 1990)

A: cancer of the liver (ICD, 9th revision, 155). B: cancer of the biliary passages (ICD, 9th revision, 156). C: cancer of the pancreas (ICD, 9th revision, 157).

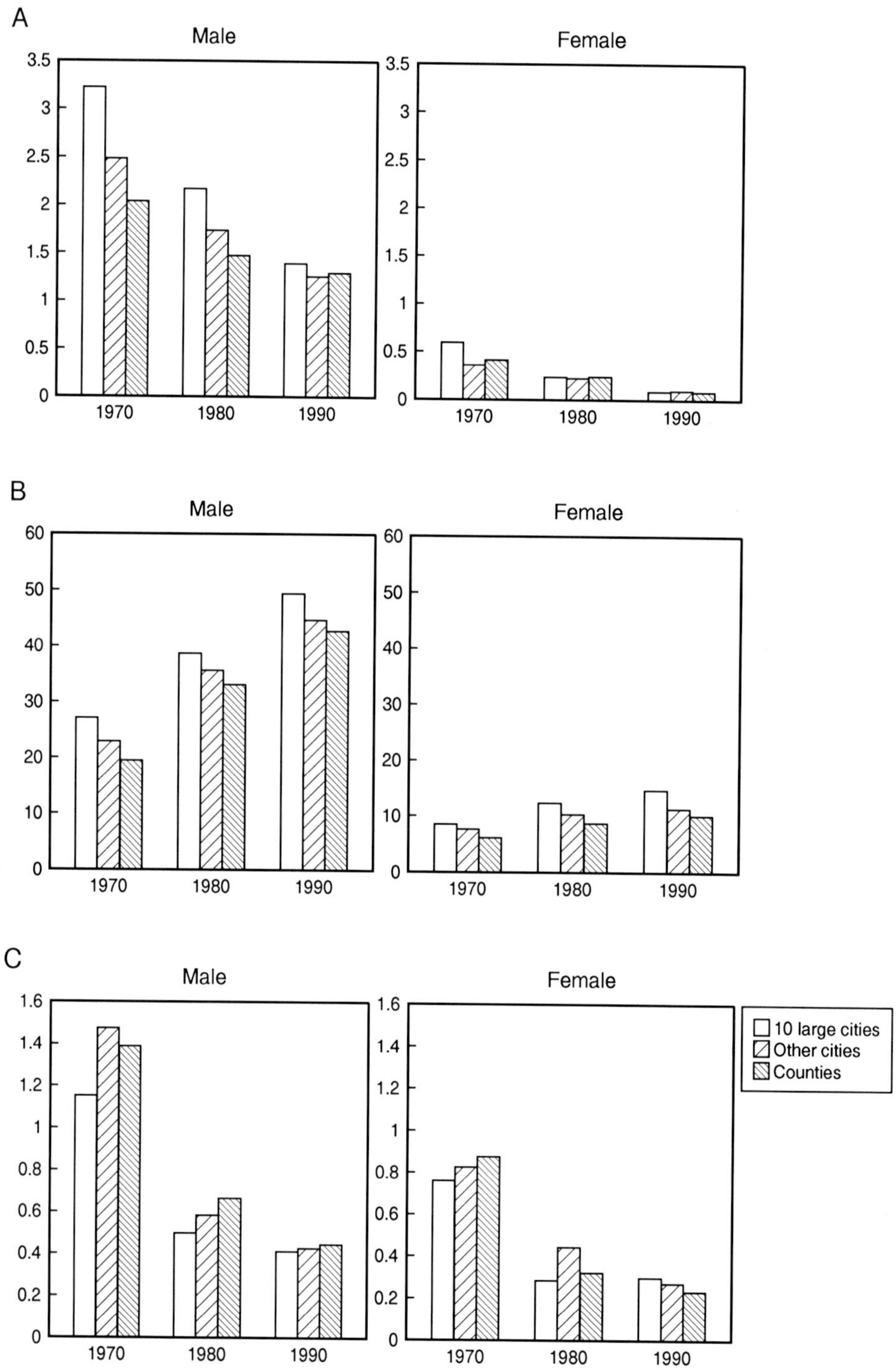

FIG. 4-4. Age-adjusted death rates for cancer for 10 large cities, other cities, and counties (1970, 1980, 1990)

A: cancer of the larynx (ICD, 9th revision, 161). B: cancer of the trachea, bronchus, and lung (ICD, 9th revision, 162). C: cancer of the bone (ICD, 9th revision, 170).

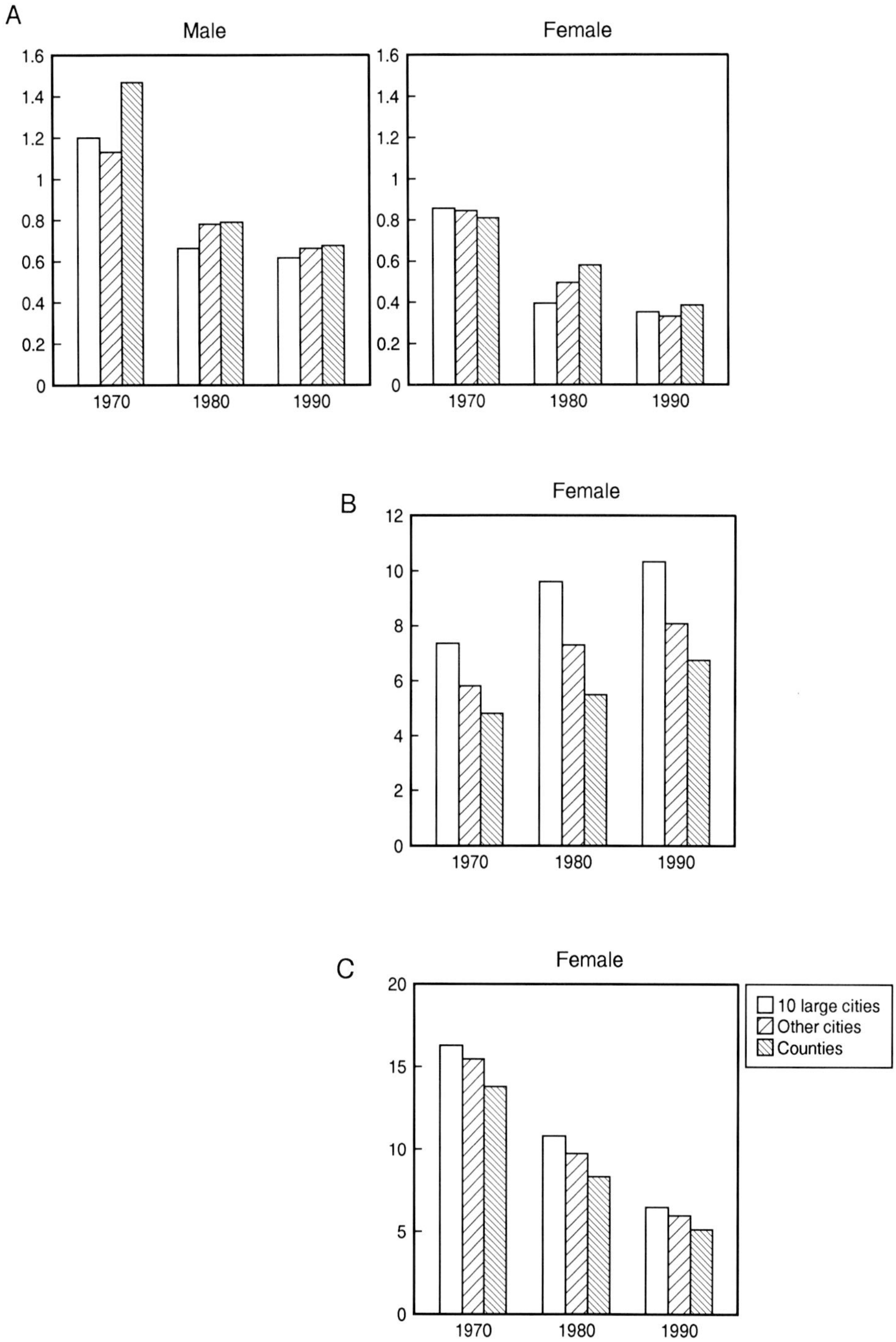

FIG. 4-5. Age-adjusted death rates for cancer for 10 large cities, other cities, and counties (1970, 1980, 1990)

A: cancer of the skin (ICD, 9th revision, 172, 173). B: cancer of the breast (ICD, 9th revision, 174). C: cancer of the uterus (ICD, 9th revision, 179–182).

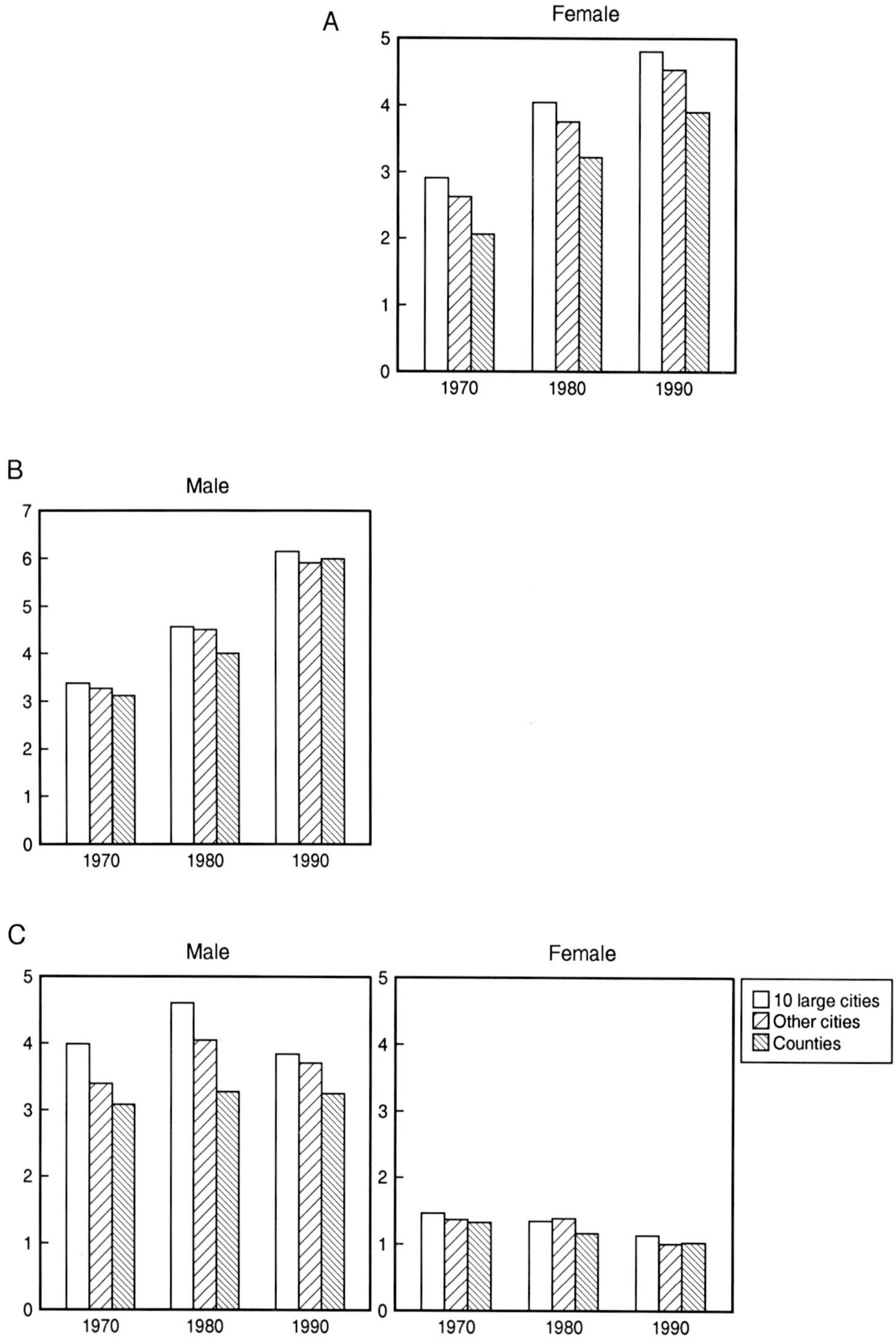

FIG. 4-6. Age-adjusted death rates for cancer for 10 large cities, other cities, and counties (1970, 1980, 1990)

A: cancer of the ovary (ICD, 9th revision, 183.0). B: cancer of the prostate (ICD, 9th revision, 185). C: cancer of the urinary bladder (ICD, 9th revision, 188).

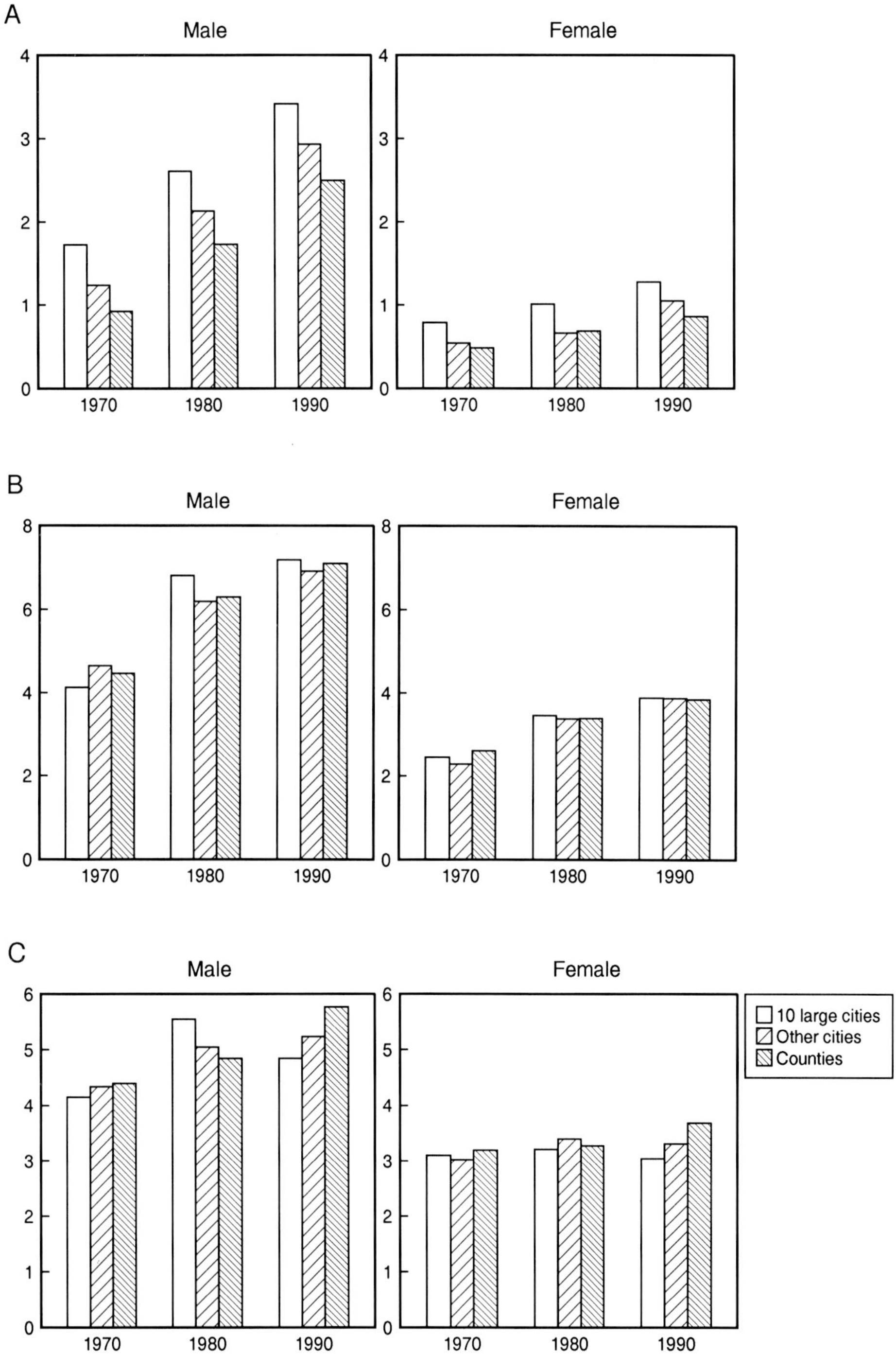

FIG. 4-7. Age-adjusted death rates for cancer for 10 large cities, other cities, and counties (1970, 1980, 1990)

A: cancer of the kidney (ICD, 9th revision, 189.0, 189.1). B: cancer of the lymphatic and hematopoietic systems other than leukemia (ICD, 9th revision, 200–203). C: leukemia (ICD, 9th revision, 204–208).

TABLE V-1. Standardized Mortality Ratio (SMR) of Cancer in Japan by Prefecture (1990)

		A. Cancer of all sites (ICD, 9th revision: 140–208)		B. Cancer of the buccal cavity and pharynx (ICD, 9th revision: 140–149)	
		Male	Female	Male	Female
1	Hokkaido	104.2	105.6	128.2	97.5
2	Aomori	108.5	97.7	91.3	73.5
3	Iwate	92.8	94.3	66.0	60.6
4	Miyagi	101.7	100.2	101.7	61.4
5	Akita	108.9	101.7	135.2	88.3
6	Yamagata	101.0	98.1	74.2	156.6
7	Fukushima	101.4	98.0	96.6	91.4
8	Ibaraki	93.6	98.4	70.3	85.7
9	Tochigi	96.0	98.0	61.0	78.7
10	Gunma	82.1	88.9	92.3	65.3
11	Saitama	97.0	100.0	90.1	101.7
12	Chiba	95.0	97.9	102.9	114.9
13	Tokyo	102.4	108.0	120.3	131.9
14	Kanagawa	98.1	102.3	102.5	116.1
15	Niigata	99.9	98.4	90.5	106.4
16	Toyama	101.3	103.0	87.7	61.7
17	Ishikawa	95.5	101.3	75.9	194.2
18	Fukui	89.5	98.0	92.8	34.4
19	Yamanashi	91.3	94.3	55.0	84.2
20	Nagano	82.8	86.9	58.5	93.2
21	Gifu	91.0	96.5	87.6	39.6
22	Shizuoka	90.0	90.0	112.7	94.9
23	Aichi	95.1	100.9	99.7	95.1
24	Mie	88.5	91.5	58.0	91.5
25	Shiga	92.3	102.0	61.0	82.5
26	Kyoto	100.8	102.5	87.8	140.2
27	Osaka	120.5	114.1	115.7	127.6
28	Hyogo	107.8	103.5	111.8	102.3
29	Nara	107.1	98.2	54.4	86.4
30	Wakayama	110.3	97.0	90.8	100.3
31	Tottori	106.6	93.3	74.2	63.0
32	Shimane	95.4	89.9	111.6	120.4
33	Okayama	91.9	90.8	88.2	129.1
34	Hiroshima	99.0	97.6	92.5	113.1
35	Yamaguchi	98.8	92.7	104.1	75.0
36	Tokushima	97.9	94.7	102.1	32.0
37	Kagawa	94.1	92.8	67.0	106.0
38	Ehime	93.9	93.9	53.3	62.3
39	Kochi	89.1	88.4	124.7	102.1
40	Fukuoka	112.2	109.0	120.1	66.1
41	Saga	111.0	107.5	124.0	61.4
42	Nagasaki	113.3	110.0	110.5	196.4
43	Kumamoto	98.1	94.5	105.8	57.6
44	Oita	95.4	92.8	74.6	76.3
45	Miyazaki	96.0	90.5	110.8	97.4
46	Kagoshima	93.5	92.1	108.0	77.2
47	Okinawa	91.1	81.0	220.8	104.3

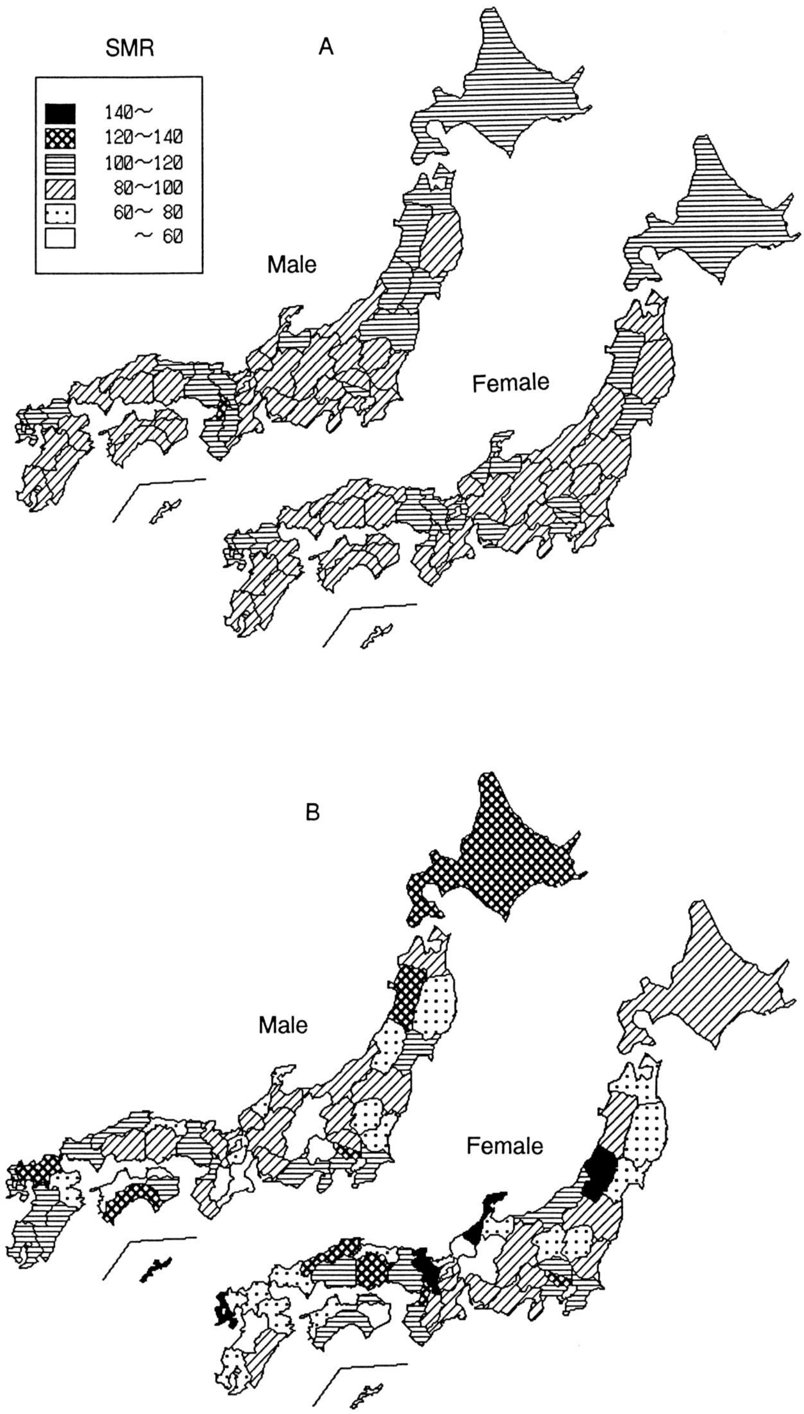

FIG. 5-1. Map of the standardized mortality ratio (SMR) of cancer in Japan by prefecture (1990)

A: cancer of all sites (ICD, 9th revision, 140–208). B: cancer of the buccal cavity and pharynx (ICD, 9th revision, 140–149).

TABLE V-2. Standardized Mortality Ratio (SMR) of Cancer in Japan by Prefecture (1990)

		A. Cancer of the esophagus (ICD, 9th revision: 150)		B. Cancer of the stomach (ICD, 9th revision: 151)	
		Male	Female	Male	Female
1	Hokkaido	135.4	104.9	97.3	91.4
2	Aomori	122.7	73.6	102.7	102.9
3	Iwate	120.1	69.9	85.0	90.2
4	Miyagi	164.8	130.8	100.5	95.0
5	Akita	154.9	127.3	124.3	123.2
6	Yamagata	132.2	130.5	119.3	131.4
7	Fukushima	117.3	100.9	115.4	102.1
8	Ibaraki	107.3	107.2	114.1	112.6
9	Tochigi	101.8	91.8	118.4	133.9
10	Gunma	107.8	70.9	86.2	92.8
11	Saitama	110.3	103.4	107.9	107.0
12	Chiba	108.0	120.7	102.1	106.3
13	Tokyo	126.5	140.9	102.1	104.8
14	Kanagawa	117.1	120.1	98.8	93.7
15	Niigata	131.3	108.6	127.5	119.3
16	Toyama	101.7	77.3	112.3	133.3
17	Ishikawa	58.0	155.9	99.6	97.9
18	Fukui	58.4	78.1	82.4	103.6
19	Yamanashi	77.1	76.4	93.9	80.8
20	Nagano	73.4	108.9	89.3	90.4
21	Gifu	66.9	87.7	105.8	103.9
22	Shizuoka	69.6	63.2	85.6	86.4
23	Aichi	69.5	81.8	102.8	100.6
24	Mie	56.5	95.4	99.5	102.4
25	Shiga	56.8	111.2	102.0	105.7
26	Kyoto	56.7	98.2	101.9	102.6
27	Osaka	102.0	133.1	111.8	111.1
28	Hyogo	95.8	121.3	97.7	101.2
29	Nara	83.5	137.4	121.0	113.9
30	Wakayama	97.1	128.3	121.2	98.8
31	Tottori	69.8	47.3	107.6	92.9
32	Shimane	78.1	50.3	89.6	96.5
33	Okayama	59.0	56.8	85.9	91.6
34	Hiroshima	86.6	89.9	86.4	94.3
35	Yamaguchi	96.4	103.9	96.7	104.8
36	Tokushima	43.2	54.4	90.9	95.0
37	Kagawa	60.8	67.6	88.3	98.2
38	Ehime	47.1	55.7	97.7	103.3
39	Kochi	86.7	24.5	94.3	94.9
40	Fukuoka	91.6	92.1	91.6	97.7
41	Saga	64.4	34.6	100.4	95.1
42	Nagasaki	84.8	96.7	88.4	102.5
43	Kumamoto	92.6	65.2	83.1	74.8
44	Oita	82.9	80.6	91.5	92.8
45	Miyazaki	110.6	20.9	83.2	73.0
46	Kagoshima	133.8	90.6	74.8	60.1
47	Okinawa	148.2	51.2	54.7	40.9

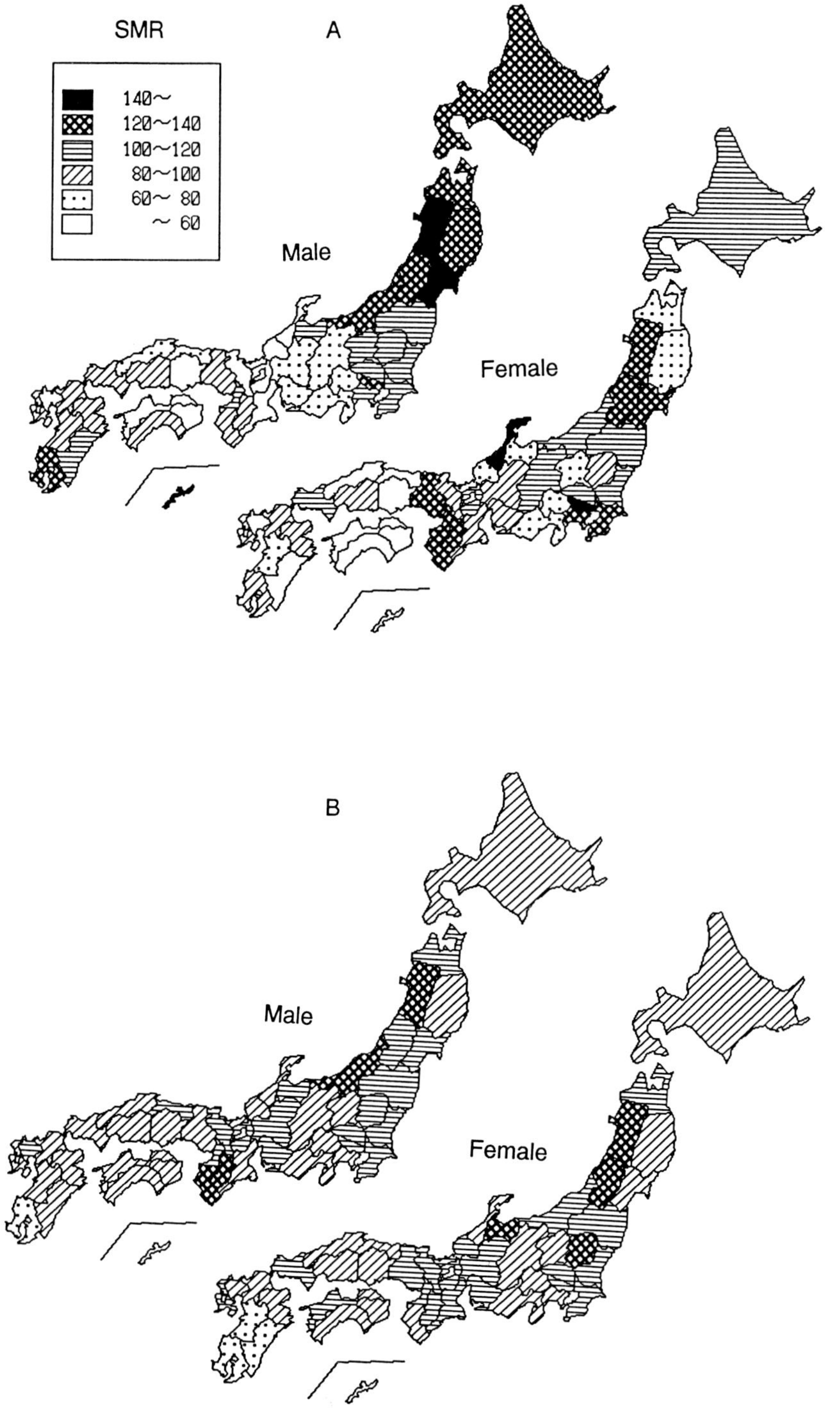

FIG. 5-2. Map of the standardized mortality ratio (SMR) of cancer in Japan by prefecture (1990)
A: cancer of the esophagus (ICD, 9th revision, 150). B: cancer of the stomach (ICD, 9th revision, 151).

TABLE V-3. Standardized Mortality Ratio (SMR) of Cancer in Japan by Prefecture (1990)

		A. Cancer of the colon (ICD, 9th revision: 153)		B. Cancer of the rectum (ICD, 9th revision: 154)	
		Male	Female	Male	Female
1	Hokkaido	110.4	111.4	101.6	122.3
2	Aomori	107.2	109.6	107.9	86.0
3	Iwate	112.5	119.3	102.6	121.0
4	Miyagi	92.3	103.2	112.0	115.3
5	Akita	118.0	111.1	107.9	96.9
6	Yamagata	115.6	104.8	106.3	85.8
7	Fukushima	92.3	93.7	132.1	121.2
8	Ibaraki	79.0	92.2	97.7	99.4
9	Tochigi	74.7	78.0	94.4	126.4
10	Gunma	78.3	88.9	100.5	81.8
11	Saitama	112.3	106.2	94.5	103.5
12	Chiba	101.5	106.8	92.2	96.2
13	Tokyo	123.3	110.1	112.9	102.5
14	Kanagawa	108.3	119.5	101.1	95.9
15	Niigata	86.1	121.6	94.8	102.2
16	Toyama	114.5	112.4	78.3	96.4
17	Ishikawa	110.5	93.7	109.3	135.1
18	Fukui	90.5	99.6	79.3	76.0
19	Yamanashi	87.4	99.1	87.8	108.3
20	Nagano	100.9	92.5	110.2	88.6
21	Gifu	94.3	107.0	101.4	114.0
22	Shizuoka	92.4	92.9	97.9	88.7
23	Aichi	100.0	105.7	90.3	93.8
24	Mie	94.3	98.4	85.6	88.4
25	Shiga	87.3	85.5	85.2	96.6
26	Kyoto	106.7	100.8	102.8	79.6
27	Osaka	106.6	98.1	104.3	104.3
28	Hyogo	97.0	104.5	107.4	95.5
29	Nara	101.4	101.0	98.1	104.0
30	Wakayama	78.1	91.7	87.7	67.9
31	Tottori	108.5	83.5	108.8	84.4
32	Shimane	86.8	119.3	90.6	84.7
33	Okayama	78.4	80.5	84.7	109.6
34	Hiroshima	95.2	95.3	99.4	82.2
35	Yamaguchi	100.0	74.4	83.2	90.3
36	Tokushima	76.9	81.9	93.4	118.7
37	Kagawa	85.5	80.5	108.8	106.5
38	Ehime	82.6	74.6	93.9	80.5
39	Kochi	68.2	70.6	97.3	79.3
40	Fukuoka	103.3	101.2	103.9	108.1
41	Saga	113.4	109.3	78.4	139.0
42	Nagasaki	102.7	95.3	96.0	91.5
43	Kumamoto	94.8	87.0	85.2	111.7
44	Oita	81.2	93.2	112.4	89.6
45	Miyazaki	88.3	67.3	100.6	95.3
46	Kagoshima	68.0	74.4	98.0	110.1
47	Okinawa	96.9	89.4	62.1	69.5

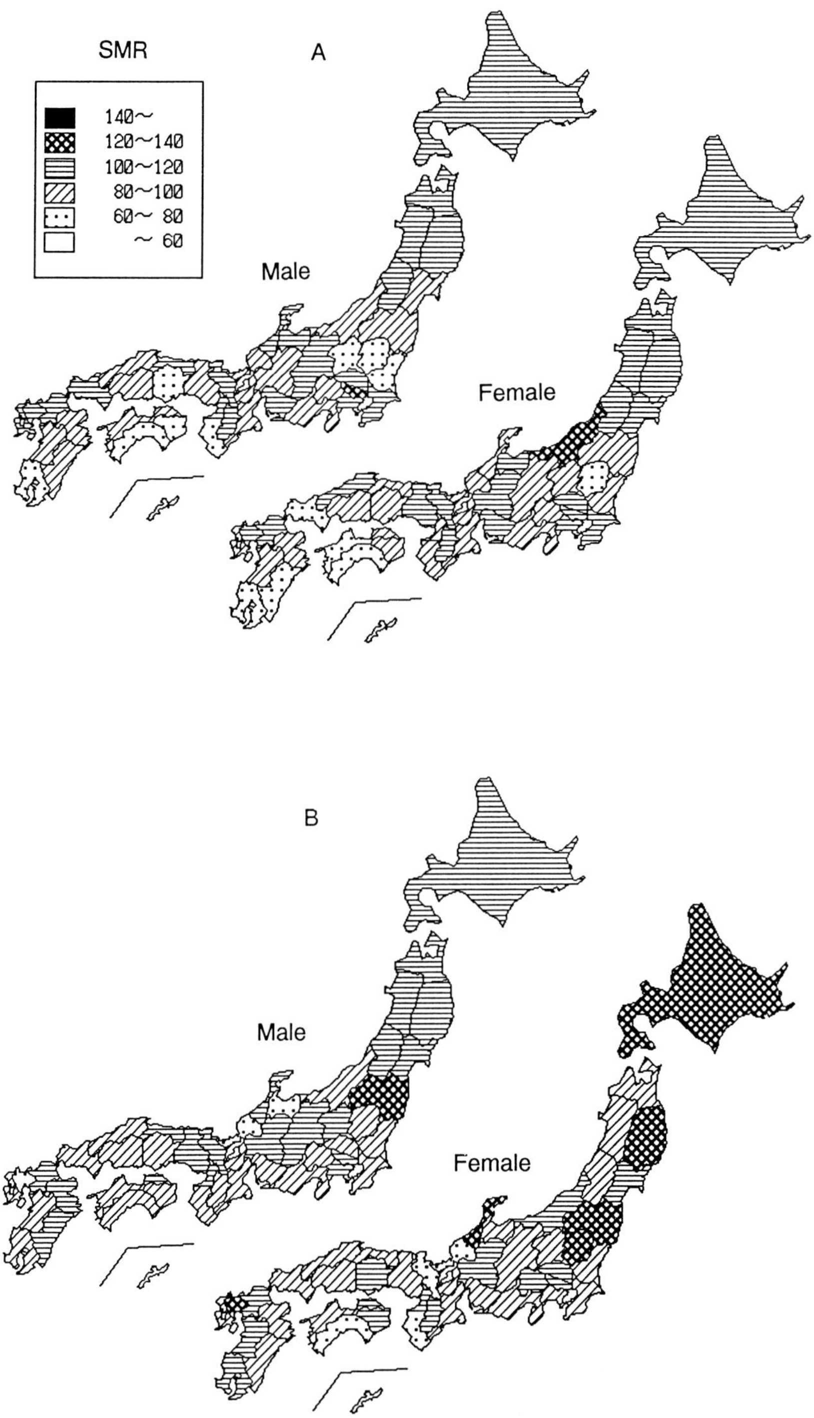

FIG. 5-3. Map of the standardized mortality ratio (SMR) of cancer in Japan by prefecture (1990)
A: cancer of the colon (ICD, 9th revision, 153). B: cancer of the rectum (ICD, 9th revision, 154).

TABLE V-4. Standardized Mortality Ratio (SMR) of Cancer in Japan by Prefecture (1990)

		A. Cancer of the liver (ICD, 9th revision: 155)		B. Cancer of the biliary passages (ICD, 9th revision: 156)	
		Male	Female	Male	Female
1	Hokkaido	74.2	82.9	123.7	105.7
2	Aomori	77.6	88.0	131.9	112.9
3	Iwate	51.8	70.2	129.2	95.3
4	Miyagi	60.3	74.1	121.8	112.5
5	Akita	45.6	69.8	131.3	107.1
6	Yamagata	61.6	72.9	92.7	102.1
7	Fukushima	61.5	65.1	124.5	124.2
8	Ibaraki	69.9	77.5	98.7	119.5
9	Tochigi	80.4	73.3	105.7	107.2
10	Gunma	60.9	88.9	98.6	113.3
11	Saitama	85.2	93.9	92.5	109.4
12	Chiba	88.0	86.3	105.1	93.7
13	Tokyo	95.5	102.0	88.8	97.9
14	Kanagawa	93.8	99.7	93.0	99.9
15	Niigata	43.3	49.5	127.2	118.4
16	Toyama	75.2	82.3	114.0	104.2
17	Ishikawa	71.6	66.1	103.3	133.4
18	Fukui	81.4	125.9	119.2	119.7
19	Yamanashi	122.9	125.2	109.9	125.9
20	Nagano	56.6	72.4	106.6	95.8
21	Gifu	80.6	95.7	93.8	87.6
22	Shizuoka	97.7	82.1	87.8	101.0
23	Aichi	86.2	84.5	93.4	103.4
24	Mie	68.7	71.0	79.2	82.6
25	Shiga	57.0	75.4	129.9	130.0
26	Kyoto	91.1	91.2	96.7	93.4
27	Osaka	179.3	159.6	94.8	98.7
28	Hyogo	138.1	137.7	85.3	88.2
29	Nara	114.8	88.8	95.9	79.6
30	Wakayama	126.5	121.7	89.9	89.9
31	Tottori	116.4	100.9	108.6	101.0
32	Shimane	88.5	80.6	103.0	78.0
33	Okayama	109.9	92.6	78.4	91.0
34	Hiroshima	146.1	124.8	78.0	84.5
35	Yamaguchi	127.6	104.6	77.0	79.3
36	Tokushima	131.0	113.2	94.8	70.8
37	Kagawa	96.1	85.4	101.7	97.8
38	Ehime	114.4	89.6	100.8	89.7
39	Kochi	86.0	100.4	82.3	59.7
40	Fukuoka	178.3	165.5	107.9	98.8
41	Saga	154.8	191.0	113.9	108.2
42	Nagasaki	131.6	122.0	131.5	114.9
43	Kumamoto	126.0	102.8	107.5	108.8
44	Oita	107.6	96.8	96.4	98.1
45	Miyazaki	103.3	93.6	96.7	98.8
46	Kagoshima	94.8	110.9	89.6	92.3
47	Okinawa	51.8	58.4	61.3	76.6

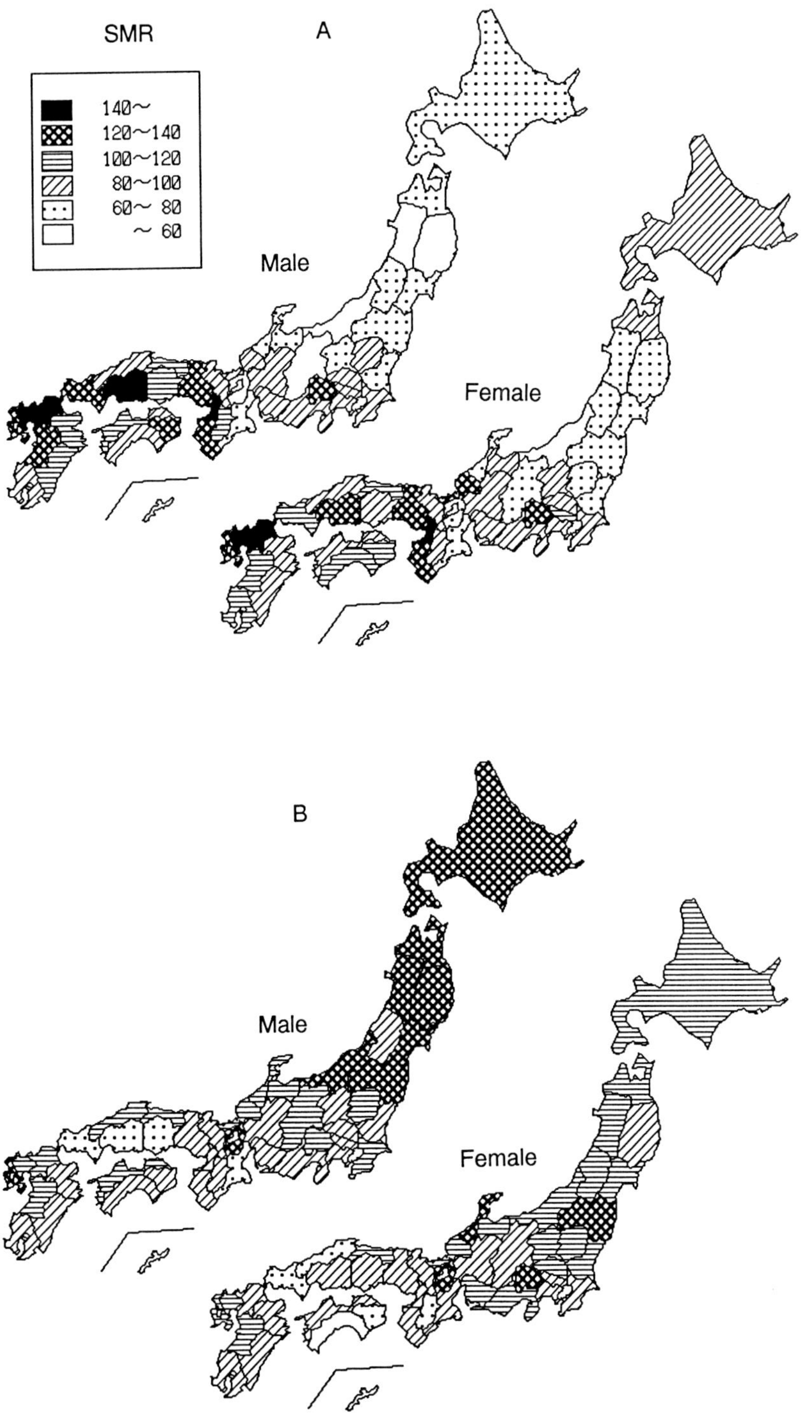

FIG. 5-4. Map of the standardized mortality ratio (SMR) of cancer in Japan by prefecture (1990)

A: cancer of the liver (ICD, 9th revision, 155). B: cancer of the biliary passages (ICD, 9th revision, 156).

TABLE V-5. Standardized Mortality Ratio (SMR) of Cancer in Japan by Prefecture (1990)

		A. Cancer of the pancreas (ICD, 9th revision: 157)		B. Cancer of the larynx (ICD, 9th revision: 161)	
		Male	Female	Male	Female
1	Hokkaido	129.3	132.3	113.5	30.0
2	Aomori	153.0	113.5	208.5	100.9
3	Iwate	90.4	108.0	96.6	0.0
4	Miyagi	131.5	91.0	65.3	74.4
5	Akita	107.6	92.0	147.3	0.0
6	Yamagata	109.3	92.5	70.3	0.0
7	Fukushima	116.9	124.0	113.2	197.5
8	Ibaraki	91.5	101.5	85.7	58.5
9	Tochigi	94.7	95.5	73.8	167.4
10	Gunma	88.8	99.6	91.0	154.6
11	Saitama	94.2	114.3	108.9	145.4
12	Chiba	89.9	91.2	102.2	112.6
13	Tokyo	93.7	108.1	102.9	62.4
14	Kanagawa	96.1	87.6	99.2	55.7
15	Niigata	102.1	91.4	86.2	51.6
16	Toyama	107.0	101.1	108.1	341.6
17	Ishikawa	100.9	95.6	114.3	120.4
18	Fukui	87.8	91.1	82.3	316.7
19	Yamanashi	93.0	77.0	63.4	309.7
20	Nagano	93.7	109.5	69.5	114.0
21	Gifu	99.7	92.5	50.3	0.0
22	Shizuoka	94.9	91.0	89.8	86.9
23	Aichi	94.9	93.3	86.3	59.1
24	Mie	102.5	108.3	32.2	0.0
25	Shiga	104.2	112.5	80.4	0.0
26	Kyoto	116.5	108.8	103.9	114.5
27	Osaka	101.2	101.6	106.4	112.3
28	Hyogo	94.8	98.1	102.6	89.6
29	Nara	113.2	81.1	84.9	0.0
30	Wakayama	118.9	101.2	160.9	115.8
31	Tottori	133.7	87.8	126.9	0.0
32	Shimane	105.5	105.6	72.8	135.7
33	Okayama	92.9	93.7	152.9	198.9
34	Hiroshima	83.9	104.2	56.9	0.0
35	Yamaguchi	73.0	90.5	131.6	0.0
36	Tokushima	97.2	84.6	93.9	442.4
37	Kagawa	91.4	81.4	38.2	122.1
38	Ehime	95.8	93.7	60.7	165.9
39	Kochi	84.3	84.1	73.8	0.0
40	Fukuoka	99.5	105.6	121.4	126.9
41	Saga	114.6	109.0	109.9	141.1
42	Nagasaki	120.9	102.8	146.0	83.3
43	Kumamoto	93.0	101.8	109.0	66.7
44	Oita	98.0	76.2	63.8	202.4
45	Miyazaki	102.1	81.3	159.4	570.9
46	Kagoshima	87.0	93.8	136.0	127.7
47	Okinawa	58.6	59.6	134.6	143.0

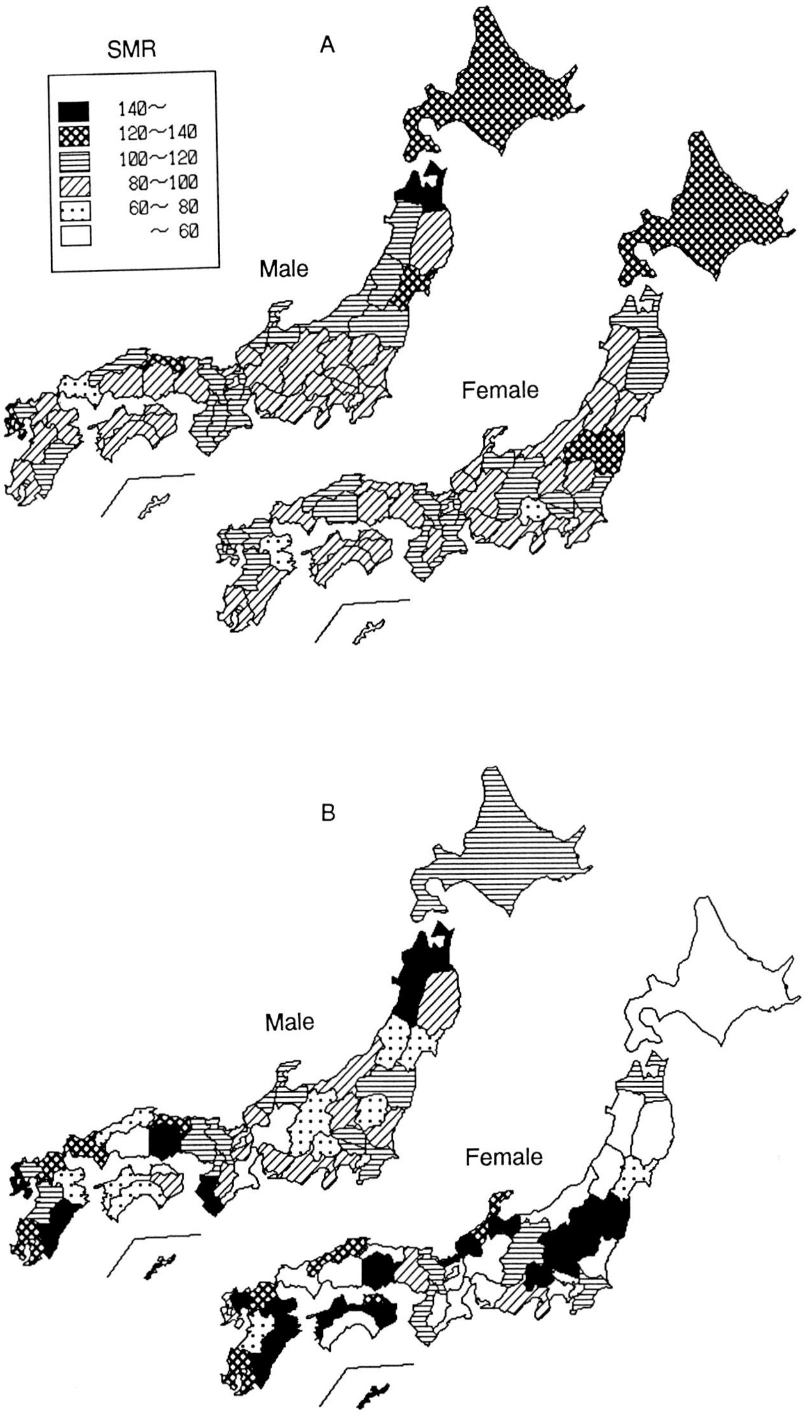

FIG. 5-5. Map of the standardized mortality ratio (SMR) of cancer in Japan by prefecture (1990)

A: cancer of the pancreas (ICD, 9th revision, 157). B: cancer of the larynx (ICD, 9th revision, 161).

TABLE V-6. Standardized Mortality Ratio (SMR) of Cancer in Japan by Prefecture (1990)

		A. Cancer of the trachea, bronchus, and lung (ICD, 9th revision: 162)		B. Cancer of the bone (ICD, 9th revision: 170)	
		Male	Female	Male	Female
1	Hokkaido	107.6	119.3	148.9	116.2
2	Aomori	112.1	83.8	95.9	125.1
3	Iwate	97.2	89.2	127.2	126.0
4	Miyagi	98.9	91.6	146.1	146.3
5	Akita	114.4	101.1	108.8	94.1
6	Yamagata	102.2	91.3	139.2	45.2
7	Fukushima	97.8	81.6	43.2	86.3
8	Ibaraki	86.7	74.1	65.4	46.5
9	Tochigi	95.1	74.4	72.1	33.8
10	Gunma	74.2	74.1	92.2	0.0
11	Saitama	92.3	89.8	115.1	70.5
12	Chiba	88.4	89.1	52.4	91.5
13	Tokyo	100.8	116.0	116.1	101.0
14	Kanagawa	95.1	100.8	78.5	75.5
15	Niigata	106.8	93.7	143.0	23.6
16	Toyama	98.5	81.2	78.7	103.9
17	Ishikawa	93.3	79.6	155.8	52.1
18	Fukui	105.7	91.0	53.9	0.0
19	Yamanashi	75.4	91.7	0.0	210.7
20	Nagano	73.1	70.3	59.5	133.3
21	Gifu	87.1	87.5	87.9	92.3
22	Shizuoka	86.5	75.3	101.5	53.1
23	Aichi	98.1	114.1	136.4	127.7
24	Mie	94.1	88.2	100.6	68.0
25	Shiga	106.4	111.3	154.3	317.6
26	Kyoto	108.3	123.1	141.3	97.3
27	Osaka	121.4	127.8	96.0	146.4
28	Hyogo	117.2	107.9	79.1	96.2
29	Nara	110.0	104.1	102.7	47.0
30	Wakayama	116.1	104.4	165.0	0.0
31	Tottori	93.5	104.3	143.4	0.0
32	Shimane	102.3	75.7	53.2	68.4
33	Okayama	93.9	84.6	113.7	121.3
34	Hiroshima	94.5	97.0	95.7	65.3
35	Yamaguchi	100.5	98.6	55.8	36.0
36	Tokushima	103.5	104.0	106.5	68.5
37	Kagawa	101.5	82.3	170.3	56.4
38	Ehime	97.2	91.4	116.8	151.3
39	Kochi	84.9	87.2	156.7	196.8
40	Fukuoka	110.5	118.5	78.7	130.8
41	Saga	109.5	82.6	51.7	0.0
42	Nagasaki	117.7	116.9	118.3	148.9
43	Kumamoto	90.4	109.0	24.4	154.9
44	Oita	88.4	97.4	71.6	138.6
45	Miyazaki	90.6	90.9	119.2	251.8
46	Kagoshima	95.3	93.9	74.6	91.5
47	Okinawa	127.9	130.7	42.2	277.5

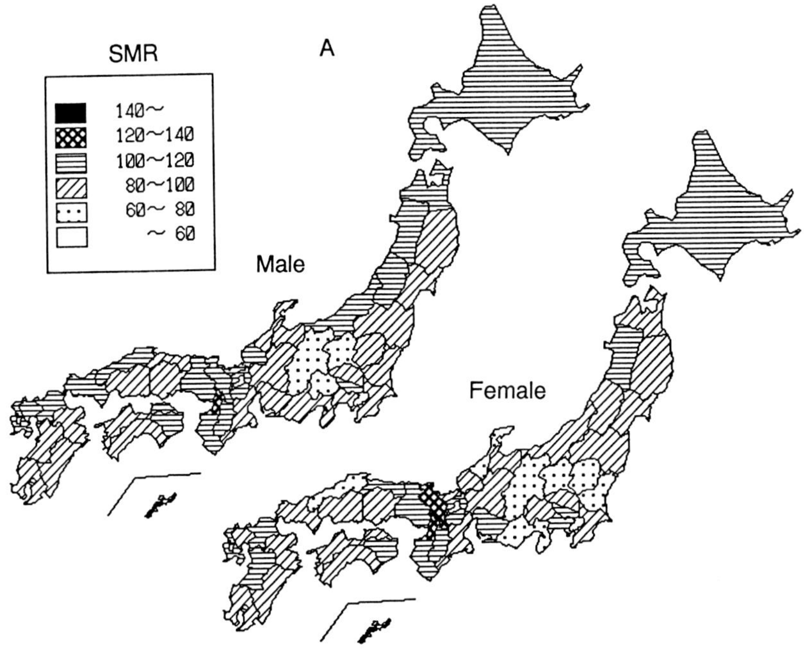

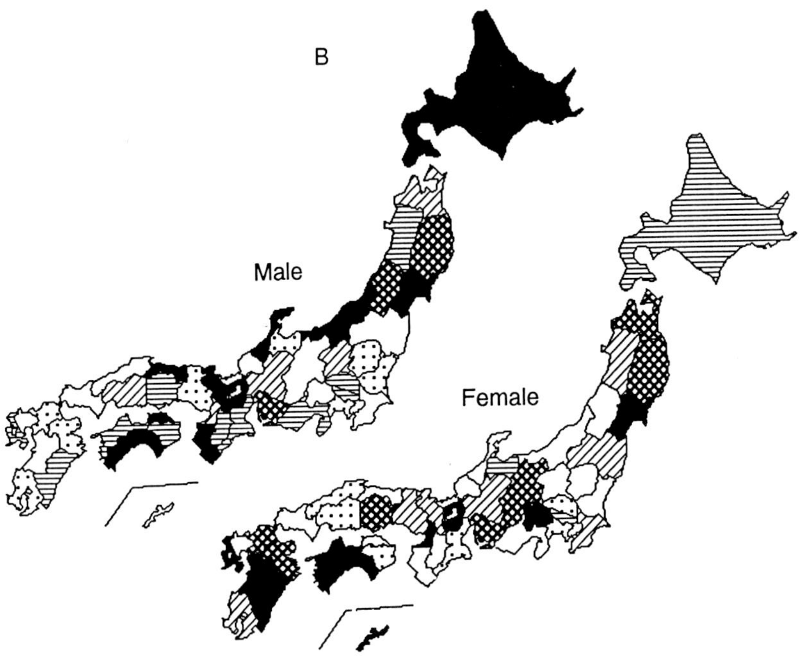

FIG. 5-6. Map of the standardized mortality ratio (SMR) of cancer in Japan by prefecture (1990)

A: cancer of the trachea, bronchus, and lung (ICD, 9th revision, 162). B: cancer of the bone (ICD, 9th revision, 170).

TABLE V-7. Standardized Mortality Ratio (SMR) of Cancer in Japan by Prefecture (1990)

		A. Cancer of the skin (ICD, 9th revision: 172–173)		B. Cancer of the breast (ICD, 9th revision: 174)
		Male	Female	Female
1	Hokkaido	113.6	129.6	113.6
2	Aomori	86.5	131.5	88.5
3	Iwate	140.5	25.0	98.2
4	Miyagi	104.5	95.8	101.6
5	Akita	133.3	83.7	85.7
6	Yamagata	168.7	102.2	70.0
7	Fukushima	125.0	208.1	76.7
8	Ibaraki	150.8	90.8	102.4
9	Tochigi	67.0	129.6	91.6
10	Gunma	92.7	40.0	99.7
11	Saitama	71.0	70.8	95.2
12	Chiba	90.1	118.9	102.7
13	Tokyo	83.1	50.3	138.0
14	Kanagawa	83.2	74.0	129.5
15	Niigata	78.4	96.4	94.1
16	Toyama	298.6	119.5	77.4
17	Ishikawa	261.6	157.6	98.9
18	Fukui	201.7	41.4	83.7
19	Yamanashi	97.5	120.7	77.7
20	Nagano	83.6	89.1	86.3
21	Gifu	87.7	136.9	86.4
22	Shizuoka	94.9	142.2	91.8
23	Aichi	110.6	89.1	104.8
24	Mie	81.5	40.1	81.3
25	Shiga	162.8	33.3	93.5
26	Kyoto	97.5	160.7	103.5
27	Osaka	87.9	44.8	114.9
28	Hyogo	121.6	98.1	87.7
29	Nara	48.7	30.0	94.6
30	Wakayama	50.9	90.4	74.7
31	Tottori	43.5	49.8	60.3
32	Shimane	0.0	105.5	74.1
33	Okayama	56.0	133.6	83.8
34	Hiroshima	62.7	140.7	91.7
35	Yamaguchi	50.6	118.5	72.0
36	Tokushima	128.3	114.7	69.2
37	Kagawa	51.7	94.3	74.2
38	Ehime	70.6	126.6	85.1
39	Kochi	29.8	133.9	94.1
40	Fukuoka	75.0	110.8	104.8
41	Saga	160.4	143.6	109.7
42	Nagasaki	169.5	84.9	110.9
43	Kumamoto	192.6	168.0	95.2
44	Oita	109.0	183.5	71.9
45	Miyazaki	50.1	145.8	72.5
46	Kagoshima	103.7	149.7	65.3
47	Okinawa	130.4	97.3	59.3

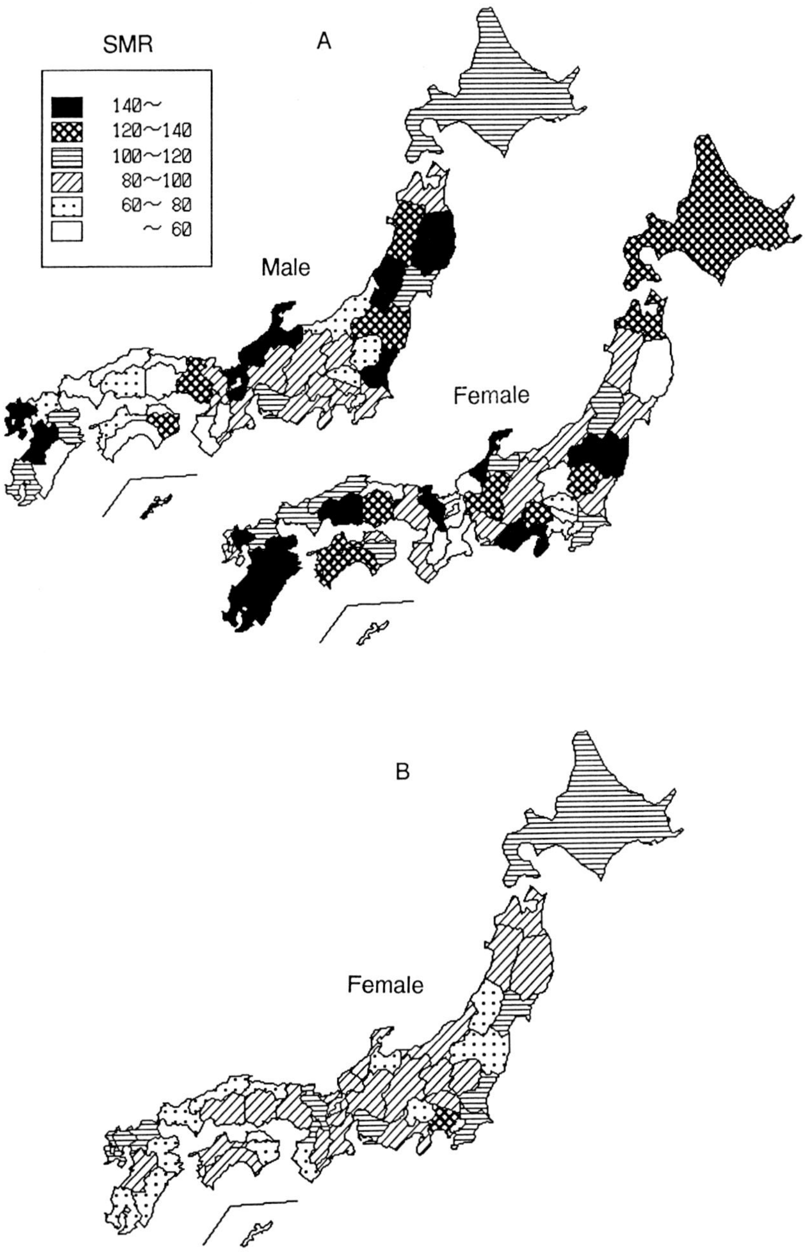

FIG. 5-7. Map of the standardized mortality ratio (SMR) of cancer in Japan by prefecture (1990)
A: cancer of the skin (ICD, 9th revision, 172, 173). B: cancer of the breast (ICD, 9th revision, 174).

TABLE V-8. Standardized Mortality Ratio (SMR) of Cancer in Japan by Prefecture (1990)

		A. Cancer of the uterus (ICD, 9th revision: 179–182)	B. Cancer of the ovary (ICD, 9th revision: 183.0)
		Female	Female
1	Hokkaido	83.2	115.5
2	Aomori	109.1	99.0
3	Iwate	76.6	105.0
4	Miyagi	88.3	135.5
5	Akita	88.7	96.8
6	Yamagata	57.9	80.5
7	Fukushima	87.7	92.6
8	Ibaraki	111.1	99.7
9	Tochigi	105.5	97.5
10	Gunma	92.3	103.2
11	Saitama	96.5	104.5
12	Chiba	111.3	103.6
13	Tokyo	98.0	125.1
14	Kanagawa	99.7	105.3
15	Niigata	56.5	79.0
16	Toyama	76.4	102.7
17	Ishikawa	103.1	88.2
18	Fukui	70.4	82.8
19	Yamanashi	74.6	101.8
20	Nagano	73.6	97.0
21	Gifu	104.3	110.8
22	Shizuoka	112.3	90.1
23	Aichi	103.6	100.3
24	Mie	94.8	80.1
25	Shiga	71.3	95.4
26	Kyoto	87.4	91.1
27	Osaka	125.5	107.2
28	Hyogo	129.8	98.5
29	Nara	93.5	77.8
30	Wakayama	86.2	90.4
31	Tottori	93.5	108.7
32	Shimane	92.6	106.6
33	Okayama	79.4	103.2
34	Hiroshima	109.9	97.2
35	Yamaguchi	102.7	52.3
36	Tokushima	133.6	92.7
37	Kagawa	84.9	83.5
38	Ehime	112.5	107.2
39	Kochi	116.7	84.1
40	Fukuoka	109.4	92.7
41	Saga	116.7	83.1
42	Nagasaki	103.9	83.6
43	Kumamoto	89.3	65.4
44	Oita	112.1	88.5
45	Miyazaki	135.1	69.3
46	Kagoshima	108.9	102.8
47	Okinawa	94.6	101.1

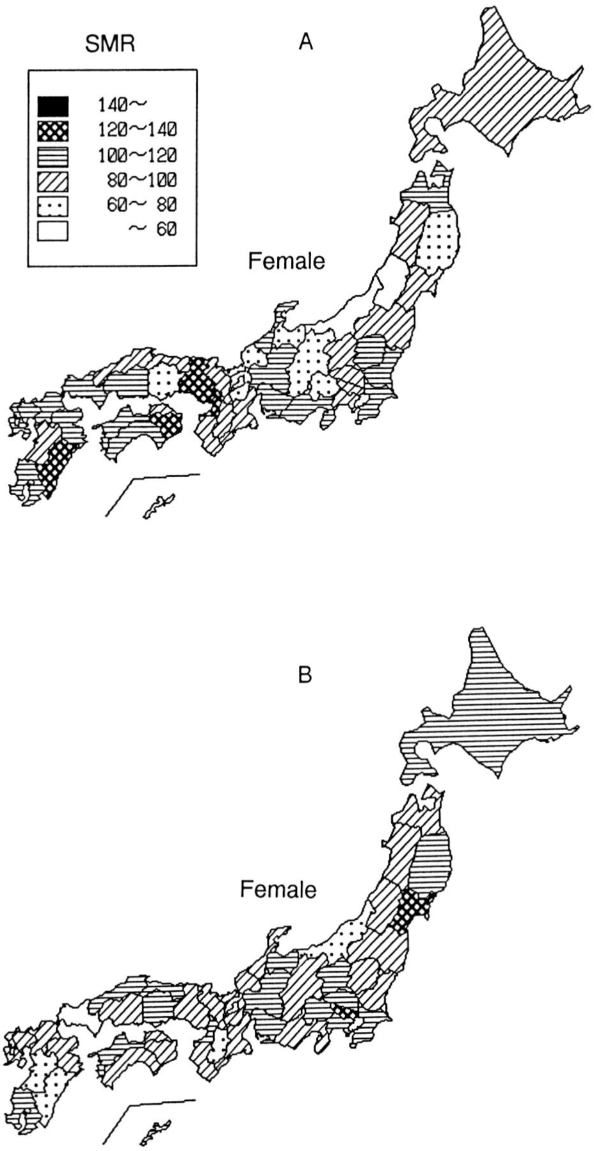

FIG. 5-8. Map of the standardized mortality ratio (SMR) of cancer in Japan by prefecture (1990)

A: cancer of the uterus (ICD, 9th revision, 179–182). B: cancer of the ovary (ICD, 9th revision, 183.0).

TABLE V-9. Standardized Mortality Ratio (SMR) of Cancer in Japan by Prefecture (1990)

		A. Cancer of the prostate (ICD, 9th revision: 185)	B. Cancer of the urinary bladder (ICD, 9th revision: 188)	
		Male	Male	Female
1	Hokkaido	109.3	113.8	108.3
2	Aomori	154.0	127.8	59.0
3	Iwate	95.9	109.1	118.5
4	Miyagi	117.6	116.1	130.4
5	Akita	113.1	104.8	182.1
6	Yamagata	107.1	83.6	78.7
7	Fukushima	85.5	73.0	130.1
8	Ibaraki	104.1	98.8	72.9
9	Tochigi	86.6	84.5	90.3
10	Gunma	131.1	87.7	57.3
11	Saitama	93.4	95.7	71.0
12	Chiba	108.2	90.8	106.3
13	Tokyo	108.4	98.5	115.1
14	Kanagawa	109.4	92.9	116.9
15	Niigata	108.8	87.6	71.9
16	Toyama	78.0	108.1	120.4
17	Ishikawa	87.9	68.5	147.7
18	Fukui	69.4	87.1	51.4
19	Yamanashi	87.2	95.4	100.2
20	Nagano	98.6	96.0	91.9
21	Gifu	78.6	116.8	119.2
22	Shizuoka	113.2	85.8	78.3
23	Aichi	101.0	107.4	116.5
24	Mie	93.3	74.7	107.6
25	Shiga	106.6	63.4	42.4
26	Kyoto	83.7	114.1	83.4
27	Osaka	97.4	122.3	112.9
28	Hyogo	88.6	91.3	80.7
29	Nara	89.6	106.6	29.3
30	Wakayama	82.1	92.7	84.2
31	Tottori	129.0	134.2	77.1
32	Shimane	65.1	120.1	75.6
33	Okayama	91.4	118.0	89.4
34	Hiroshima	95.9	143.1	98.5
35	Yamaguchi	78.1	101.6	123.9
36	Tokushima	89.6	94.3	142.8
37	Kagawa	100.3	75.5	98.1
38	Ehime	79.3	57.5	79.8
39	Kochi	90.2	50.7	105.3
40	Fukuoka	91.3	108.2	95.1
41	Saga	124.7	115.7	134.8
42	Nagasaki	104.3	147.3	120.8
43	Kumamoto	108.4	108.9	84.8
44	Oita	116.0	78.5	106.7
45	Miyazaki	107.8	78.6	74.1
46	Kagoshima	110.9	80.5	138.7
47	Okinawa	50.8	89.6	76.8

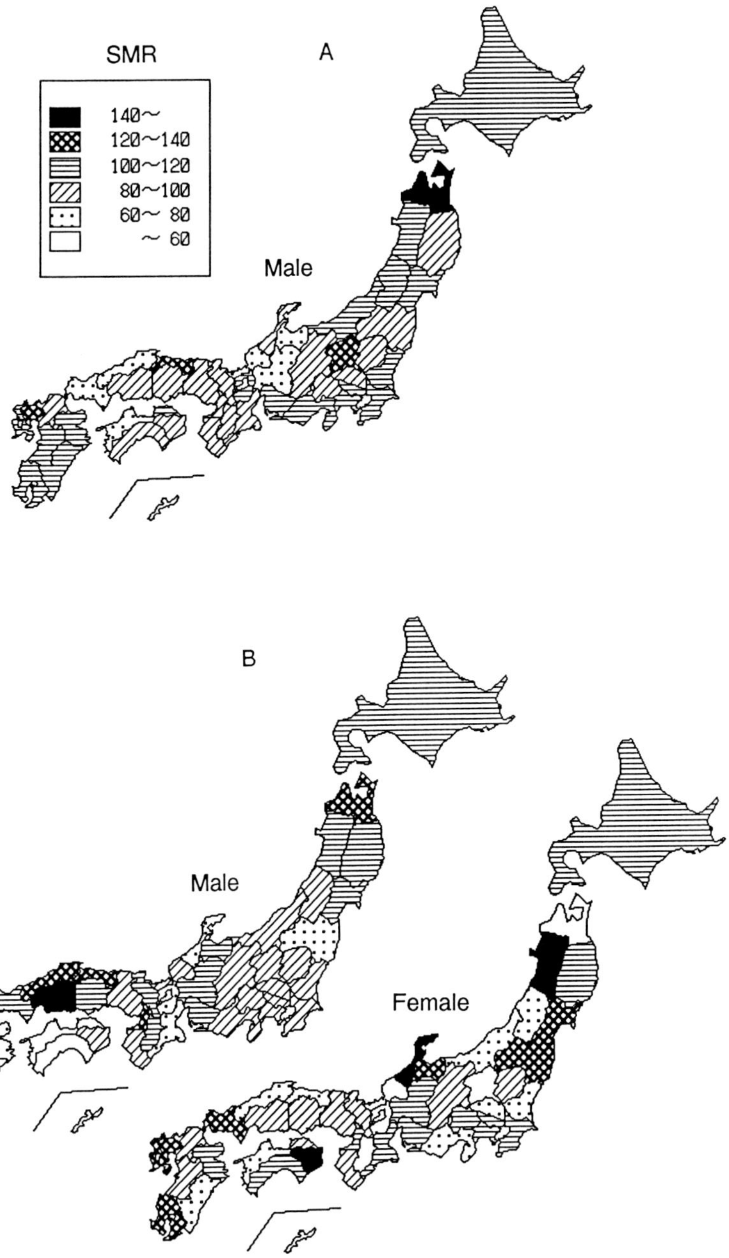

FIG. 5-9. Map of the standardized mortality ratio (SMR) of cancer in Japan by prefecture (1990)
A: cancer of the prostate (ICD, 9th revision, 185). B: cancer of the urinary bladder (ICD, 9th revision, 188).

Table V-10. Standardized Mortality Ratio (SMR) of Cancer in Japan by Prefecture (1990)

		A. Cancer of the kidney (ICD, 9th revision: 189.0, 189.1)		B. Cancer of the lymphoid tissue (ICD, 9th revision: 200–202)	
		Male	Female	Male	Female
1	Hokkaido	113.6	173.1	91.6	102.2
2	Aomori	145.8	81.8	70.4	62.3
3	Iwate	119.7	61.0	111.2	91.3
4	Miyagi	94.8	133.2	114.1	111.0
5	Akita	135.1	113.7	72.7	73.0
6	Yamagata	98.3	134.2	84.6	89.3
7	Fukushima	106.1	114.8	94.9	85.0
8	Ibaraki	111.7	84.9	79.0	81.2
9	Tochigi	100.0	75.8	96.2	95.4
10	Gunma	60.0	77.7	87.2	100.8
11	Saitama	104.5	74.9	72.3	100.4
12	Chiba	84.9	98.5	92.6	80.8
13	Tokyo	110.7	109.3	98.2	96.0
14	Kanagawa	111.8	151.3	81.8	97.2
15	Niigata	93.4	110.4	93.2	103.5
16	Toyama	181.0	159.3	106.9	94.0
17	Ishikawa	73.0	133.9	114.3	104.4
18	Fukui	139.8	88.8	67.4	110.7
19	Yamanashi	92.1	72.5	97.3	96.4
20	Nagano	62.5	96.2	97.0	81.6
21	Gifu	98.2	68.7	92.2	107.3
22	Shizuoka	78.4	74.9	99.9	107.2
23	Aichi	98.6	117.4	90.6	98.3
24	Mie	117.6	57.6	116.9	77.6
25	Shiga	105.3	59.5	79.7	120.9
26	Kyoto	129.8	111.3	106.9	90.4
27	Osaka	109.9	106.5	111.2	93.0
28	Hyogo	96.1	94.6	113.4	100.8
29	Nara	63.3	64.8	113.5	100.4
30	Wakayama	71.8	32.4	110.9	140.8
31	Tottori	123.5	180.4	135.1	125.6
32	Shimane	106.3	64.6	111.6	115.9
33	Okayama	131.2	99.6	96.1	93.5
34	Hiroshima	103.3	75.1	109.5	102.3
35	Yamaguchi	62.7	72.1	97.3	126.2
36	Tokushima	49.1	55.1	164.4	137.5
37	Kagawa	126.1	125.8	114.7	98.4
38	Ehime	97.6	77.1	97.9	100.6
39	Kochi	114.0	38.0	112.3	124.1
40	Fukuoka	99.4	92.4	101.9	104.1
41	Saga	77.7	92.8	109.0	92.3
42	Nagasaki	105.9	131.3	136.1	124.3
43	Kumamoto	62.3	62.4	108.1	109.6
44	Oita	100.4	84.6	96.0	91.2
45	Miyazaki	43.7	73.7	123.1	145.9
46	Kagoshima	45.2	72.3	147.5	139.3
47	Okinawa	44.1	79.2	158.1	107.0

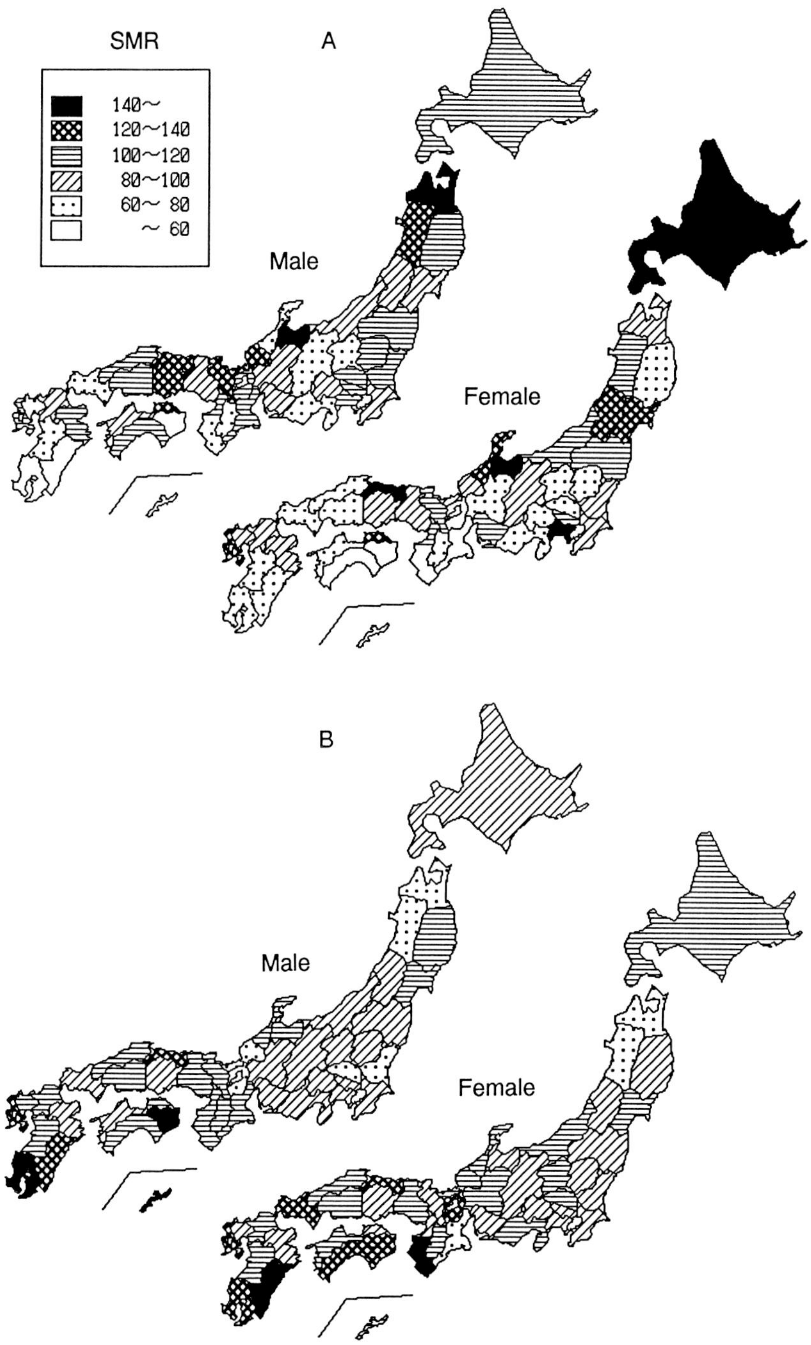

FIG. 5-10. Map of the standardized mortality ratio (SMR) of cancer in Japan by prefecture (1990)

A: cancer of the kidney (ICD, 9th revision, 189.0, 189.1). B: cancer of the lymphatic and hematopoietic systems other than leukemia (ICD, 9th revision, 200–203).

TABLE V-11. Standardized Mortality Ratio (SMR) of Cancer in Japan by Prefecture (1990)

		A. Leukemia (ICD, 9th revision: 204–208)	
		Male	Female
1	Hokkaido	103.6	87.1
2	Aomori	97.6	94.0
3	Iwate	137.6	94.0
4	Miyagi	100.0	118.1
5	Akita	97.8	71.6
6	Yamagata	99.4	90.6
7	Fukushima	97.2	103.7
8	Ibaraki	100.7	79.8
9	Tochigi	88.0	88.5
10	Gunma	89.6	81.6
11	Saitama	95.2	82.6
12	Chiba	84.1	85.9
13	Tokyo	92.4	94.8
14	Kanagawa	91.0	96.4
15	Niigata	85.7	106.6
16	Toyama	78.1	125.5
17	Ishikawa	127.4	78.4
18	Fukui	89.9	73.5
19	Yamanashi	86.3	83.0
20	Nagano	99.7	87.5
21	Gifu	46.4	80.4
22	Shizuoka	96.5	101.8
23	Aichi	65.2	78.5
24	Mie	77.0	85.5
25	Shiga	92.1	140.0
26	Kyoto	89.0	104.3
27	Osaka	104.1	101.1
28	Hyogo	93.0	89.4
29	Nara	97.0	131.2
30	Wakayama	88.0	91.4
31	Tottori	152.3	56.9
32	Shimane	123.3	52.9
33	Okayama	93.0	90.8
34	Hiroshima	95.9	87.7
35	Yamaguchi	88.1	92.2
36	Tokushima	70.7	90.5
37	Kagawa	118.2	110.2
38	Ehime	99.4	94.4
39	Kochi	126.1	76.2
40	Fukuoka	110.9	112.5
41	Saga	160.9	138.3
42	Nagasaki	191.3	157.7
43	Kumamoto	156.6	145.0
44	Oita	119.1	122.2
45	Miyazaki	138.9	197.0
46	Kagoshima	192.4	233.5
47	Okinawa	193.3	179.4

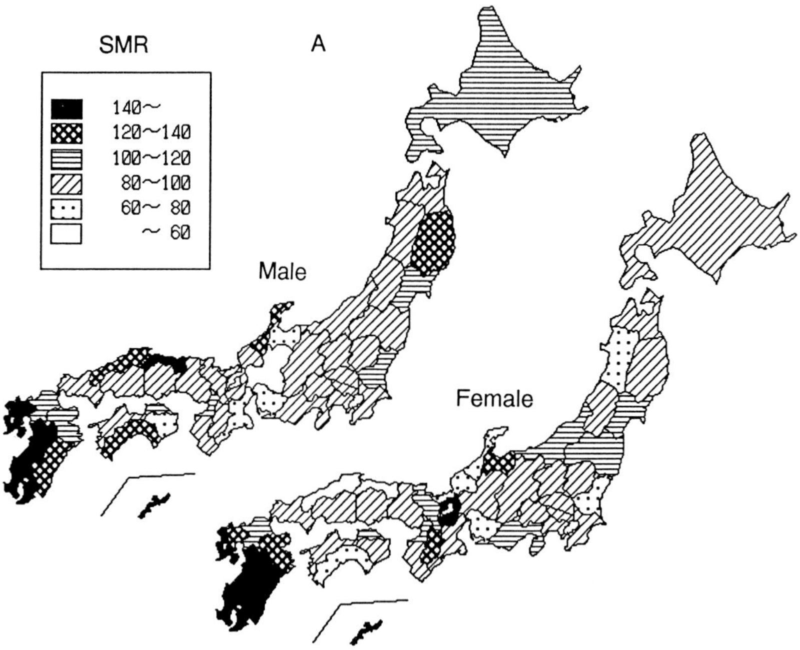

FIG. 5-11. Map of the standardized mortality ratio (SMR) of cancer in Japan by prefecture (1990)
A: leukemia (ICD, 9th revision, 204–208).

CANCER INCIDENCE IN JAPAN

The Research Group for Population-Based Cancer Registration in Japan*1,*2

The Research Group for Population-Based Cancer Registration in Japan has been conducting a cooperative study to estimate cancer incidence in Japan. Annual incidence has been estimated for the 14 years from 1975 to 1988. This report presents the age-specific, crude, and age-standardized incidence rates, as well as the number of incident cases by sex and site for each of the years 1975–1984 and for 1988.

Long-term trends are also noted utilizing the data from four registries: Miyagi, Osaka, Hiroshima City, and Nagasaki City. These registries showed largely consistent trends in cancer occurrence, though with some minor variations between their respective areas.

Annual cancer incidence rates in Japan have been estimated with reasonable reliability since 1975, though they are based on data from a limited number of registries (*1, 5*).

In general, prefectural governments have set up their own population-based cancer registries and requested all medical institutions located in the prefecture, as well as medical doctors, to participate in the programs on a voluntary basis.

The Research Group for Population-Based Cancer Registration in Japan has been operating since 1975 with a research grant from the Japanese Ministry of Health and Welfare. Since its inception, the Research Group has been conducting a cooperative study for the purpose of estimating cancer incidence in Japan, and estimates have been accumulated for 14 years (*7*). Cancer data is passively collected in most cancer registries in Japan. As few hospitals have a central record library, cancer notifications are sent from hospital doctors intermittently to cancer registries. Even after incidence rates for a certain year were calculated, notifications for that year are routinely accumulated in the registry during successive years. In 1988–1990 registries recalculated the incidence for each year of 1974–1985. Definitive incidence estimates in Japan in 1975–1984 were also recalculated based on these data.

However, estimates for the more recent 4-year period of 1985–1988 are still tentative and will be comprehensively recalculated in the future. Therefore, in this

*1 This report was prepared by Aya Hanai, Ph.D. and Isaburo Fujimoto, M.D., Ph.D., Osaka Cancer Registry, Department of Field Research, Center for Adult Diseases, Osaka, 1-3-3 Nakamichi, Higashinari-ku, Osaka 537, Japan (花井　彩, 藤本伊三郎).

*2 The Research Group study personnel included: Isaburo Fujimoto (Chairman, 1975–1980, and 1987–1992), Seigo Fukuma (Chairman, 1981–1986), Aya Hanai (Chairman, 1993–), Junkichi Atsuya (Hokkaido Cancer Registry), Akira Takano (Miyagi Cancer Registry), Yukio Sato (Yamagata Cancer Registry), Motoi Murata (Chiba Cancer Registry), Naoyuki Okamoto (Kanagawa Cancer Registry), Yutaka Kurosawa (Toyama Cancer Registry), Shin Yamasaki (Fukui Cancer Registry), Seishi Yoshimura (Shiga Cancer Registry), Masatoshi Furuya (Kyoto Cancer Registry), Teruko Ishida (Hyogo Cancer Registry), Hideaki Nakayama (Tottori Cancer Registry), Takeo Yoshida (Okayama Morbidity Survey), Kiyohiko Mabuchi (Hiroshima City Tumor Registry), Masaharu Nakajima (Yamaguchi Cancer Registry), Tsunehisa Nagata (Fukuoka Cancer Registry), Kenya Hiura (Saga Cancer Registry), Takayoshi Ikeda (Nagasaki City Tumor Registry), and Tetsuo Kuroishi (Aichi Cancer Center).

report, definitive estimates for the years 1975–1984 and estimates for the most recent year 1988, even though these are tentative, are described with their reliability and a brief explanation of the estimation procedures.

The first section of this paper lists the population-based cancer registries in Japan who belonged to the Research Group as of 1992 and the tentative estimates of incidence for 1988, which were calculated in 1992. The second section presents 10-year trends of definitive estimated annual incidence in Japan for the period 1975 to 1984. The third section shows, by way of charts, 25 or 30-year trends of incidence from four cancer registries: Miyagi, Osaka, Hiroshima City, and Nagasaki City.

Population-Based Cancer Registries in Japan

1. Cancer registries in Japan

Nineteen population-based cancer registries were participating in the Research Group as of 1992, each of which has been calculating cancer incidence annually. Their annual populations, number of incidence and of deaths (*2*) are shown on average for 1987–1989 in Table I together with indices of their registration reliability. As the incidence data from Fukuoka was only available up until 1987, the data for 1985–1987 from this registry is shown in Table I.

Both Chiba and Kanagawa prefectures had a large population, 8.0 and 5.6 million, respectively, making complete reporting difficult. It was therefore decided to designate a district with the best reporting rate to provide the representative incidence for each of these prefectures. The Nagasaki City Cancer Registry is one of the oldest registries in Japan, and has been a part of the Nagasaki Prefectural Registry since 1985. The total population covered by the nineteen registries in Table I was 49.0 million, which was equivalent to 40% of the population in Japan that year.

2. Reliability of registry data

The four indices showing reliability of registry data are shown in the right column of Table I.

The proportions of cases registered by death certificate only (DCO), the inverse index of completeness of reporting, are widely distributed from 2.4 to 63.2%. The average was 26.6%. The ratio of incidence to deaths also showed wide variation from 1.25–2.16, with an average of 1.59. The International Association of Cancer Registries (IACR) uses an inverse index: deaths *vs.* incidence, but the objective of evaluating the quantity of obtained incidence (*3*) is the same.

The proportion of cases verified histologically to incidence or to reported cases has been used to express the accuracy of diagnosis of registered tumors. The proportion to incidence varied from 23.6 to 81.4% and the average was 54.2%, while the proportion to reported cases varied from 44.9 to 88.4% and the average was 73.2%.

3. Incidence rates in each registry

Annual age-standardized incidence rates to world population in 1987–1989 are shown according to registry, sex, and primary site in Table II. A comparison is possible among registries with the similar level of completeness of reporting.

Estimated Incidence and Incidence Rates in Japan in 1988

1. Selection of registry data

Registry data which satisfied the following two standards were selected: (1) proportion of cases registered by DCO for all sites for both sexes was 30% or less, and (2) the ratio of cancer incidence to cancer deaths of all sites for both sexes was 1.4 or over. Incidence data in 1987–1989 from the following ten registries met the standards and was used to estimate incidence in Japan in 1988: Miyagi, Yamagata, Chiba, Kanagawa, Fukui, Osaka, Tottori, Saga, and Nagasaki Prefectures, and Hiroshima City. The population covered by these ten registries was 19.3 million, which corresponded to 15.7% of the entire population of Japan in 1988.

2. Estimation of cancer incidence in Japan

The arithmetic mean of incidence rates from the ten qualifying registries was calculated according to sex, primary site, and 5-year age group.* These were regarded as the estimates (pre-correction) of age-specific incidence rates in Japan in 1988 (Tables III-1 and III-2). The estimates of number of incident cases, crude rates, and age-standardized rates were further calculated from these age-specific rates and are shown in the left column of Tables IV-1 and IV-2.

3. Correction of estimates

To minimize regional bias caused by the selection of registries, the following correction was made to the crude estimates obtained above.

Cancer mortality in Japan was estimated by the same methods using mortality data from the above mentioned ten registries. The correction coefficient was then calculated according to site and sex by dividing cancer mortality in Vital Statistics (*2*) by the estimated cancer mortality in Japan. These figures are shown in the center column of Tables IV-1 and IV-2. Correction coefficient for all sites of cancer was 0.97 in males and 0.99 in females. The smallest was 0.88 for lymphatic tissue and the largest was 1.32 for thyroid, both in males.

The estimated number of incidence, the crude rate, and the age-standardized rate were multiplied by the correction coefficient according to sex and site to obtain the corrected estimates which are shown in the right column of Tables IV-1 and IV-2.

Cancer incidence in Japan for all sites in 1988 was estimated as 199,492 for males and 155,668 for females, a total of 355,160 for both sexes. The age-standardized rates to world population were 248.2 and 158.6 for males and females, respectively.

Correction has not yet been made for the age-specific incidence rates in Table II. As reliable and statistically stable correction coefficients were not obtained for some age groups with a small number of deaths in many cancer sites, correction coefficients for all ages should also be applied for correcting all age-specific rates.

4. Reliability of estimated incidence

Reliability of the estimated incidence is as follows. The proportion of DCO cases for all sites of cancer was 17.6% in males and 16.3% in females as shown in the

* An alternative method would be to divide the total number of incidence by the total population of the qualified registries. However, if this method were chosen, a significant influence on the results from a large population-sized registry would be unavoidable.

third column from the far right in Tables IV-1 and IV-2. The ratios of incidence to deaths were 1.63 in males and 1.87 in females, as shown in the second column from the right in these two tables. The proportion of cases verified histologically to incidence was 63.6% and 67.1% in males and in females, respectively. It can therefore be said that these estimates show a sufficient level of qualified reliability of registration.

Estimated Cancer Incidence and Incidence Rates in Japan from 1975 to 1984

1. Qualified registries for estimation of incidence in 1975–1984 and registry data reliability

Tables V-1, V-2, and V-3 show the reliability of registry data used for the re-estimation of incidence in 1975–1984 according to registry. For the re-estimation (*6*) of incidence through the first 5-year period, Miyagi, Yamagata, Osaka, Hiroshima City, and Nagasaki City were qualified, and for the second 5-year period, Chiba and Saga were also qualified.

2. Trends of incidence and incidence rates in Japan from 1975 to 1984

Tables VI–IX indicate trends in the number of incident cases, crude rates, and age-standardized rates to the world population and to the Japanese model population (*3, 4*) in 1985.

The number of incident cases for all sites increased 1.48 times in males and 1.33 times in females during the period from 1975 to 1984 as shown in Tables VI-1 and VI-2. When observed according to primary site, it decreased in the uterine cervix, non-Hodgkin's lymphoma, and myeloid leukemia while it increased in many other sites. As observed in Tables VIII-1 and VIII-2, age-standardized incidence rates to the world population for all sites of cancer increased gradually during the period from 205.6 to 234.5 (1.14 times) in males, while it increased only slightly or almost leveled off, from 152.1 to 155.5 (1.02 times) in females. When observed according to primary site, the rates increased noticeably in many sites such as the colon (1.88 and 1.48 times in males and in females, respectively), liver (1.75 in males), gallbladder (1.43 and 1.37 in males and in females, respectively), lung (1.37 and 1.32), and prostate (1.35), while the rates decreased in the sites of esophagus (0.95 and 0.88 times in males and in females, respectively), stomach (0.89 and 0.85), myeloid leukemia (0.93 and 0.80), total uterus (invasive) (0.66), and uterine cervix (0.66).

3. Trends of reliability of the estimated incidence from 1975 to 1984

Proportions of cases registered with DCO are shown in Table X. A slight decrease in DCO was observed only in the first 5-year period, with no noticeable change for the latest 4 years. Incidence trends for 10 years did not, therefore, seem to be influenced by changes in the completeness of reporting.

The ratio of incidence to deaths was low for the first 5-year period but rose over the next 5 years (Table XI). Considering that there were no specific trends in the proportion of DCO during these years, this rise might have been caused by improvements in the survival of cancer patients.

The proportion of cases verified histologically rose markedly in the first 5 years, then leveled off in the successive 5 years. It was 68.3% in 1984, as shown in Table XII.

In Tables XIII-1 and XIII-2, correction coefficients used to obtain corrected estimates are shown by sex, primary site, and year.

4. *Age-specific incidence rates (pre-correction) in Japan during the observation period*
Age-specific incidence rates for each year from 1975 to 1984 are tabulated in Tables XIV-1 to XXIII-2. The rates are uncorrected as described above.

Long-Term Time Trends of Incidence in Four Regional Cancer Registries

Incidence trends for a period as long as 25 or 30 years were available from registries in Miyagi, Osaka, Hiroshima City, and Nagasaki City. The data presented by each registry are illustrated in Figs. 1–4 for eight major sites for males: all sites, stomach, colon, rectum, liver, pancreas, lung, and bladder, and ten major sites for females: the same sites as in males and breast and uterus. Fourteen-year trends of estimated incidence in Japan are also shown in Fig. 5.

Incidence rates were prepared for each 5-year period between 1958–1987 in the registries of Hiroshima City and Nagasaki City and between 1963–1987 in the registries of Miyagi and Osaka. The sum of primary liver cancer and liver cancer not specified as primary or secondary is shown as "liver cancer" in these charts, with the exception of the data from Miyagi for the first to the third periods which indicates liver cancer specified as primary only.

For males, the incidence rate for all sites of cancer increased from the period 1968–1972 in Miyagi and Osaka, from the period of 1973–1977 in Hiroshima City, and from 1958–1962 in Nagasaki City. A steep increase in liver cancer started in nearly the same period in most registries. Colon and lung cancers increased from the beginning of the observation period in all four registries. The incidence rate for stomach cancer decreased throughout the periods in three registries, although this decrease only began in 1973–1977 in Nagasaki City.

For females, the cancer incidence rate for all sites decreased slightly in the earlier period, then increased slightly in Miyagi, Osaka, and Hiroshima City, while it leveled off in Nagasaki City. Incidence rates for breast, lung, and colon cancers increased throughout the periods in most registries, while that of liver cancer decreased until 1973–1977, after which it showed a rising trend in all four registries. Stomach cancer decreased throughout all periods in Osaka, however, in other districts the decrease began after 1968–1972 or 1973–1977. The incidence rate for total uterus declined in all registries throughout all periods.

The observed trends seemed rather consistent among these four registries with the occasional exception of Nagasaki City. However, each registry showed the characteristic starting point of increasing or decreasing trends and a characteristic high or low incidence rate for some sites. Estimated incidence rates for Japan as a whole indicate similar but milder changes than those in the four registries observed above. Discontinuity in trends was observed in some sites for the year 1985. As mentioned above, estimates after 1985 are tentative, and these will be re-estimated in the near future.

Acknowledgments

The authors would like to thank all of the following concerned registries and persons: prefectural cancer registries of Hokkaido, Miyagi, Yamagata, Chiba, Kanagawa, Toyama, Fukui, Aichi, Shiga, Kyoto, Osaka, Hyogo, Tottori, Yamaguchi, Kochi, Fukuoka, Saga, Nagasaki, and the city registry of Hiroshima, as well as one morbidity survey from Okayama which jointly contributed to this cooperative study. The Research Group for Population-Based Cancer Registration in Japan has been supported by a grant-in-aid from the Ministry of Health and Welfare (2-5 & 5-3). The registries of Miyagi, Hiroshima City, Nagasaki City, and Osaka prepared the long-term data for this report. Computer programming and operation were done by Mr. Kenzo Kawai, Ms. Takako Kitagawa, Mr. Hiroshi Matsumoto, and Mr. Seiki Kozono, and data illustration was prepared by Mr. Masanori Sakamoto and Dr. Hideaki Tsukuma from the Osaka Cancer Registry.

REFERENCES

1. Fujimoto, I., Hanai, A., Nakai, K., Oshima, A., Chiba, S., Takano, A., *et al.* Cancer incidence in Japan—Data from population-based cancer registries in Japan. *Jpn. J. Cancer Clin.*, **27**, 517–533 (1981) (in Japanese).
2. Health and Welfare Statistics and Information Department, Minister's Secretariat, Ministry of Health and Welfare. Vital Statistics 1987–1989 (1989–1991). Health and Welfare Statistics Association, Tokyo (in Japanese).
3. Parkin, D.M. and Muir, C.S. Comparability and quality of data. *In* "Cancer Incidence in Five Continents, Vol. VI," eds. D.M. Parkin, C.S. Muir, S.L. Whelan, Y.T. Gao, I. Ferlay, and J. Powell, pp.45–173 (1992). IARC, Lyon.
4. Statistics and Information Department, Minister's Secretariat, Ministry of Health and Welfare. Age-Adjusted Death Rates by Prefecture, Special Report on Vital Statistics 1990, 9 pp. (1992). Health and Welfare Statistics Association, Tokyo (in Japanese).
5. The Research Group for Population-Based Cancer Registration in Japan. Cancer incidence in Japan, 1975—Cancer registry statistics. *In* "Cancer Mortality and Morbidity Statistics—Japan and the World," Gann Monograph on Cancer Research, No. 26, eds. M. Segi, S. Tominaga, K. Aoki, and I. Fujimoto, pp.92–116 (1981). Japan Scientific Societies Press, Tokyo.
6. The Research Group for Population-Based Cancer Registration in Japan. Cancer Incidence in Japan, 1975–1979, pp.iv–xiii (1984). The Research Group, Osaka.
7. The Research Group for Population-Based Cancer Registration in Japan. Cancer incidence and incidence rates in Japan in 1987. *Jpn. J. Clin. Oncol.*, **22**, 437–442 (1993).

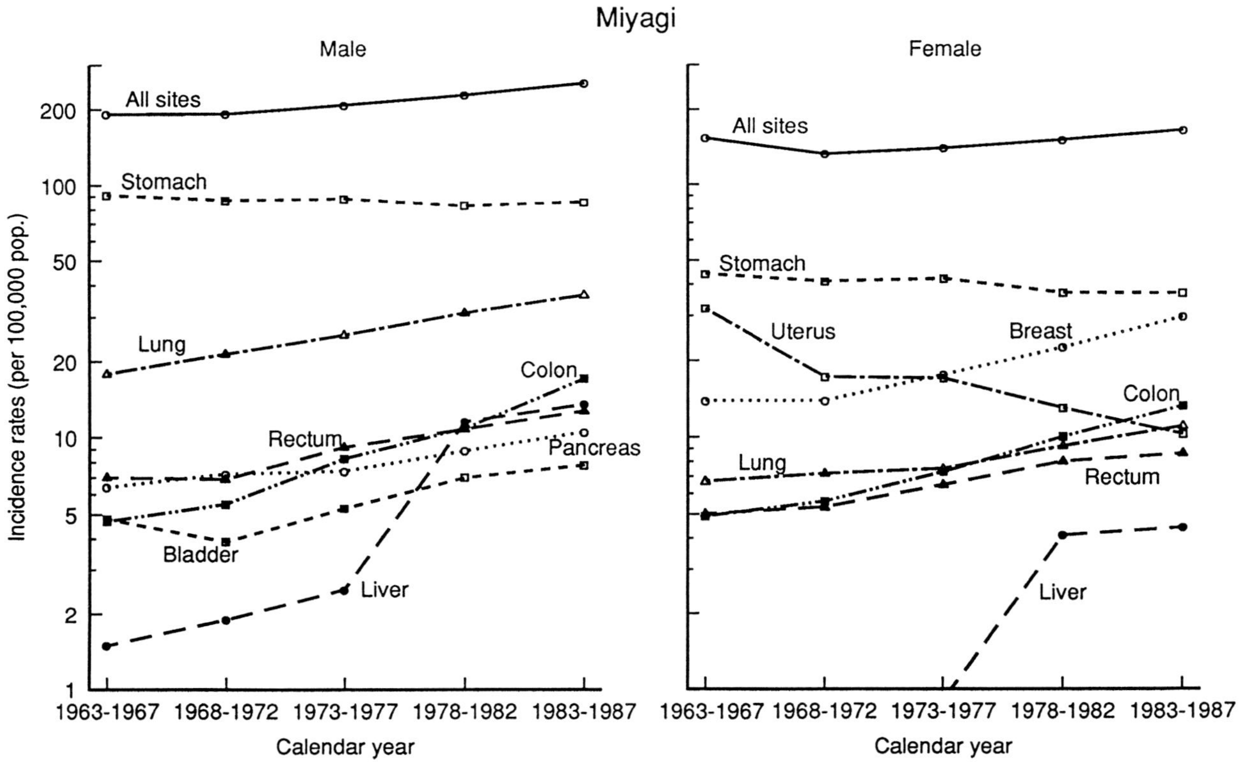

FIG. 1. Time trends in age-standardized incidence rates in Miyagi according to sex and primary site for 1963–1987: prepared by A. Takano *et al.* (Miyagi Cancer Registry)

Time trends in age-standardized incidence rates to world population in Miyagi Prefecture are illustrated from 1963–1967 to 1983–1987. Rates for liver cancer for the first to the third periods represent those specified as primary only and the data for the latter two periods show the sum of primary liver cancer and liver cancer not specified as primary or secondary. The decreasing trend in stomach cancer was very slow in both sexes while the incidence rate of uterine cancer declined very rapidly compared with other registries.

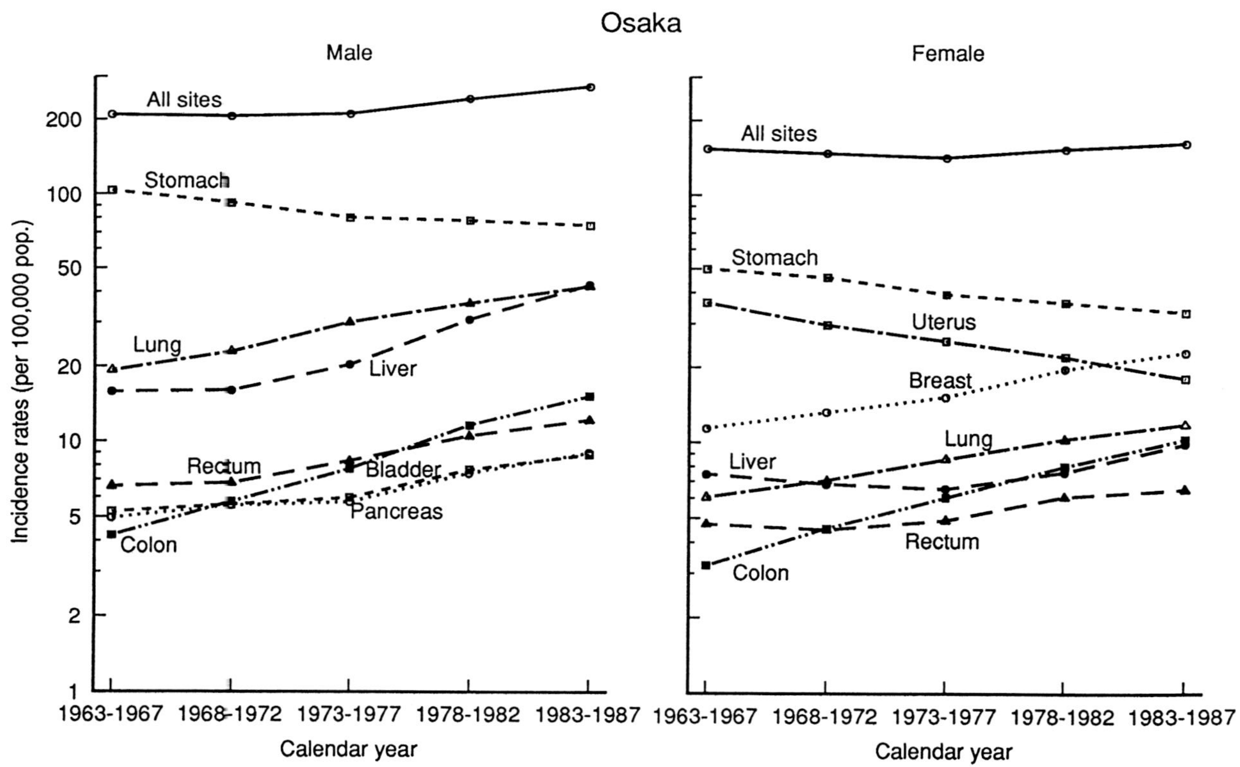

FIG. 2. Time trends in age-standardized incidence rates in Osaka according to sex and primary site for 1963–1987: prepared by A. Hanai *et al.* (Osaka Cancer Registry)

Time trends in age-standardized incidence rates to world population in Osaka Prefecture are illustrated from 1963–1967 to 1983–1987. The decline of stomach and uterine cancers and the increase of all other cancers appeared in clear and smooth trends in Osaka. Both incidence rates for the liver and the lung among males in Osaka were the highest among the four registries and showed the same high rates for the latest period. Breast and uterine cancer incidence rates were shown as the lowest among the four registries.

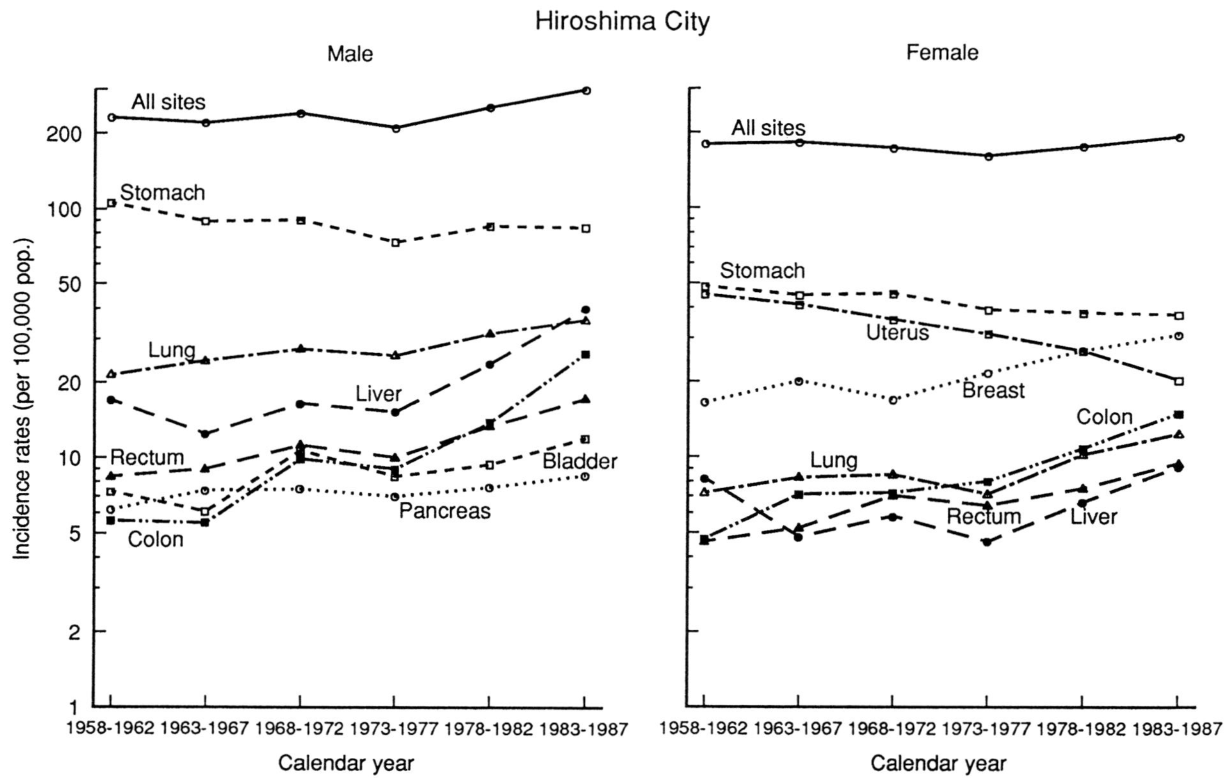

FIG. 3. Time trends in age-standardized incidence rates in Hiroshima City according to sex and primary site for 1958–1987: prepared by K. Mabuchi *et al.* (Hiroshima City Cancer Registry)

Curves of time trends in age-standardized incidence rates in Hiroshima City are illustrated by sex and site in this chart. The curves in both Hiroshima City and Nagasaki City start from 1958–1962 which is 5 years earlier than the starting year in Miyagi and Osaka. Rising trends in many sites seemed similar to Miyagi and Osaka, but appeared slower compared with Nagasaki City.

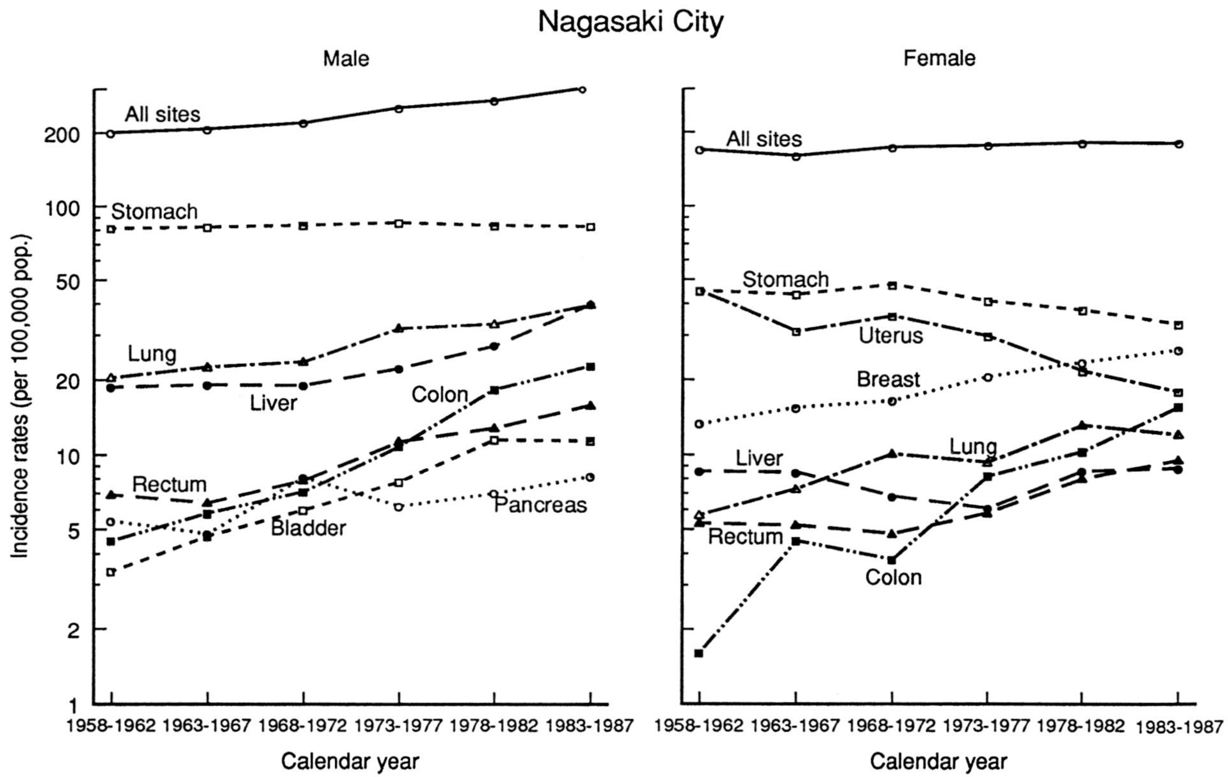

FIG. 4. Time trends in age-standardized incidence rates in Nagasaki City according to sex and primary site for 1958–1987: prepared by T. Ikeda *et al.* (Nagasaki City Cancer Registry)

Colon cancer showed the most rapid increase among the four registries in both sexes. Liver cancer among males in Nagasaki City showed a higher incidence rate than in Hiroshima City from the start, and the rate rapidly increased. As a result, the liver cancer incidence rate was as high as that for the lung in the latest period.

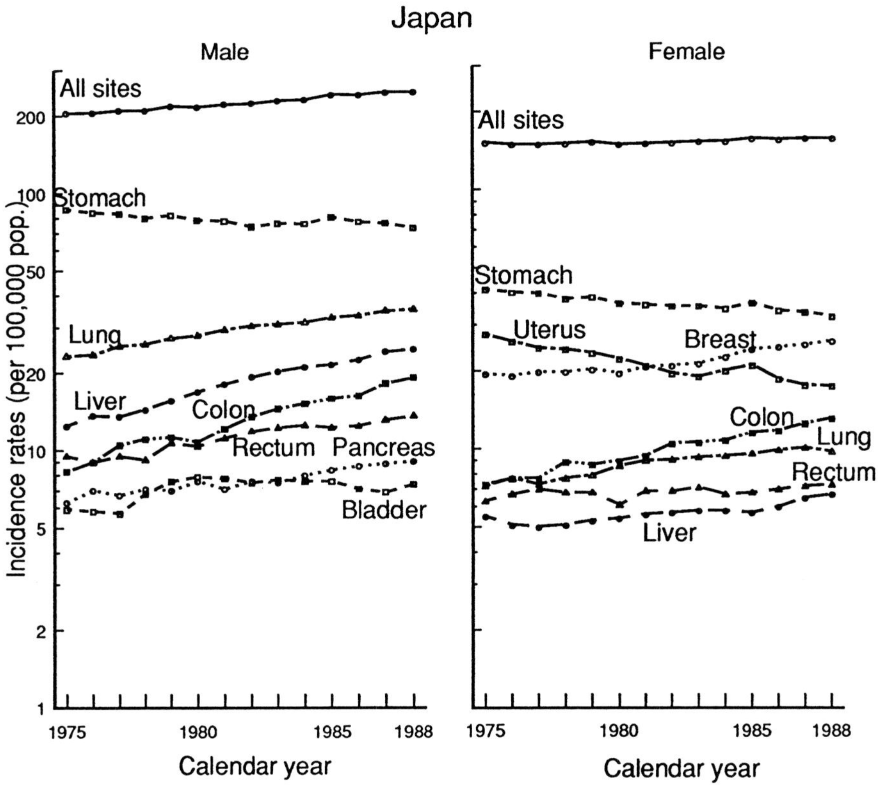

FIG. 5. Time trends in estimated age-standardized incidence rates in Japan according to sex and primary site for 1975–1988: prepared by the Research Group for Population-Based Cancer Registration in Japan

This chart shows trends of annual incidence rates instead of an average of the 5-year data as seen in Figs.1–4. These 14-year trends were largely consistent with those observed in the four registries in Figs. 1–4, although the incidence rate of liver cancer among males was substantially lower than that of the lung.

TABLE I. Cancer Registries in Japan
— The Populations, Incident Cases, Deaths, and Reliability of the Data — (1987–1989)

Registry	Population	Number of: Incident cases	Number of: Deaths	Reliability of the data — Completeness of reporting: Proportion of cases with death certificate only to incidence (%) DCO/I	Completeness of reporting: Ratio of incidence to deaths I/D	Accuracy of diagnosis — Proportion of histologically verified cases: to incidence (%) H/I	Accuracy of diagnosis — Proportion of histologically verified cases: to reported cases (%) H/R
	(Average annual in period)						
Hokkaido	5,657,964	13,116	9,965	63.2	1.32	23.6	64.3
Miyagi	2,219,653	6,796	3,632	8.3	1.87	75.5	82.3
Yamagata	1,259,699	4,399	2,636	17.1	1.67	64.2	77.4
Chiba[a]	1,068,445	2,089	1,393	29.9	1.50	51.9	74.0
Kanagawa[a]	1,054,361	2,434	1,498	27.8	1.62	52.1	72.1
Toyama	1,119,444	3,471	2,188	52.9	1.59	32.0	67.8
Fukui	821,204	2,709	1,486	2.4	1.82	73.1	74.8
Aichi	6,595,210	14,811	9,417	33.2	1.57	50.4	75.5
Shiga	1,195,784	2,479	1,913	6.5	1.30	42.0	44.9
Kyoto	2,596,106	6,063	4,537	46.6	1.34	36.9	69.1
Osaka	8,707,948	23,009	14,555	22.3	1.58	65.8	84.7
Hyogo	5,354,244	13,580	9,434	35.8	1.44	47.7	74.3
Tottori	615,843	2,215	1,277	24.8	1.73	54.8	72.9
Hiroshima City	1,069,070	3,394	1,569	7.8	2.16	81.4	88.4
Yamaguchi	1,584,220	4,897	3,186	32.1	1.54	49.0	72.1
Kouchi	829,029	2,609	1,635	34.7	1.60	47.7	73.1
Fukuoka[b]	4,752,418	10,748	8,606	29.5	1.25	47.9	67.9
Saga	878,716	2,975	1,884	15.1	1.58	57.9	68.1
Nagasaki	1,575,363	5,643	3,319	14.7	1.70	74.4	87.2
Total	48,954,721	127,437	84,130	—	—	—	—
Average	—	—	—	26.6	1.59	54.2	73.2

[a] A district in the prefecture.
[b] Data from Fukuoka is only available for 1985–1987.

TABLE II-1. Age-Standardized (World Population) Annual Incidence Rates According to Sex, Primary Site, and Registry (1987–1989), Male

Site	All sites	All sites	Mouth and pharynx	Esophagus	Stomach	Colon	Rectum	Liver	Gallbladder etc.	Pancreas	Larynx	Lung, trachea	Skin	Breast	Uterus	Overy	Prostate	Bladder	Kidney etc.	Brain, nervous system	Thyroid	Malignant lymphoma	Multiple myeloma	Leukemia	Cervix *in situ*
Registry	140–208 2330 2331	140–208	140–149	150	151	153	154	155	156	157	161	162	172–173 2330	174–175 2331	179–182	1830	185	188	189	191–192	193	200–202	203	204–208	2331
Hokkaido	210.6	210.6	3.6	10.9	54.5	15.5	10.6	19.4	7.1	11.5	1.3	38.9	0.6	0.1			4.9	3.8	3.6	2.4	0.9	3.1	1.0	3.4	
Miyagi	275.6	275.6	5.7	13.9	82.8	23.9	16.4	14.2	6.9	12.4	3.8	39.0	2.5	0.2			8.1	8.6	6.8	2.4	1.9	6.7	1.3	5.4	
Yamagata	245.8	245.8	3.2	11.5	93.9	17.9	12.9	13.1	7.4	9.7	2.8	33.2	1.3	0.1			6.9	6.8	3.1	2.4	0.6	5.2	1.5	4.3	
Chiba[a]	218.0	218.0	4.0	10.5	53.4	15.1	9.8	22.7	7.6	7.6	2.7	36.4	2.2	0.2			8.6	7.8	6.7	0.9	0.7	4.6	2.3	4.9	
Kanagawa[a]	226.0	226.0	6.7	10.3	54.3	19.1	13.0	23.7	4.5	9.6	2.9	39.3	0.5	0.1			8.1	5.0	5.0	1.6	0.7	7.0	1.6	4.6	
Toyama	241.4	241.4	4.6	8.3	81.1	15.0	10.2	18.7	7.4	9.7	3.0	34.8	2.3	0.2			6.2	7.7	5.1	2.3	1.3	4.2	0.9	7.9	
Fukui	237.8	237.8	2.8	3.6	80.9	20.5	12.6	18.4	9.0	8.9	3.4	34.7	1.0	0.2			6.7	8.1	4.0	1.8	1.5	6.0	1.4	4.7	
Aichi	214.2	214.2	4.0	5.5	54.1	18.1	13.7	21.3	6.7	8.3	2.6	36.3	1.1	0.2			6.9	6.9	4.4	2.1	1.0	5.9	1.5	4.6	
Shiga	175.9	175.9	1.2	6.0	45.6	12.3	9.0	13.5	7.9	7.7	1.8	38.1	1.2	0.0			5.2	4.6	2.6	3.3	0.7	2.5	1.2	4.3	
Kyoto	176.6	176.6	2.2	5.9	41.6	12.7	8.5	22.6	5.7	7.8	1.7	34.4	2.0	0.0			5.5	4.5	4.0	2.1	1.0	3.7	1.1	2.7	
Osaka	265.6	265.6	6.0	9.1	65.3	18.6	13.1	43.0	5.3	9.1	3.6	41.8	1.8	0.2			6.5	8.4	5.2	4.0	0.9	5.8	1.4	5.6	
Hyogo	220.1	220.1	4.4	6.8	55.7	14.7	11.6	32.0	4.9	8.4	3.1	36.8	2.1	0.1			6.0	6.5	4.2	2.5	1.0	4.6	1.3	4.1	
Tottori	264.3	264.3	5.7	5.5	95.6	18.2	16.4	31.3	4.6	11.1	3.3	29.5	1.6	0.2			5.6	6.6	3.1	4.7	1.7	3.0	1.5	2.7	
Hiroshima City	303.1	303.1	6.5	10.2	73.3	32.4	19.1	38.6	7.2	9.1	3.1	35.9	5.3	0.2			10.1	12.5	7.9	1.7	3.0	6.4	1.7	5.1	
Yamaguchi	212.8	212.8	4.0	8.9	57.1	8.1	19.5	28.2	4.6	7.1	1.3	37.4	0.7	0.2			5.6	6.2	3.4	1.6	0.9	4.1	0.9	5.0	
Kouchi	205.5	205.5	4.8	6.8	59.3	14.8	9.6	21.9	4.4	8.1	3.3	26.1	3.4	0.2			6.7	7.4	3.9	2.1	2.3	5.0	1.8	3.6	
Saga	271.7	271.7	5.4	6.8	74.4	17.4	9.7	42.0	7.3	9.5	3.4	39.1	3.9	0.0			7.8	11.5	5.6	1.7	1.2	7.5	1.4	8.1	
Nagasaki	284.3	284.3	7.0	7.9	75.2	22.9	16.1	29.9	8.8	9.1	3.1	37.7	5.6	0.4			9.2	11.6	5.6	2.8	1.9	11.2	1.2	5.4	
Nagasaki City	318.3	318.3	8.1	6.9	78.5	31.5	18.3	31.7	7.5	10.6	1.8	42.2	5.5	0.2			12.8	15.3	6.8	3.9	2.1	9.9	1.9	7.2	

[a] A district in the prefecture.

TABLE II-2. Age-Standardized (World Population) Annual Incidence Rates According to Sex, Primary Site, and Registry (1987–1989), Female

Site / Registry	All sites 140–208 2330 2331	All sites 140–208	Mouth and pharynx 140–149	Esophagus 150	Stomach 151	Colon 153	Rectum 154	Liver 155	Gall-bladder etc. 156	Pancreas 157	Larynx 161	Lung, trachea 162	Skin 172–173 2330	Breast 174–175 2331	Uterus 179–182	Overy 1830	Prostate 185	Bladder 188	Kidney etc. 189	Brain, nervous system 191–192	Thyroid 193	Malignant lymphoma 200–202	Multiple myeloma 203	Leukemia 204–208	Cervix *in situ* 2331
Hokkaido	122.3	122.3	0.8	1.6	23.0	11.4	5.8	5.5	5.7	6.6	0.1	10.4	0.6	14.1	11.5	4.3		1.1	1.5	1.7	3.9	1.4	0.6	2.5	0.0
Miyagi	175.0	168.0	1.4	2.2	36.6	15.2	8.0	4.6	6.7	6.0	0.2	9.8	1.6	34.5	14.3	5.4		2.3	2.5	2.0	8.4	2.6	1.1	3.3	4.6
Yamagata	150.0	145.7	0.7	1.7	41.9	12.8	8.8	3.9	7.9	5.1	0.0	7.7	1.4	19.7	12.8	4.2		1.1	1.7	2.4	4.4	2.6	0.7	4.3	4.3
Chiba[a]	116.2	114.7	1.2	1.6	19.3	9.0	3.7	4.3	5.2	7.9	0.5	9.3	1.5	19.7	9.9	5.1		0.5	2.7	0.9	2.1	2.6	0.5	2.4	0.8
Kanagawa[a]	152.7	151.4	1.2	2.0	26.0	12.4	7.0	8.0	5.7	5.3	0.3	8.3	1.5	27.9	14.3	8.4		2.7	2.3	1.2	1.8	3.6	1.5	4.4	1.3
Toyama	152.0	152.0	1.3	1.4	29.9	15.0	8.0	5.9	7.6	5.1	0.2	7.7	0.6	19.4	14.7			1.4	2.1	1.6	7.8	2.5	1.8	5.3	
Fukui	157.8	154.6	1.1	1.3	42.6	13.7	8.3	7.4	9.4	5.3	0.0	7.6	1.0	20.5	12.8	2.9		1.4	2.0	1.1	5.4	3.5	1.3	3.4	2.7
Aichi	149.4	145.9	1.6	1.1	26.8	13.5	6.9	5.6	6.2	5.0	0.2	11.6	1.0	26.4	15.4	5.5		1.7	1.7	1.6	3.8	3.4	1.0	4.0	3.1
Shiga	112.1	106.8	1.1	1.1	22.8	8.9	5.7	3.6	7.1	4.1	0.1	8.3	0.2	12.6	13.9	3.6		1.0	1.5	5.4	0.9	2.4	0.9	3.0	5.3
Kyoto	110.7	108.2	0.7	1.2	18.9	8.5	5.2	6.2	5.0	5.4	0.2	9.0	0.7	17.1	14.5	5.3		0.9	1.1	1.5	2.6	1.5	0.9	1.2	1.8
Osaka	153.6	149.5	1.9	1.6	26.7	11.9	6.0	10.7	5.8	5.2	0.4	11.8	1.1	23.5	16.6	5.0		1.9	1.8	3.2	3.0	3.6	0.9	3.7	3.5
Hyogo	132.5	130.0	2.0	1.4	24.3	10.8	5.1	7.8	4.9	4.8	0.1	9.7	1.4	20.2	15.0	5.0		1.4	1.8	1.9	4.1	2.3	0.8	2.7	2.5
Tottoi	158.0	155.1	1.1	1.1	41.4	11.5	8.1	7.9	4.4	6.6	0.6	8.2	1.2	19.0	16.0	6.5		1.6	0.9	3.4	6.1	1.8	1.1	3.3	2.9
Hiroshima City	202.0	187.3	1.3	1.4	35.7	22.2	11.6	9.4	5.1	3.9	0.2	10.2	5.3	33.5	29.8	6.4		2.8	2.3	2.0	7.0	4.1	0.7	2.8	12.6
Yamaguchi	127.3	127.3	1.4	1.4	27.7	6.3	11.3	6.6	4.4	3.8	0.0	10.4	1.0	18.2	11.9			1.1	1.2	1.8	2.1	3.2	0.9	2.7	
Kouchi	147.9	145.3	1.9	1.2	25.0	8.9	5.7	6.0	3.8	4.4	0.0	9.7	0.9	25.7	26.1	5.3		1.5	1.2	2.2	7.8	2.7	0.7	2.0	2.6
Saga	145.8	140.8	1.4	0.5	29.2	11.9	5.4	10.1	8.4	6.5	0.0	9.8	1.8	16.0	17.2	4.0		1.8	1.8	2.4	2.8	2.8	1.4	4.6	4.9
Nagasaki	178.8	171.1	2.2	1.1	33.8	13.8	8.8	6.8	6.5	4.9	0.1	12.1	4.2	26.0	22.6	5.4		2.3	2.2	2.4	5.7	5.1	1.3	4.7	7.4
Nagasaki City	186.2	180.7	1.9	0.8	29.4	15.5	7.0	7.1	5.6	5.9	0.2	14.2	5.1	33.0	20.5	5.3		3.1	2.1	3.2	6.2	5.8	0.4	5.4	5.1

[a] A district in the prefecture.

TABLE III-1. Age-Specific Incidence Rates per 100,000 Population (Uncorrected Estimates) in Japan According to Sex and Primary Site (1988), Male

Primary site	ICD, 9th	Age group																		All ages
		0–	5–	10–	15–	20–	25–	30–	35–	40–	45–	50–	55–	60–	65–	70–	75–	80–	85–	
All sites	140–208, 233	23.8	11.1	11.1	10.7	12.9	18.3	36.8	65.1	108.3	202.5	391.0	709.7	1070.6	1365.8	1939.6	2451.9	2699.2	3031.3	353.5
All sites	140–208	23.8	11.1	11.1	10.7	12.9	18.3	36.8	65.1	108.3	202.5	391.0	709.7	1070.6	1365.8	1939.4	2451.9	2699.2	3031.3	353.5
Mouth	140–145	0.1	0.1	0.1	0.2	0.4	0.6	0.9	1.2	2.4	3.8	6.2	9.5	13.1	15.7	15.9	19.6	22.0	20.5	4.1
Pharynx	146–149	0.4	0.2	0.1	0.2	0.2	0.1	0.5	1.1	1.5	3.2	4.0	7.6	7.7	10.2	14.4	14.6	8.6	11.2	2.8
Esophagus	150	0.8	0.4	0.2	0.1	0.1	0.1	0.1	0.5	1.9	6.6	14.1	29.0	47.5	51.1	67.3	83.7	77.2	73.7	12.1
Stomach	151	1.1	1.0	1.0	1.3	1.4	3.0	10.3	22.7	40.4	73.2	129.6	213.5	319.1	403.0	565.6	682.3	719.2	746.4	105.2
Colon	153	0.6	0.3	0.5	0.2	0.4	0.8	2.1	4.5	7.6	17.6	36.2	54.3	82.0	102.7	137.3	179.8	189.6	269.4	26.4
Rectum	154	0.1	0.1	0.3	0.1	0.4	0.5	1.0	3.5	8.3	14.4	24.5	47.3	55.1	67.6	100.1	110.9	125.4	150.8	18.8
Liver	155	1.3	0.2	0.3	0.1	0.1	0.2	1.9	4.0	10.8	20.6	63.1	123.1	148.8	149.1	166.7	166.7	173.1	194.5	37.3
Gallbladder *etc.*	156	0.1	0.1	0.0	0.2	0.1	0.0	0.3	1.1	1.6	3.5	6.7	12.4	22.7	39.4	66.3	98.2	115.3	123.2	10.0
Pancreas	157	0.3	0.5	0.2	0.1	0.2	0.1	0.4	1.1	2.6	6.2	11.4	22.0	40.0	56.5	80.5	106.4	123.0	118.7	13.3
Nose, sinuses	160	0.1	0.0	0.0	0.0	0.1	0.3	0.0	0.1	0.9	1.0	1.9	4.0	4.0	5.4	7.4	9.4	5.6	9.9	1.5
Larynx	161	0.0	0.0	0.1	0.0	0.0	0.0	0.0	0.3	0.4	2.1	3.6	12.4	18.0	22.7	23.5	24.1	28.3	24.9	4.4
Lung, trachea	162	2.4	1.0	0.6	0.8	0.4	0.3	1.4	3.6	6.8	14.6	31.4	76.7	151.0	219.9	345.5	451.3	494.9	506.2	50.6
Connective tissue	171	1.1	0.3	0.4	0.3	0.4	0.0	0.6	0.8	0.5	0.6	0.9	1.6	2.3	3.1	3.9	4.0	3.1	9.7	1.0
Skin	172,173	0.2	0.1	0.0	0.1	0.2	0.5	0.5	0.9	1.3	2.1	3.5	5.6	9.8	11.1	18.3	26.6	43.5	47.5	3.5
Other skin	173	0.1	0.1	0.0	0.1	0.1	0.5	0.4	0.7	0.8	1.5	2.8	4.9	8.6	9.4	16.5	22.8	38.7	45.9	3.0
Prostate	185	0.1	0.1	0.1	0.1	0.2	0.1	0.0	0.0	0.1	0.4	1.7	6.3	18.7	37.1	84.0	156.6	195.4	283.3	11.6
Testis	186	1.2	0.0	0.1	0.5	1.6	3.9	4.4	2.3	1.2	1.4	0.9	0.8	0.8	0.3	1.4	0.3	1.1	1.4	1.4
Bladder	188	0.0	0.1	0.1	0.0	0.2	0.3	0.8	2.0	3.2	4.4	9.6	19.2	30.5	43.7	67.8	93.7	119.8	180.5	11.6
Kidney *etc.*	189	1.0	0.2	0.0	0.1	0.2	0.6	0.9	1.3	2.1	4.8	10.3	14.6	20.4	33.0	40.3	41.6	48.6	36.6	7.1
Brain, nervous system	191–192	2.3	1.4	1.5	1.2	1.1	1.3	2.2	2.1	1.5	2.9	4.3	5.1	5.3	6.6	8.9	10.4	13.3	4.1	3.0
Thyroid	193	0.0	0.1	0.1	0.2	0.4	0.5	0.8	1.3	2.4	1.8	3.3	4.5	5.2	4.0	3.5	5.6	6.3	10.3	1.8
Lymphatic tissue	200–203	1.3	1.0	1.4	1.3	1.2	1.9	2.2	4.0	3.8	6.6	9.5	18.7	29.8	37.3	53.3	69.4	71.9	73.4	10.5
Non-Hodgkin's lymphoma	200,202	1.3	0.7	1.4	1.3	1.1	1.6	1.9	3.7	3.3	5.4	7.6	15.4	22.5	26.6	35.9	49.1	48.2	50.9	7.9
Multiple myeloma	203	0.0	0.0	0.0	0.0	0.0	0.0	0.1	0.2	0.3	1.0	1.5	2.9	6.5	9.4	16.1	19.1	21.2	21.2	2.2
Leukemia	204–208	4.6	3.2	2.7	2.5	1.6	2.0	2.9	4.8	4.6	4.9	6.0	8.7	13.8	16.6	22.5	29.8	28.7	37.3	6.4
Lymphoid leukemia	204	2.9	2.5	1.6	1.7	0.4	0.3	0.5	0.9	0.7	1.4	2.0	2.1	2.7	2.2	3.3	4.1	5.8	7.1	1.7
Myeloid leukemia	205	1.0	0.6	0.9	0.6	1.0	1.5	1.9	3.1	2.7	2.9	3.5	4.9	7.9	9.8	14.7	16.9	14.7	18.2	3.4

ICD: International Classification of Diseases.

TABLE III-2. Age-Specific Incidence Rates per 100,000 Population (Uncorrected Estimates) in Japan According to Sex and Primary Site (1988), Female

Primary site	ICD, 9th	Age group																		All ages
		0–	5–	10–	15–	20–	25–	30–	35–	40–	45–	50–	55–	60–	65–	70–	75–	80–	85–	
All sites	140–208, 233	17.4	9.9	8.4	9.8	14.2	28.6	63.1	124.2	182.1	246.9	299.7	386.6	523.4	676.1	914.1	1122.8	1344.0	1451.2	259.3
All sites	140–208	17.4	9.9	8.4	9.7	13.7	25.6	52.3	107.1	162.7	231.7	292.3	381.0	517.1	669.4	909.9	1120.5	1342.1	1449.4	252.7
Mouth	140–145	0.0	0.0	0.0	0.1	0.2	0.5	0.7	0.5	0.9	1.6	2.5	1.8	3.9	5.6	7.6	8.4	11.2	10.2	1.9
Pharynx	146–149	0.1	0.0	0.0	0.0	0.0	0.1	0.0	0.5	0.3	1.3	0.8	1.6	1.7	1.8	2.2	2.7	3.2	5.2	0.8
Esophagus	150	0.1	0.0	0.0	0.0	0.0	0.1	0.0	0.1	0.3	0.9	2.8	2.6	5.7	8.1	13.4	16.5	22.9	28.1	2.7
Stomach	151	0.3	0.8	0.3	0.5	1.7	4.7	9.6	21.1	31.1	44.3	58.9	76.3	114.9	166.1	222.5	281.8	328.4	339.4	57.6
Colon	153	0.3	0.3	0.2	0.3	0.6	1.1	2.1	4.7	8.3	14.7	23.3	35.1	49.5	64.9	92.2	120.5	148.6	168.0	22.9
Rectum	154	0.1	0.1	0.1	0.1	0.3	0.2	0.9	2.9	5.4	10.3	15.0	20.8	30.5	36.0	48.7	60.7	55.3	71.6	12.5
Liver	155	0.8	0.4	0.2	0.2	0.4	0.1	0.3	0.8	1.8	3.8	9.0	19.5	31.8	47.0	59.9	68.6	78.9	74.3	12.6
Gallbladder *etc.*	156	0.1	0.1	0.0	0.2	0.1	0.1	0.3	1.4	1.5	3.9	8.2	13.8	23.8	34.3	61.7	79.2	107.7	115.1	12.8
Pancreas	157	0.0	0.1	0.3	0.3	0.4	0.0	0.4	0.9	1.3	3.8	6.1	11.4	16.7	30.3	49.6	68.1	79.6	97.6	10.1
Nose, sinuses	160	0.0	0.0	0.0	0.1	0.0	0.1	0.1	0.4	0.4	0.9	0.6	1.4	2.3	1.2	3.9	3.7	5.2	2.5	0.8
Larynx	161	0.0	0.0	0.0	0.1	0.0	0.1	0.1	0.0	0.2	0.1	0.3	0.5	1.1	1.1	1.7	1.4	2.0	2.3	0.4
Lung, trachea	162	0.0	0.2	0.3	0.2	0.4	0.8	0.7	2.4	4.4	7.8	14.2	23.7	34.8	60.0	82.6	110.0	143.8	136.3	18.3
Connective tissue	171	1.5	0.5	0.2	0.2	0.7	0.3	0.5	0.2	0.8	0.5	1.2	1.8	1.1	1.6	1.2	2.1	3.5	4.1	0.9
Skin	172,173	0.0	0.2	0.2	0.7	0.2	0.8	0.6	1.0	1.5	1.6	1.6	4.8	4.3	6.0	11.2	19.3	26.1	55.3	3.4
Other skin	173	0.0	0.1	0.1	0.5	0.1	0.7	0.3	0.6	1.0	1.2	1.1	3.8	3.7	4.5	10.1	18.0	22.5	52.3	2.9
Breast	174–175, 2330	0.1	0.2	0.4	0.2	0.8	4.1	14.7	35.8	58.3	78.2	63.4	62.2	69.4	62.0	63.4	54.6	50.3	45.5	33.5
Uterus	179–182, 2331	0.3	0.2	0.1	0.2	1.2	6.1	17.3	31.5	36.1	34.3	37.5	43.0	50.8	45.6	51.1	57.3	66.7	70.1	24.6
Uterus	179–182	0.3	0.2	0.1	0.1	0.7	3.3	7.0	15.6	19.0	21.6	32.0	38.1	45.8	40.6	48.0	55.6	64.9	68.6	18.9
Cervix uteri	180	0.3	0.1	0.1	0.1	0.3	2.4	5.9	13.3	14.8	15.5	18.9	21.8	28.1	27.2	31.4	36.2	38.1	32.9	12.3
Corpus uteri	182	0.0	0.0	0.0	0.0	0.2	0.4	0.8	1.7	3.6	5.1	10.7	14.1	14.5	10.6	9.8	8.0	9.5	6.8	4.5
Uterus, unspecified	179	0.0	0.1	0.0	0.0	0.1	0.0	0.1	0.5	0.4	0.8	2.3	2.1	3.3	2.8	6.8	11.4	17.2	28.9	2.0
Ovary *etc.*	183	0.2	0.8	0.7	1.2	2.1	2.0	3.3	5.1	8.2	10.5	13.9	17.1	15.6	14.8	18.2	18.2	23.1	24.5	7.7
Bladder	188	0.1	0.1	0.0	0.1	0.1	0.0	0.2	0.2	0.5	1.1	2.4	4.0	5.0	10.1	15.9	22.0	35.0	42.0	3.7
Kidney *etc.*	189	0.6	0.1	0.0	0.1	0.1	0.2	0.2	0.7	1.1	2.7	2.8	4.3	8.0	10.6	15.1	17.4	18.0	20.9	3.3
Brain, nervous system	191–192	1.8	1.5	2.0	0.8	0.6	1.4	1.2	0.9	1.1	1.6	3.3	2.9	4.2	6.3	7.8	6.8	5.8	6.7	2.5
Thyroid	193	0.1	0.0	0.2	0.3	1.5	1.7	5.0	7.2	9.9	10.1	12.9	13.1	14.4	14.9	15.1	14.9	16.0	12.9	7.1
Lymphatic tissue	200–203	0.3	0.5	0.5	1.4	0.3	1.3	1.1	1.8	3.1	4.4	7.2	10.8	14.6	18.8	26.9	38.6	41.8	33.8	7.1
Non-Hodgkin's lymphoma	200,202	0.3	0.5	0.5	1.0	0.1	1.2	1.1	1.5	2.9	3.5	5.4	7.4	9.4	11.2	18.2	25.4	22.2	23.2	4.8
Multiple myeloma	203	0.0	0.0	0.0	0.1	0.2	0.0	0.0	0.2	0.2	0.6	1.5	2.9	4.5	7.2	8.2	12.5	17.7	9.9	2.0
Leukemia	204–208	6.5	2.7	1.7	1.5	1.7	1.9	2.3	2.5	2.7	4.0	5.6	4.6	5.6	9.1	13.6	14.1	16.1	13.2	4.5
Lymphoid leukemia	204	4.3	2.0	0.8	0.6	0.7	0.5	0.6	0.6	0.9	1.2	1.3	1.9	1.8	1.9	2.4	2.3	3.5	1.8	1.4
Myeloid leukemia	205	1.1	0.6	0.8	0.9	0.8	1.4	1.3	1.6	1.5	2.2	3.2	1.8	3.1	5.8	7.0	8.5	8.3	7.5	2.3

TABLE IV-1. Uncorrected and Corrected Estimates of Incident Cases, Crude, and Age-Standardized Incidence Rates per 100, 000 Population in Japan with Correction Coefficient and Reliability of the Estimates, According to Sex and Primary Site (1988), Male

Estimated based on the data from cancer registries: Miyagi, Yamagata, Chiba,[a] Kanagawa,[a] Fukui, Osaka, Tottori, Nagasaki Prefectures, and Hiroshima City

Primary site	ICD, 9th	Uncorrected estimates in Japan				Deaths	Observed deaths in Japan	Correction coefficient	Corrected estimates in Japan				Completeness of reporting		Accuracy of diagnosis
		Incidence	Crude rates	Age-standardized rates					Incidence	Crude rates	Age-standardized rates				
				World population	Japanese 1985 model population						World population	Japanese 1985 model population	DCO/I (%)[b]	I/D	H/I (%)[b]
		(A)	(B)	(C)	(D)	(E)	(F)	(F/E)	(A*F/E)	(B*F/E)	(C*F/E)	(D*F/E)			
All sites	140–208, 233	206,485	353.5	256.9	358.4	126,292	122,015	0.97	199,492	341.6	248.2	346.2	17.6	1.63	63.6
All sites	140–208	206,483	353.5	256.9	358.4	126,292	122,015	0.97	199,490	341.6	248.2	346.2	17.6	1.63	63.6
Mouth, Pharynx	140–149	4,071	6.8	5.2	6.9	1,831	1,787	0.98	3,973	6.7	5.0	6.7	10.2	2.22	81.1
Esophagus	150	7,200	12.1	9.0	12.4	5,559	5,625	1.01	7,285	12.3	9.1	12.5	14.9	1.30	72.5
Stomach	151	60,672	105.2	74.9	104.8	30,583	30,009	0.98	59,533	103.3	73.5	102.8	13.9	1.98	77.9
Colon	153	15,616	26.4	19.3	27.0	6,749	6,747	1.00	15,611	26.4	19.3	27.0	13.9	2.31	74.0
Rectum	154	11,032	18.8	13.6	19.0	5,032	5,070	1.01	11,115	19.0	13.7	19.1	11.2	2.19	78.2
Liver	155	22,293	37.3	27.8	37.6	18,175	16,238	0.89	19,917	33.3	24.9	33.6	27.0	1.23	22.8
Gallbladder *etc.*	156	5,724	10.0	6.9	10.2	4,903	4,655	0.95	5,434	9.5	6.5	9.7	25.2	1.17	43.1
Pancreas	157	7,651	13.3	9.4	13.5	7,093	6,906	0.97	7,449	13.0	9.1	13.1	29.3	1.08	31.3
Larynx	161	2,583	4.4	3.2	4.5	764	760	0.99	2,569	4.4	3.2	4.4	5.6	3.38	86.5
Lung, trachea	162	29,334	50.6	35.9	52.0	24,609	24,333	0.99	29,005	50.0	35.5	51.4	22.9	1.19	50.2
Skin	172, 173	2,114	3.5	2.6	3.7	362	359	0.99	2,096	3.5	2.6	3.7	3.1	5.84	90.7
Prostate	185	6,800	11.6	7.9	12.5	3,184	3,035	0.95	6,482	11.0	7.6	11.9	15.5	2.14	70.4
Bladder	188	6,774	11.6	8.3	12.0	2,074	1,851	0.89	6,046	10.3	7.4	10.7	10.8	3.27	78.4
Kidney *etc.*	189	4,188	7.1	5.3	7.3	1,833	1,777	0.97	4,060	6.8	5.1	7.0	13.4	2.28	68.3
Brain, nervous system	191–192	1,765	3.0	2.6	3.0	612	596	0.97	1,719	2.9	2.5	2.9	18.2	2.88	66.9
Thyroid	193	1,070	1.8	1.4	1.8	227	300	1.32	1,414	2.4	1.8	2.3	6.8	4.71	83.8
Lymphatic tissue	200–203	4,787	8.3	6.2	8.2	3,226	2,845	0.88	4,222	7.3	5.5	7.2	18.1	1.48	72.4
Multiple myeloma	203	1,275	2.2	1.6	2.3	955	978	1.02	1,306	2.3	1.6	2.3	28.3	1.34	53.0
Leukemia	204–208	3,768	6.4	5.4	6.4	3,538	3,223	0.91	3,433	5.8	4.9	5.8	25.1	1.07	56.3

[a] A district in the prefecture. [b] Average of proportion of each registry.
DCO/I: proportion of cases registered with death certificate only to incidence.
I/D: incidence to deaths.
H/I: proportion of cases verified histologically to incidence.

Table IV-2. Uncorrected and Corrected Estimates of Incident Cases, Crude, and Age-Standardized Incidence Rates per 100, 000 Population in Japan with Correction Coefficient and Reliability of the Estimates, According to Sex and Primary Site (1988), Female

Estimated based on the data from cancer registries: Miyagi, Yamagata, Chiba,[a] Kanagawa,[a] Fukui, Osaka, Tottori, Nagasaki Prefectures, and Hiroshima City

Primary site	ICD, 9th	Uncorrected estimates in Japan				Deaths	Observed deaths in Japan	Correction coefficient	Corrected estimates in Japan				Completeness of reporting		Accuracy of diagnosis
		Incidence	Crude rates	Age-standardized rates					Incidence	Crude rates	Age-standardized rates		DCO/I (%)[b]	I/D	H/I (%)[b]
				World population	Japanese 1985 model population						World population	Japanese 1985 model population			
		(A)	(B)	(C)	(D)	(E)	(F)	(F/E)	(A*F/E)	(B*F/E)	(C*F/E)	(D*F/E)			
All sites	140–208, 233	157,270	259.3	160.3	216.7	84,314	83,455	0.99	155,668	256.6	158.6	214.5	16.3	1.87	67.1
All sites	140–208	153,158	252.7	155.1	210.2	84,314	83,455	0.99	151,598	250.1	153.5	208.0	16.6	1.82	66.5
Mouth, Pharynx	140–149	1,616	2.6	1.7	2.2	614	659	1.07	1,734	2.8	1.8	2.4	9.6	2.63	79.2
Esophagus	150	1,680	2.7	1.5	2.2	1,255	1,199	0.96	1,605	2.6	1.4	2.1	19.8	1.34	60.2
Stomach	151	34,146	57.6	33.2	46.2	18,379	17,995	0.98	33,433	56.4	32.5	45.2	15.6	1.86	75.2
Colon	153	13,884	22.9	13.2	18.5	6,885	6,893	1.00	13,900	23.0	13.2	18.5	15.8	2.02	71.7
Rectum	154	7,466	12.5	7.3	10.1	3,606	3,589	1.00	7,431	12.4	7.3	10.1	13.2	2.07	76.4
Liver	155	7,604	12.6	7.2	10.1	6,212	5,830	0.94	7,136	11.9	6.7	9.4	32.2	1.22	19.4
Gallbladder *etc.*	156	7,493	12.8	6.6	9.6	6,481	6,445	0.99	7,451	12.7	6.5	9.6	27.1	1.16	39.1
Pancreas	157	6,107	10.1	5.4	7.9	5,678	5,649	0.99	6,076	10.1	5.3	7.8	30.9	1.08	25.7
Larynx	161	219	0.4	0.2	0.3	79	96	1.22	266	0.4	0.3	0.4	9.2	2.77	73.5
Lung, trachea	162	11,098	18.3	10.1	14.5	9,286	9,055	0.98	10,822	17.8	9.8	14.1	25.9	1.20	47.0
Skin	172, 173	2,074	3.4	1.9	2.7	303	277	0.91	1,896	3.1	1.7	2.4	4.4	6.84	88.5
Breast	174, 2330	20,994	33.5	24.3	31.3	5,201	5,602	1.08	22,613	36.1	26.2	33.7	5.4	4.04	86.1
Uterus	179–182, 2331	15,204	24.6	17.1	22.3	4,577	4,724	1.03	15,692	25.4	17.6	23.0	8.0	3.32	81.5
Ovary *etc.*	179	4,591	7.4	5.3	6.7	3,082	3,118	1.01	4,645	7.4	5.3	6.8	17.7	1.49	65.4
Bladder	183	2,162	3.7	1.9	2.8	932	874	0.94	2,027	3.4	1.8	2.6	15.9	2.32	70.9
Kidney *etc.*	189	2,037	3.3	2.0	2.7	911	884	0.97	1,977	3.2	2.0	2.7	15.5	2.24	62.7
Brain, nervous system	191–192	1,486	2.5	2.0	2.2	494	484	0.98	1,456	2.4	1.9	2.2	17.9	3.01	66.3
Thyroid	193	4,388	7.1	5.0	6.5	583	611	1.05	4,599	7.4	5.3	6.8	4.4	7.53	85.8
Lymphatic tissue	200–203	3,054	5.1	3.2	4.2	2,005	1,918	0.96	2,921	4.8	3.0	4.0	18.2	1.52	73.3
Multiple myeloma	203	1,207	2.0	1.1	1.6	988	936	0.95	1,143	1.9	1.0	1.5	33.2	1.22	51.1
Leukemia	204–208	2,775	4.5	3.9	4.2	2,511	2,358	0.94	2,606	4.2	3.6	3.9	22.4	1.11	57.7

[a] A district in the prefecture. [b] Average of proportion of each registry.

DCO/I: proportion of cases registered with death certificate only to incidence.

I/D: incidence to deaths.

H/I: proportion of cases verified histologically to incidence.

TABLE V. Reliability of the Data from Cancer Registries Whose Data Were Used in Estimation of Incidence in Japan

1. Proportion of Cases Registered with Death Certificate Only to Incidence According to Registry and Period, All Sites, Both Sexes

Registry	1974–76	1975–77	1976–78	1977–79	1978–80	1979–81	1980–82	1981–83	1982–84	1983–85
Miyagi	20.3	19.5	17.9	16.7	14.8	14.0	13.6	13.5	12.2	10.9
Yamagata	27.0	24.1	18.7	14.8	15.3	16.1	15.8	13.5	14.1	15.3
Chiba[a]	—	—	—	—	—	26.0	21.5	22.9	24.5	26.3
Osaka	25.1	24.7	24.0	23.1	22.1	20.9	20.7	19.5	19.3	19.2
Hiroshima City	6.2	6.7	6.3	5.2	6.5	7.1	8.0	7.3	8.0	9.6
Saga	—	—	—	—	—	35.2	22.8	19.9	15.4	15.2
Nagasaki City	6.6	7.5	6.6	7.1	6.3	7.5	6.4	7.0	7.9	8.2

2. Ratios of Incidence to Deaths According to Registry and Period, All Sites, Both Sexes

Registry	1974–76	1975–77	1976–78	1977–79	1978–80	1979–81	1980–82	1981–83	1982–84	1983–85
Miyagi	1.58	1.56	1.56	1.56	1.60	1.61	1.64	1.68	1.71	1.73
Yamagata	1.49	1.42	1.40	1.44	1.42	1.43	1.45	1.50	1.54	1.56
Chiba[a]	—	—	—	—	—	1.44	1.44	1.41	1.42	1.39
Osaka	1.45	1.47	1.49	1.53	1.56	1.59	1.60	1.61	1.63	1.61
Hiroshima City	1.73	1.71	1.77	1.80	1.88	1.97	2.06	2.06	2.02	1.92
Saga	—	—	—	—	—	1.43	1.45	1.50	1.57	1.60
Nagasaki City	1.71	1.71	1.72	1.64	1.62	1.60	1.62	1.66	1.68	1.71

3. Proportion of Cases Verified Histologically to Incidence According to Registry and Period, All Sites, Both Sexes

Registry	1974–76	1975–77	1976–78	1977–79	1978–80	1979–81	1980–82	1981–83	1982–84	1983–85
Miyagi	62.0	62.7	64.2	65.0	67.4	69.1	70.5	71.1	72.1	73.1
Yamagata	40.4	45.3	51.8	55.5	56.0	56.6	59.1	62.5	61.9	62.0
Chiba[a]	—	—	—	—	—	48.7	51.8	51.5	52.0	52.2
Osaka	48.6	52.4	55.9	59.3	61.7	63.7	64.7	66.7	67.4	67.7
Hiroshima City	75.5	75.3	78.0	80.9	80.8	80.8	80.6	82.3	82.6	82.7
Saga	—	—	—	—	—	47.2	58.3	61.5	63.6	62.4
Nagasaki City	75.1	75.7	78.2	77.9	78.0	76.0	78.0	78.0	77.7	77.7

[a] A district in prefecture.

Table VI-1. Trends of Number of Incident Cases (Corrected Estimates) in Japan According to Sex, Primary Site, and Year (1975–1984), Male

Primary site	ICD, 9th	Year									
		1975	1976	1977	1978	1979	1980	1981	1982	1983	1984
All sites	140–208, 233	112,787	116,144	122,583	126,314	134,736	137,290	145,119	151,056	159,429	167,403
All sites	140–208	112,787	116,144	122,583	126,314	134,736	137,290	145,119	151,056	159,429	167,403
Mouth	140–145	1,349	1,356	1,372	1,579	1,807	1,579	1,869	1,835	2,238	2,083
Pharynx	146–149	605	602	633	600	784	900	1,083	923	1,034	1,116
Esophagus	150	4,470	4,356	4,617	4,995	5,191	5,166	5,264	5,527	5,758	5,672
Stomach	151	47,737	47,869	48,896	48,526	50,962	50,035	51,151	50,242	53,271	55,061
Colon	153	4,636	5,113	6,110	6,648	7,086	6,913	8,063	9,202	10,271	11,228
Rectum	154	5,258	5,092	5,532	5,553	6,632	6,582	7,296	8,005	8,594	9,213
Liver	155	6,884	7,784	7,897	8,650	9,571	10,712	11,851	13,080	14,165	15,731
Gallbladder *etc.*	156	2,269	2,431	2,723	2,766	2,972	3,230	3,431	3,744	4,138	4,307
Pancreas	157	3,406	3,926	3,899	4,284	4,357	4,826	4,738	5,164	5,268	5,783
Nose, sinuses	160	1,038	1,002	951	942	982	1,097	1,057	1,052	951	817
Larynx	161	1,447	2,018	2,120	2,225	2,425	2,135	2,203	2,192	2,193	2,475
Lung, trachea	162	12,715	13,240	14,759	15,627	17,026	17,998	19,596	20,832	21,783	23,105
Connective tissue	171	424	440	559	374	417	504	532	558	558	474
Skin	172, 173	1,424	1,606	1,539	1,751	1,751	1,908	2,266	2,212	1,990	2,392
Other skin	173	1,331	1,424	1,402	1,766	1,580	1,879	2,176	2,481	2,040	2,062
Prostate	185	2,747	2,793	3,380	3,813	4,112	3,944	4,032	4,362	4,735	5,201
Testis	186	564	719	792	603	635	835	766	861	749	836
Bladder	188	3,165	3,232	3,330	4,108	4,701	4,959	5,106	5,097	5,386	5,469
Kidney *etc.*	189	1,641	1,782	1,825	1,845	1,711	1,834	1,883	2,085	2,328	2,813
Brain, nervous system	191–192	1,238	1,069	1,619	2,090	1,913	1,662	1,973	1,589	1,578	1,412
Thyroid	193	418	418	579	737	728	821	934	900	892	837
Lymphatic tissue	200–203	3,290	3,409	3,791	3,563	3,787	3,883	4,370	4,286	4,653	4,351
Non-Hodgkin's lymphoma	200,202	2,261	2,298	2,551	2,418	2,644	2,603	2,938	3,003	3,236	2,993
Multiple myeloma	203	548	689	804	762	773	1,036	1,243	1,013	1,147	1,104
Leukemia	204–208	2,907	3,031	2,846	2,871	2,942	3,240	3,459	3,721	3,405	3,456
Lymphoid leukemia	204	569	606	530	568	662	807	821	922	926	871
Myeloid leukemia	205	1,662	1,842	1,853	1,883	1,876	1,809	1,976	2,075	1,868	1,848

TABLE VI-2. Trends of Number of Incident Cases (Corrected Estimates) in Japan According to Sex, Primary Site, and Year (1975–1984), Female

Primary site	ICD, 9th	Year									
		1975	1976	1977	1978	1979	1980	1981	1982	1983	1984
All sites	140–208,233	102,069	103,667	106,776	110,695	115,682	116,536	120,708	125,299	130,560	135,811
All sites	140–208	99,428	101,188	104,278	108,256	113,311	113,751	117,825	122,024	127,318	132,166
Mouth	140–145	748	714	826	972	1,029	1,340	993	1,082	992	1,261
Pharynx	146–149	181	200	279	279	268	284	260	456	385	432
Esophagus	150	1,301	1,344	1,268	1,421	1,462	1,553	1,402	1,436	1,690	1,626
Stomach	151	28,230	28,374	29,165	28,604	30,014	29,370	29,899	30,493	31,332	31,754
Colon	153	4,998	5,447	5,619	6,704	6,757	7,223	7,869	9,079	9,473	9,996
Rectum	154	4,341	4,757	5,143	5,135	5,296	4,875	5,615	5,835	6,224	6,105
Liver	155	3,798	3,669	3,730	3,929	4,240	4,425	4,718	5,015	5,250	5,557
Gallbladder *etc.*	156	3,235	3,366	3,531	3,721	3,995	4,507	5,050	5,377	5,977	6,115
Pancreas	157	2,680	2,646	2,626	2,872	3,207	3,536	3,790	3,955	4,301	4,414
Nose, sinuses	160	659	753	688	556	442	525	593	609	641	507
Larynx	161	208	237	257	198	173	210	179	244	235	382
Lung, trachea	162	5,008	5,503	5,400	5,877	6,206	6,979	7,545	7,968	8,618	9,182
Connective tissue	171	344	320	356	374	382	416	394	471	445	488
Skin	172,173	1,206	1,136	1,954	2,347	2,372	2,372	2,463	2,561	1,979	2,030
Other skin	173	988	940	1,986	2,594	2,252	2,177	2,216	2,371	1,508	1,601
Breast	174–175,2330	12,798	12,948	13,679	13,988	14,628	14,447	15,635	16,221	16,850	18,411
Uterus	179–182,2331	18,481	17,703	17,231	17,485	17,410	16,777	16,127	15,485	15,430	16,523
Uterus	179–182	15,715	15,120	14,641	14,988	15,033	14,142	13,436	12,474	12,429	13,123
Cervix uteri	180	10,987	11,998	10,474	11,998	11,585	11,552	10,482	9,417	8,751	9,240
Corpus uteri	182	1,885	1,205	1,844	1,568	2,419	1,826	2,287	2,177	2,541	2,670
Uterus, unspecified	179	2,090	1,916	1,746	1,538	1,424	1,388	1,268	1,232	1,233	1,224
Ovary *etc.*	183	2,589	2,596	2,804	3,269	3,726	3,433	3,650	3,592	3,811	4,204
Bladder	188	1,184	1,270	1,213	1,340	1,264	1,618	1,472	1,677	1,804	1,679
Kidney *etc.*	189	652	757	875	1,173	1,111	975	1,168	1,388	1,254	1,207
Brain, nervous system	191–192	1,035	1,247	1,338	1,371	1,225	1,444	1,386	1,066	1,008	962
Thyroid	193	2,096	2,074	2,983	2,670	2,419	2,175	2,320	2,560	3,040	2,950
Lymphatic tissue	200–203	2,226	2,379	2,565	2,598	2,762	2,633	2,890	3,109	3,402	3,578
Non-Hodgkin's lymphoma	200,202	1,412	1,563	1,778	1,699	1,629	1,640	1,944	2,244	2,383	2,370
Multiple myeloma	203	523	572	563	664	885	784	759	735	839	1,050
Leukemia	204–208	2,337	2,119	2,110	1,980	2,326	2,343	2,421	2,453	2,444	2,714
Lymphoid leukemia	204	334	353	360	302	475	679	640	698	601	781
Myeloid leukemia	205	1,423	1,311	1,240	1,170	1,376	1,262	1,278	1,262	1,314	1,439

TABLE VII-1. Trends of Crude Incidence Rates per 100,000 Population (Corrected Estimates) in Japan According to Sex and Primary Site (1975–1984), Male

Primary site	ICD, 9th	Year									
		1975	1976	1977	1978	1979	1980	1981	1982	1983	1984
All sites	140–208, 233	198.92	202.97	211.67	216.94	229.27	234.39	246.26	255.20	267.80	279.53
All sites	140–208	198.92	202.97	211.67	216.94	229.27	234.39	246.26	255.20	267.80	279.53
Mouth	140–145	2.32	2.30	2.33	2.64	3.01	2.65	3.15	3.05	3.70	3.43
Pharynx	146–149	1.08	1.06	1.09	0.99	1.31	1.51	1.81	1.52	1.69	1.78
Esophagus	150	7.93	7.73	8.17	8.81	9.09	8.80	8.98	9.33	9.71	9.47
Stomach	151	85.77	84.97	85.50	84.46	88.07	86.65	88.06	86.12	90.59	93.28
Colon	153	8.06	8.87	10.49	11.39	12.00	11.60	13.45	15.37	17.11	18.54
Rectum	154	9.29	8.94	9.60	9.57	11.28	11.13	12.29	13.44	14.35	15.30
Liver	155	11.88	13.38	13.32	14.52	15.84	18.07	19.74	21.66	23.38	25.86
Gallbladder *etc.*	156	4.01	4.25	4.77	4.81	5.14	5.62	5.93	6.39	7.02	7.26
Pancreas	157	6.10	6.94	6.82	7.38	7.44	8.29	8.16	8.83	8.91	9.70
Nose, sinuses	160	1.81	1.76	1.66	1.66	1.71	1.93	1.82	1.79	1.60	1.35
Larynx	161	2.45	3.39	3.54	3.72	4.00	3.58	3.67	3.67	3.65	4.09
Lung, trachea	162	21.89	22.65	24.90	26.32	28.46	30.71	33.24	35.28	36.74	38.69
Connective tissue	171	0.74	0.77	0.98	0.66	0.71	0.87	0.90	0.94	0.93	0.78
Skin	172,173	2.41	2.66	2.54	2.88	2.86	3.17	3.82	3.74	3.36	3.98
Other skin	173	2.24	2.35	2.30	2.88	2.56	3.12	3.68	4.19	3.44	3.41
Prostate	185	4.63	4.70	5.67	6.40	6.84	6.45	6.58	7.07	7.68	8.40
Testis	186	1.03	1.31	1.45	1.10	1.13	1.44	1.33	1.48	1.28	1.41
Bladder	188	5.39	5.48	5.59	6.84	7.71	8.13	8.39	8.32	8.78	8.85
Kidney *etc.*	189	2.88	3.10	3.16	3.14	2.90	3.09	3.11	3.44	3.82	4.65
Brain, nervous system	191–192	2.25	1.91	2.85	3.65	3.32	2.86	3.36	2.72	2.66	2.37
Thyroid	193	0.71	0.72	0.99	1.26	1.24	1.36	1.55	1.47	1.47	1.38
Lymphatic tissue	200–203	5.77	5.94	6.61	6.18	6.49	6.72	7.46	7.27	7.81	7.31
Non-Hodgkin's lymphoma	200, 202	3.96	4.01	4.43	4.20	4.53	4.55	5.04	5.12	5.43	5.03
Multiple myeloma	203	0.96	1.19	1.43	1.32	1.31	1.72	2.08	1.69	1.94	1.86
Leukemia	204–208	5.19	5.34	4.98	4.98	5.06	5.54	5.89	6.33	5.76	5.85
Lymphoid leukemia	204	1.03	1.09	0.95	1.01	1.15	1.42	1.43	1.59	1.59	1.48
Myeloid leukemia	205	2.95	3.21	3.21	3.22	3.22	3.08	3.33	3.49	3.12	3.11

TABLE VII-2. Trends of Crude Incidence Rates per 100,000 Population (Corrected Estimates) in Japan According to Sex and Primary Site (1975–1984), Female

Primary site	ICD, 9th	Year									
		1975	1976	1977	1978	1979	1980	1981	1982	1983	1984
All sites	140–208, 233	175.17	176.01	179.74	185.19	191.67	192.25	198.06	204.55	212.13	219.83
All sites	140–208	170.52	171.70	175.49	181.12	187.76	187.65	193.30	199.20	206.89	213.95
Mouth	140–145	1.27	1.20	1.35	1.57	1.64	2.16	1.63	1.78	1.61	2.00
Pharynx	146–149	0.32	0.34	0.47	0.47	0.45	0.46	0.42	0.73	0.61	0.69
Esophagus	150	2.22	2.25	2.14	2.42	2.43	2.53	2.26	2.31	2.70	2.60
Stomach	151	48.95	48.64	49.58	48.39	50.34	49.10	49.75	50.54	51.79	52.22
Colon	153	8.51	9.18	9.46	11.24	11.20	11.91	12.92	14.87	15.44	16.29
Rectum	154	7.56	8.24	8.81	8.76	8.91	8.09	9.26	9.54	10.17	9.93
Liver	155	6.41	6.15	6.15	6.43	6.84	7.30	7.69	8.16	8.59	9.10
Gallbladder *etc.*	156	5.57	5.83	6.12	6.43	6.81	7.57	8.37	8.91	9.86	10.10
Pancreas	157	4.63	4.46	4.41	4.83	5.40	5.98	6.36	6.54	7.05	7.19
Nose, sinuses	160	1.12	1.27	1.16	0.93	0.72	0.84	0.93	0.97	1.03	0.82
Pharynx	161	0.34	0.37	0.40	0.31	0.27	0.32	0.27	0.38	0.37	0.63
Lung, trachea	162	8.39	9.16	8.96	9.65	10.09	11.30	12.15	12.74	13.73	14.63
Connective tissue	171	0.59	0.56	0.63	0.62	0.63	0.69	0.66	0.77	0.72	0.80
Skin	172, 173	2.04	1.88	3.19	3.82	3.80	3.84	3.99	4.15	3.21	3.29
Other skin	173	1.67	1.55	3.24	4.17	3.58	3.51	3.57	3.84	2.47	2.61
Breast	174–175, 2330	22.18	22.13	23.07	23.38	24.21	23.69	25.54	26.32	27.09	29.37
Uterus	179–182, 2331	31.50	29.74	28.66	28.87	28.44	27.35	26.18	24.96	24.64	26.25
Uterus	179–182	26.63	25.25	24.25	24.70	24.53	23.01	21.73	20.05	19.79	20.74
Cervix uteri	180	18.54	19.96	17.33	19.71	18.87	18.67	16.84	15.05	13.88	14.56
Corpus uteri	182	3.16	2.00	3.06	2.62	3.97	2.93	3.68	3.48	4.05	4.22
Uterus, unspecified	179	3.62	3.25	2.89	2.53	2.32	2.39	2.15	2.06	2.01	1.99
Ovary *etc.*	183	4.44	4.41	4.75	5.50	6.18	5.61	5.91	5.80	6.06	6.73
Bladder	188	2.01	2.08	1.97	2.14	2.03	2.59	2.36	2.69	2.88	2.68
Kidney *etc.*	189	1.11	1.27	1.46	1.94	1.84	1.61	1.91	2.24	2.01	1.93
Brain, nervous system	191–192	1.82	2.17	2.28	2.32	2.05	2.40	2.28	1.75	1.66	1.58
Thyroid	193	3.54	3.48	4.99	4.46	4.01	3.59	3.81	4.18	4.90	4.67
Lymphatic tissue	200–203	3.73	3.98	4.29	4.32	4.55	4.39	4.75	5.07	5.51	5.83
Non-Hodgkin's lymphoma	200, 202	2.38	2.61	2.95	2.82	2.69	2.75	3.23	3.67	3.84	3.84
Multiple myeloma	203	0.87	0.97	0.96	1.10	1.43	1.28	1.22	1.18	1.36	1.73
Leukemia	204–208	4.02	3.58	3.54	3.32	3.92	3.91	4.05	4.06	4.06	4.49
Lymphoid leukemia	204	0.59	0.60	0.61	0.51	0.79	1.14	1.07	1.17	1.02	1.31
Myeloid leukemia	205	2.44	2.22	2.08	1.96	2.32	2.09	2.13	2.07	2.15	2.35

TABLE VIII-1. Trends of Age-Standardized Incidence Rates (World Population) per 100,000 Population (Corrected Estimates) in Japan According to Sex and Primary Site (1975–1984), Male

Primary site	ICD, 9th	Year									
		1975	1976	1977	1978	1979	1980	1981	1982	1983	1984
All sites	140–208, 233	205.61	205.92	210.97	210.86	218.65	216.93	222.37	224.27	229.90	234.52
All sites	140–208	205.61	205.92	210.97	210.86	218.65	216.93	222.37	224.27	229.90	234.52
Mouth	140–145	2.43	2.37	2.32	2.61	2.87	2.44	2.82	2.68	3.17	2.87
Pharynx	146–149	1.11	1.09	1.12	1.02	1.31	1.44	1.68	1.36	1.48	1.53
Esophagus	150	8.34	7.85	8.07	8.47	8.56	8.25	8.11	8.15	8.30	7.93
Stomach	151	86.60	84.30	83.47	80.31	82.44	78.85	78.24	74.29	76.47	76.86
Colon	153	8.26	9.02	10.55	11.09	11.33	10.75	12.20	13.56	14.55	15.49
Rectum	154	9.46	8.96	9.48	9.23	10.68	10.39	11.14	11.85	12.33	12.89
Liver	155	12.47	13.73	13.55	14.50	15.72	16.97	18.19	19.36	20.40	21.88
Gallbladder *etc.*	156	4.17	4.28	4.66	4.62	4.79	5.03	5.15	5.48	5.95	5.96
Pancreas	157	6.28	7.04	6.74	7.12	7.02	7.55	7.14	7.64	7.53	8.08
Nose, sinuses	160	1.89	1.74	1.60	1.55	1.57	1.72	1.61	1.60	1.41	1.16
Larynx	161	2.71	3.69	3.70	3.73	3.92	3.38	3.40	3.29	3.20	3.51
Lung, trachea	162	23.28	23.63	25.53	26.02	27.36	28.05	29.59	30.59	31.08	31.99
Connective tissue	171	0.75	0.78	0.95	0.63	0.70	0.85	0.88	0.87	0.85	0.71
Skin	172, 173	2.58	2.88	2.70	3.03	2.86	2.99	3.42	3.24	2.86	3.35
Other skin	173	2.38	2.56	2.43	3.07	2.57	2.97	3.31	3.65	2.94	2.89
Prostate	185	5.18	4.96	5.81	6.36	6.62	6.10	6.01	6.21	6.57	6.97
Testis	186	0.98	1.22	1.34	1.02	1.03	1.33	1.23	1.39	1.19	1.34
Bladder	188	5.94	5.78	5.69	6.82	7.60	7.89	7.78	7.50	7.72	7.64
Kidney *etc.*	189	3.04	3.23	3.21	3.15	2.80	2.98	2.98	3.23	3.45	4.09
Brain, nervous system	191–192	2.27	1.97	2.90	3.64	3.23	2.78	3.20	2.56	2.50	2.21
Thyroid	193	0.72	0.71	0.95	1.18	1.13	1.23	1.38	1.28	1.27	1.19
Lymphatic tissue	200–203	5.92	6.06	6.64	5.98	6.11	6.16	6.77	6.53	6.91	6.24
Non-Hodgkin's lymphoma	200, 202	4.07	4.13	4.54	4.13	4.27	4.15	4.55	4.59	4.81	4.33
Multiple myeloma	203	0.98	1.17	1.33	1.20	1.22	1.58	1.89	1.52	1.69	1.54
Leukemia	204–208	5.41	5.50	5.09	5.06	5.15	5.60	5.87	6.10	5.41	5.40
Lymphoid leukemia	204	1.19	1.24	1.06	1.16	1.32	1.60	1.54	1.65	1.59	1.47
Myeloid leukemia	205	2.99	3.25	3.20	3.14	3.15	2.98	3.17	3.19	2.81	2.77

TABLE VIII-2. Trends of Age-Standardized Incidence Rates (World Population) per 100,000 Population (Corrected Estimates) in Japan According to Sex and Primary Site (1975–1984), Female

Primary site	ICD, 9th	Year									
		1975	1976	1977	1978	1979	1980	1981	1982	1983	1984
All sites	140–208, 233	152.06	150.05	150.05	151.00	153.27	149.89	151.04	152.00	153.61	155.45
All sites	140–208	148.08	146.36	146.41	147.52	150.00	146.10	147.15	147.65	149.37	150.73
Mouth	140–145	1.10	1.05	1.17	1.30	1.32	1.73	1.24	1.32	1.16	1.49
Pharynx	146–149	0.27	0.29	0.41	0.40	0.36	0.38	0.34	0.60	0.49	0.54
Esophagus	150	1.85	1.80	1.67	1.80	1.83	1.87	1.62	1.57	1.75	1.62
Stomach	151	41.44	40.32	39.99	38.05	38.54	36.49	36.07	35.66	35.64	35.15
Colon	153	7.32	7.68	7.72	8.89	8.70	8.95	9.38	10.47	10.58	10.82
Rectum	154	6.26	6.66	6.97	6.75	6.82	6.09	6.90	6.94	7.08	6.73
Liver	155	5.48	5.10	4.98	5.09	5.33	5.38	5.57	5.73	5.82	5.94
Gallbladder *etc.*	156	4.64	4.72	4.80	4.89	5.04	5.46	5.84	5.95	6.41	6.34
Pancreas	157	3.95	3.75	3.62	3.73	4.03	4.28	4.43	4.43	4.63	4.53
Nose, sinuses	160	0.97	1.08	0.96	0.74	0.57	0.65	0.73	0.74	0.75	0.57
Larynx	161	0.31	0.33	0.32	0.25	0.21	0.25	0.19	0.28	0.26	0.43
Lung, trachea	162	7.18	7.67	7.28	7.74	7.89	8.60	8.95	9.05	9.31	9.50
Connective tissue	171	0.56	0.53	0.61	0.62	0.61	0.60	0.57	0.68	0.63	0.70
Skin	172, 173	1.76	1.61	2.66	3.18	3.04	2.91	2.86	2.91	2.19	2.18
Other skin	173	1.44	1.32	2.67	3.47	2.87	2.64	2.54	2.64	1.63	1.69
Breast	174–175, 2330	19.50	19.24	19.79	19.81	20.27	19.60	20.75	21.01	21.42	22.93
Uterus	179–182, 2331	27.81	26.01	24.64	24.31	23.51	22.25	20.96	19.62	19.12	20.07
Uterus	179–182	23.65	22.17	20.87	20.75	20.23	18.66	17.33	15.62	15.20	15.66
Cervix uteri	180	16.59	17.65	14.95	16.63	15.63	15.32	13.57	11.87	10.78	11.13
Corpus uteri	182	2.86	1.80	2.72	2.25	3.31	2.44	3.00	2.79	3.19	3.26
Uterus, unspecified	179	3.05	2.71	2.37	2.02	1.81	1.70	1.50	1.39	1.33	1.27
Ovary *etc.*	183	4.06	3.99	4.17	4.69	5.20	4.71	4.93	4.72	4.87	5.30
Bladder	188	1.69	1.74	1.60	1.70	1.56	1.91	1.68	1.86	1.92	1.74
Kidney *etc.*	189	0.98	1.13	1.25	1.66	1.54	1.32	1.52	1.73	1.50	1.38
Brain, nervous system	191–192	1.79	2.14	2.27	2.29	1.97	2.29	2.21	1.70	1.55	1.39
Thyroid	193	3.11	3.00	4.22	3.70	3.33	2.98	3.07	3.29	3.86	3.68
Lymphatic tissue	200–203	3.39	3.54	3.73	3.68	3.82	3.46	3.70	3.89	4.17	4.25
Non-Hodgkin's lymphoma	200, 202	2.16	2.36	2.65	2.47	2.33	2.20	2.54	2.86	2.99	2.93
Multiple myeloma	203	0.80	0.84	0.76	0.85	1.10	0.96	0.91	0.86	0.93	1.12
Leukemia	204–208	4.05	3.58	3.55	3.27	3.76	3.73	3.78	3.78	3.60	3.85
Lymphoid leukemia	204	0.68	0.72	0.71	0.59	0.90	1.26	1.14	1.22	1.00	1.23
Myeloid leukemia	205	2.35	2.10	1.96	1.79	2.04	1.84	1.84	1.77	1.77	1.88

TABLE IX-1. Trends of Age-Standardized Incidence Rates (Japanese 1985 Model Population) per 100,000 Population (Corrected-Estimates) in Japan According to Sex and Primary Site (1975–1984), Male

Primary site	ICD, 9th	Year									
		1975	1976	1977	1978	1979	1980	1981	1982	1983	1984
All sites	140–208, 233	285.12	286.27	292.61	292.39	303.47	302.30	310.45	313.76	321.40	328.30
All sites	140–208	285.12	286.27	292.61	292.39	303.47	302.30	310.45	313.76	321.40	328.30
Mouth	140–145	3.31	3.20	3.19	3.61	3.98	3.39	3.84	3.67	4.33	3.98
Pharynx	146–149	1.48	1.45	1.47	1.35	1.73	1.90	2.24	1.86	2.02	2.13
Esophagus	150	11.77	11.25	11.52	12.05	12.13	11.73	11.47	11.58	11.73	11.20
Stomach	151	120.36	117.58	116.30	111.68	114.14	109.50	108.97	103.76	106.93	107.41
Colon	153	11.69	12.63	14.71	15.49	16.04	15.33	17.35	19.23	20.66	22.03
Rectum	154	13.35	12.65	13.27	12.89	14.76	14.50	15.59	16.62	17.28	18.00
Liver	155	17.20	18.76	18.30	19.49	21.19	23.17	24.79	26.42	27.72	29.91
Gallbladder *etc.*	156	6.05	6.34	6.79	6.60	6.91	7.37	7.61	8.08	8.68	8.76
Pancreas	157	8.68	9.72	9.33	9.90	9.84	10.65	10.20	10.85	10.75	11.54
Nose, sinuses	160	2.58	2.44	2.24	2.13	2.13	2.32	2.17	2.13	1.87	1.59
Larynx	161	3.85	5.14	5.12	5.15	5.41	4.70	4.72	4.60	4.47	4.88
Lung, trachea	162	33.37	33.94	36.61	37.51	39.75	40.97	43.32	44.69	45.29	46.61
Connective tissue	171	0.89	0.91	1.14	0.76	0.85	0.99	1.04	1.05	1.05	0.87
Skin	172, 173	3.73	4.22	3.95	4.38	4.20	4.39	5.01	4.69	4.10	4.77
Other skin	173	3.51	3.76	3.58	4.44	3.80	4.36	4.84	5.29	4.21	4.10
Prostate	185	8.20	7.98	9.33	10.02	10.38	9.75	9.60	10.00	10.41	11.10
Testis	186	0.98	1.23	1.41	1.09	1.12	1.43	1.30	1.48	1.29	1.44
Bladder	188	8.61	8.49	8.37	10.00	11.06	11.37	11.21	10.79	11.14	11.01
Kidney *etc.*	189	3.95	4.27	4.35	4.30	3.86	3.97	3.97	4.28	4.65	5.48
Brain, nervous system	191–192	2.44	2.10	3.05	3.87	3.54	3.11	3.63	2.87	2.81	2.47
Thyroid	193	0.98	0.95	1.26	1.55	1.48	1.65	1.85	1.76	1.69	1.56
Lymphatic tissue	200–203	7.73	7.90	8.63	7.86	8.12	8.23	9.04	8.75	9.24	8.40
Non-Hodgkin's lymphoma	200, 202	5.18	5.21	5.70	5.26	5.58	5.43	5.99	6.08	6.37	5.73
Multiple myeloma	203	1.41	1.72	1.94	1.78	1.75	2.32	2.70	2.16	2.39	2.22
Leukemia	204–208	6.04	6.17	5.61	5.66	5.81	6.31	6.68	7.06	6.39	6.35
Lymphoid leukemia	204	1.04	1.09	0.87	0.93	1.13	1.44	1.47	1.66	1.66	1.53
Myeloid leukemia	205	3.52	3.80	3.76	3.85	3.85	3.60	3.88	3.99	3.55	3.45

TABLE IX-2. Trends of Age-Standardized Incidence Rates (Japanese 1985 Model Population) per 100,000 Population (Corrected Estimates) in Japan According to Sex and Primary Site (1975–1984), Female

Primary site	ICD, 9th	Year									
		1975	1976	1977	1978	1979	1980	1981	1982	1983	1984
All sites	140–208, 233	204.10	201.92	201.57	203.22	206.40	202.22	203.66	205.06	207.71	210.26
All sites	140–208	199.13	197.32	197.02	198.84	202.26	197.42	198.76	199.59	202.37	204.33
Mouth	140–145	1.51	1.41	1.58	1.80	1.84	2.34	1.68	1.76	1.56	1.95
Pharynx	146–149	0.36	0.38	0.53	0.51	0.48	0.49	0.44	0.75	0.62	0.69
Esophagus	150	2.73	2.73	2.47	2.67	2.65	2.70	2.35	2.31	2.61	2.42
Stomach	151	56.98	55.69	55.37	52.69	53.62	50.89	50.30	49.66	49.53	48.80
Colon	153	10.20	10.83	10.78	12.45	12.12	12.54	13.24	14.76	14.90	15.24
Rectum	154	8.83	9.42	9.83	9.51	9.50	8.48	9.49	9.54	9.86	9.40
Liver	155	7.81	7.34	7.15	7.29	7.61	7.68	7.91	8.11	8.22	8.42
Gallbladder *etc.*	156	6.65	6.68	6.78	6.90	7.19	7.82	8.46	8.67	9.31	9.21
Pancreas	157	5.48	5.23	5.02	5.31	5.75	6.13	6.34	6.39	6.71	6.63
Nose, sinuses	160	1.34	1.49	1.31	1.03	0.79	0.91	0.99	1.00	1.01	0.77
Larynx	161	0.42	0.47	0.49	0.36	0.30	0.36	0.30	0.40	0.37	0.60
Lung, trachea	162	10.29	10.98	10.37	10.91	11.15	12.13	12.66	12.90	13.46	13.85
Connective tissue	171	0.67	0.61	0.65	0.66	0.66	0.71	0.67	0.78	0.73	0.78
Skin	172, 173	2.48	2.28	3.77	4.38	4.29	4.12	4.12	4.13	3.08	3.07
Other skin	173	2.04	1.89	3.84	4.84	4.08	3.78	3.71	3.80	2.34	2.42
Breast	174–175, 2330	24.96	24.67	25.41	25.48	26.03	25.23	26.72	27.07	27.56	29.51
Uterus	179–182, 2331	36.42	34.06	32.28	31.93	30.96	29.16	27.38	25.65	25.00	26.22
Uterus	179–182	31.20	29.26	27.55	27.46	26.81	24.63	22.80	20.62	20.06	20.69
Cervix uteri	180	21.76	23.18	19.70	21.97	20.65	20.10	17.78	15.57	14.15	14.62
Corpus uteri	182	3.80	2.36	3.49	2.87	4.31	3.19	3.91	3.62	4.13	4.24
Uterus, unspecified	179	4.25	3.79	3.36	2.87	2.58	2.42	2.13	1.99	1.93	1.85
Ovary *etc.*	183	5.03	4.93	5.23	5.95	6.60	5.95	6.21	5.96	6.19	6.69
Bladder	188	2.46	2.57	2.34	2.50	2.27	2.79	2.45	2.69	2.80	2.52
Kidney *etc.*	189	1.32	1.47	1.64	2.13	1.98	1.69	1.96	2.27	1.99	1.85
Brain, nervous system	191–192	1.87	2.21	2.36	2.40	2.13	2.47	2.34	1.77	1.65	1.54
Thyroid	193	4.06	3.92	5.49	4.81	4.26	3.76	3.92	4.23	4.94	4.70
Lymphatic tissue	200–203	4.42	4.58	4.81	4.75	4.94	4.57	4.88	5.10	5.42	5.55
Non-Hodgkin's lymphoma	200, 202	2.79	2.98	3.31	3.09	2.91	2.85	3.29	3.69	3.81	3.71
Multiple myeloma	203	1.05	1.12	1.07	1.23	1.59	1.36	1.27	1.20	1.32	1.58
Leukemia	204–208	4.28	3.83	3.73	3.44	4.02	3.99	4.06	4.03	3.94	4.28
Lymphoid leukemia	204	0.56	0.58	0.60	0.50	0.79	1.12	1.06	1.15	0.98	1.24
Myeloid leukemia	205	2.67	2.42	2.24	2.09	2.41	2.17	2.15	2.07	2.12	2.27

TABLE X. Trends of Proportions (%) of Cases Registered by Death Certificate Only to Incidence, According to Primary Site (1975–1984), Both Sexes

Primary site	ICD, 9th	Year									
		1975	1976	1977	1978	1979	1980	1981	1982	1983	1984
All sites	140–208, 233	17.05	16.50	14.73	13.39	13.03	18.11	15.54	14.77	14.46	14.65
All sites	140–208	17.25	16.69	14.89	13.53	13.17	18.34	15.72	14.94	14.61	14.82
Mouth	140–145	11.06	11.94	9.18	8.35	6.78	7.78	5.96	6.51	7.09	7.36
Pharynx	146–149	11.49	10.52	8.22	7.34	8.60	8.91	6.14	5.70	6.42	5.38
Esophagus	150	20.58	19.36	17.27	15.41	14.06	18.02	15.85	15.61	15.45	15.42
Stomach	151	16.19	15.19	13.59	12.11	12.27	18.10	15.38	14.49	13.47	13.34
Colon	153	14.78	14.85	12.65	11.78	11.85	18.19	15.52	13.36	12.47	12.10
Rectum	154	15.84	14.18	12.61	10.67	10.55	15.91	13.05	11.26	11.19	11.59
Liver	155	36.24	35.84	33.39	30.46	27.90	32.65	28.97	28.45	28.44	27.48
Gallbladder *etc.*	156	26.89	24.82	20.78	17.03	16.51	24.61	22.52	21.55	20.53	21.71
Pancreas	157	23.54	24.89	22.40	23.07	21.05	28.28	24.51	24.26	23.97	23.87
Nose, sinuses	160	13.04	13.44	15.37	13.82	14.30	13.54	10.05	8.79	9.26	9.83
Larynx	161	10.75	6.62	7.42	6.22	6.08	8.58	6.71	5.72	4.83	5.65
Lung, trachea	162	21.59	21.82	20.04	17.90	17.72	23.50	20.49	19.55	19.81	20.21
Connective tissue	171	13.98	11.92	7.68	6.26	4.47	9.74	8.40	9.22	9.67	9.58
Skin	172, 173	8.11	8.19	7.39	7.80	7.76	6.36	4.98	4.80	5.53	5.37
Other skin	173	7.61	7.70	6.48	5.57	6.34	5.48	4.61	3.81	4.76	4.60
Breast	174–175, 2330	6.52	5.63	4.26	3.55	3.58	6.63	5.27	3.87	4.15	4.51
Uterus	179–182, 2331	8.15	8.36	6.01	5.30	4.59	7.43	6.27	6.19	5.36	5.21
Uterus	179–182	9.60	9.75	7.07	6.24	5.37	8.77	7.45	7.59	6.60	6.49
Cervix uteri	180	3.08	3.33	2.29	2.23	2.14	3.21	3.15	2.67	2.20	2.37
Corpus uteri	182	3.63	2.73	2.03	1.75	1.86	3.75	2.63	2.92	2.73	2.53
Uterus, unspecified	179	40.82	42.98	35.79	32.32	32.50	47.30	43.41	47.50	45.14	48.96
Ovary *etc.*	183	14.63	15.50	13.40	11.16	11.08	15.12	13.02	12.06	11.43	13.38
Prostate	185	15.08	13.21	11.73	10.22	10.11	15.24	14.10	14.08	12.31	11.75
Testis	186	5.00	5.07	3.40	5.50	4.95	4.64	5.52	5.46	2.90	0.82
Bladder	188	13.88	13.55	12.64	12.95	11.27	12.04	9.41	9.23	9.46	9.37
Kidney *etc.*	189	15.83	14.50	12.68	10.90	10.46	14.97	13.29	11.98	12.43	12.20
Brain, nervous system	191–192	17.49	14.19	9.87	9.18	10.23	13.02	11.60	13.02	15.05	16.44
Thyroid	193	9.71	7.14	5.34	4.73	4.85	7.05	5.91	5.37	4.57	4.84
Lymphatic tissue	200–203	16.17	15.23	13.87	13.12	13.09	16.51	13.81	13.49	14.25	16.39
Non-Hodgkin's lymphoma	200, 202	14.57	13.58	11.40	11.17	10.00	14.15	10.56	11.10	11.31	14.07
Multiple myeloma	203	24.47	22.12	22.81	19.37	21.97	22.49	23.28	21.90	24.51	24.20
Leukemia	204–208	21.62	22.11	20.38	18.46	15.08	21.09	17.52	18.47	18.51	20.33
Lymphoid leukemia	204	11.63	12.78	11.44	9.78	9.52	12.55	9.57	8.70	9.99	13.26
Myeloid leukemia	205	19.91	19.86	18.24	16.40	13.56	19.12	16.13	17.22	16.67	17.40

TABLE XI. Trends of Ratios of Incidence to Deaths According to Primary Site (1975–1984), Both Sexes

Primary site	ICD, 9th	Year									
		1975	1976	1977	1978	1979	1980	1981	1982	1983	1984
All sites	140–208, 233	1.58	1.56	1.58	1.58	1.60	1.56	1.60	1.62	1.65	1.66
All sites	140–208	1.56	1.54	1.56	1.56	1.58	1.54	1.58	1.61	1.63	1.64
Mouth	140–145	2.12	2.15	2.32	2.58	2.42	2.37	2.42	2.42	2.61	2.65
Pharynx	146–149	1.69	1.54	1.67	1.53	1.68	1.84	2.00	2.00	1.83	1.94
Esophagus	150	1.16	1.12	1.13	1.20	1.21	1.16	1.18	1.19	1.24	1.22
Stomach	151	1.52	1.52	1.56	1.56	1.60	1.56	1.62	1.65	1.71	1.74
Colon	153	1.73	1.73	1.81	1.88	1.89	1.77	1.85	1.98	2.02	2.01
Rectum	154	1.63	1.63	1.70	1.67	1.73	1.64	1.77	1.90	1.94	1.95
Liver	155	1.03	1.02	1.00	1.00	1.03	1.07	1.12	1.14	1.15	1.19
Gallbladder *etc.*	156	1.23	1.18	1.17	1.16	1.16	1.17	1.20	1.21	1.24	1.18
Pancreas	157	1.08	1.11	1.03	1.05	1.05	1.06	1.03	1.04	1.03	1.08
Nose, sinuses	160	1.55	1.71	1.51	1.45	1.42	1.65	1.92	1.89	1.83	1.63
Larynx	161	1.94	2.54	2.77	2.76	2.93	2.69	2.77	2.91	3.03	3.25
Lung, trachea	162	1.20	1.18	1.17	1.16	1.17	1.17	1.19	1.19	1.19	1.18
Connective tissue	171	2.75	2.82	3.03	2.29	1.88	1.84	1.94	2.07	1.96	1.71
Skin	172, 173	3.72	3.67	4.29	5.24	6.45	6.68	7.35	7.62	6.73	6.85
Other skin	173	4.49	4.42	5.53	7.40	9.64	10.42	11.25	12.81	9.88	10.23
Breast	174–175, 2330	3.97	3.89	3.85	3.70	3.76	3.41	3.58	3.76	3.83	3.84
Uterus	179–182, 2331	3.05	3.01	3.03	3.06	3.09	3.04	3.01	2.99	3.00	3.33
Uterus	179–182	2.59	2.57	2.57	2.63	2.67	2.57	2.51	2.41	2.42	2.64
Cervix uteri	180	7.16	7.34	6.41	7.02	6.44	6.57	6.06	5.43	5.08	5.27
Corpus uteri	182	8.16	5.88	7.51	5.90	7.71	5.39	5.98	5.93	6.44	6.44
Uterus, unspecified	179	0.50	0.49	0.47	0.42	0.41	0.42	0.40	0.41	0.42	0.44
Ovary *etc.*	183	1.68	1.48	1.54	1.65	1.78	1.59	1.56	1.51	1.55	1.63
Prostate	185	2.17	2.16	2.34	2.56	2.48	2.25	2.17	2.13	2.20	2.27
Testis	186	2.89	3.71	3.88	2.92	3.62	4.93	4.91	4.83	4.20	5.93
Bladder	188	2.41	2.30	2.26	2.61	2.65	2.73	2.77	2.81	2.89	2.91
Kidney *etc.*	189	2.10	2.27	2.34	2.18	2.00	1.77	1.89	1.91	1.85	1.88
Brain, nervous system	191–192	3.66	3.38	4.05	4.03	3.99	3.48	3.63	2.96	2.70	2.57
Thyroid	193	4.17	4.27	5.03	5.09	4.91	4.22	4.32	4.65	5.02	5.13
Lymphatic tissue	200–203	1.48	1.49	1.54	1.44	1.43	1.32	1.41	1.40	1.44	1.37
Non-Hodgkin's lymphoma	200, 202	1.48	1.45	1.53	1.40	1.36	1.27	1.38	1.42	1.46	1.34
Multiple myeloma	203	1.30	1.45	1.42	1.41	1.53	1.43	1.50	1.30	1.29	1.37
Leukemia	204–208	1.26	1.19	1.12	1.11	1.16	1.21	1.25	1.27	1.20	1.18
Lymphoid leukemia	204	2.13	1.91	1.71	1.68	1.85	2.20	2.18	1.82	1.48	1.48
Myeloid leukemia	205	1.36	1.34	1.30	1.26	1.29	1.25	1.30	1.33	1.31	1.27

TABLE XII. Trends of The Proportions (%) of Cases Verified Histologically to Incidence According to Primary Site (1975–1984), Both Sexes

Primary site	ICD, 9th	Year									
		1975	1976	1977	1978	1979	1980	1981	1982	1983	1984
All sites	140–208,233	60.32	62.29	65.64	67.70	68.75	63.16	66.14	67.64	68.24	68.13
All sites	140–208	59.87	61.89	65.31	67.40	68.48	62.75	65.80	67.32	67.94	67.81
Mouth	140–145	79.48	80.56	83.09	85.07	85.10	82.27	84.73	84.63	82.75	81.21
Pharynx	146–149	81.51	83.06	84.98	84.18	82.46	81.58	86.20	85.87	85.13	85.29
Esophagus	150	48.58	50.91	57.30	64.57	67.63	62.23	65.37	68.92	69.07	71.40
Stomach	151	58.97	62.80	67.44	70.59	72.43	66.94	71.04	73.70	75.94	77.10
Colon	153	61.74	63.50	67.63	69.60	69.96	63.99	67.45	71.34	73.04	73.66
Rectum	154	62.71	64.97	69.16	72.22	72.87	68.40	72.71	76.19	77.15	77.99
Liver	155	25.01	26.20	28.96	31.09	32.13	26.50	27.65	27.43	26.85	25.22
Gallbladder *etc.*	156	47.52	49.66	52.36	53.51	51.44	43.81	46.35	48.74	47.09	45.38
Pancreas	157	39.09	40.55	41.99	40.28	42.80	36.20	38.92	38.79	38.92	37.95
Nose, sinuses	160	77.42	79.91	79.78	80.87	78.15	75.76	80.83	82.79	83.26	81.89
Larynx	161	75.98	81.60	82.30	83.52	85.59	81.47	83.88	83.75	82.07	82.08
Lung, trachea	162	44.54	45.26	48.31	49.69	49.18	46.50	49.99	52.52	52.01	52.36
Connective tissue	171	84.08	86.91	90.48	90.99	93.74	85.84	85.64	85.70	85.21	86.43
Skin	172, 173	85.37	85.25	84.95	83.57	85.05	85.44	86.39	84.17	84.19	85.14
Other skin	173	85.61	85.26	86.47	85.34	86.40	86.79	86.92	84.87	84.84	86.22
Breast	174–175, 2330	83.62	85.48	88.10	88.62	89.06	84.62	87.06	89.10	89.55	89.49
Uterus	179–182,2331	83.09	83.53	85.17	86.26	86.84	83.16	85.60	85.53	86.54	86.57
Uterus	179–182	80.34	81.07	83.13	84.54	85.18	80.63	83.45	83.12	84.20	84.12
Cervix uteri	180	90.61	90.85	91.73	91.92	92.25	88.00	90.22	90.24	91.04	90.33
Corpus uteri	182	92.62	92.39	91.65	92.33	89.37	87.71	89.57	91.80	91.98	91.13
Uterus, unspecified	179	25.31	26.18	30.02	35.11	31.31	27.30	31.70	28.96	29.46	28.31
Ovary *etc.*	183	70.79	72.64	74.05	73.25	73.02	68.72	71.43	71.90	71.63	70.47
Prostate	185	65.17	67.71	72.68	76.18	76.79	69.69	72.27	74.69	75.83	75.74
Testis	186	88.88	92.08	90.11	88.73	89.39	93.76	92.86	89.34	85.83	88.80
Bladder	188	70.44	72.05	74.71	75.16	78.74	76.12	79.06	80.14	80.12	80.45
Kidney *etc.*	189	65.10	65.70	68.20	72.15	74.21	67.02	67.85	69.40	69.10	68.75
Brain, nervous system	191–192	67.71	72.44	76.53	78.56	78.30	73.32	74.84	75.24	73.55	70.82
Thyroid	193	79.50	81.96	85.74	88.26	88.55	79.67	81.51	84.30	86.57	87.84
Lymphatic tissue	200–203	73.11	73.31	76.76	79.38	82.46	75.19	78.40	77.50	77.32	74.86
Non-Hodgkin's lymphoma	200, 202	77.38	79.40	83.62	85.74	88.79	81.62	84.74	83.24	82.64	79.87
Multiple myeloma	203	54.15	49.92	51.87	59.19	62.43	56.38	58.10	56.98	56.90	59.80
Leukemia	204–208	56.67	58.34	61.63	64.26	63.97	53.05	56.42	55.33	57.10	59.40
Lymphoid leukemia	204	58.28	57.47	62.00	69.05	71.18	61.55	63.95	63.17	65.58	66.04
Myeloid leukemia	205	62.42	65.14	69.65	70.26	65.71	54.65	56.57	56.31	58.31	62.18

TABLE XIII-1. Trends of Correction Coefficients Used for Correction of Estimated Incidence in Japan According to Sex and Primary Site (1975–1984), Male

Primary site	ICD, 9th	Year									
		1975	1976	1977	1978	1979	1980	1981	1982	1983	1984
All sites	140–208, 233	0.91	0.92	0.94	0.92	0.93	0.94	0.94	0.92	0.93	0.93
All sites	140–208	0.91	0.92	0.94	0.92	0.93	0.94	0.94	0.92	0.93	0.93
Mouth	140–145	0.88	0.88	0.86	0.93	0.97	0.90	0.99	0.91	1.04	0.96
Pharynx	146–149	0.90	0.80	0.85	0.72	0.82	0.90	1.00	0.81	0.87	0.83
Esophagus	150	0.89	0.86	0.88	0.90	0.92	0.95	0.91	0.89	0.91	0.90
Stomach	151	0.97	0.98	1.00	0.97	0.98	0.96	0.96	0.92	0.95	0.97
Colon	153	0.94	0.98	1.01	1.02	0.99	0.97	0.97	0.96	0.94	0.95
Rectum	154	0.89	0.89	0.97	0.94	1.01	0.97	0.99	0.99	1.03	1.03
Liver	155	0.82	0.83	0.81	0.81	0.83	0.84	0.82	0.82	0.81	0.81
Gallbladder *etc.*	156	0.92	0.95	0.92	0.87	0.92	0.95	0.94	0.90	0.98	0.94
Pancreas	157	0.95	1.00	0.95	0.94	0.90	0.94	0.92	0.97	0.97	0.98
Nose, sinuses	160	1.23	1.01	0.96	0.89	1.00	1.19	1.15	1.16	1.06	0.92
Larynx	161	0.89	1.16	1.13	1.16	1.19	1.07	1.01	0.92	0.89	0.98
Lung, trachea	162	0.83	0.84	0.91	0.90	0.91	0.93	0.95	0.94	0.93	0.95
Connective tissue	171	0.98	0.89	1.05	0.82	0.83	0.94	0.82	0.87	0.76	0.75
Skin	172, 173	0.93	1.00	0.89	0.99	0.95	1.11	1.16	1.07	0.97	1.06
Other skin	173	1.00	1.00	0.92	1.18	1.00	1.27	1.27	1.35	1.11	1.01
Prostate	185	0.87	0.82	0.93	0.95	1.01	0.96	0.95	0.91	0.92	0.91
Testis	186	1.07	1.34	1.33	1.09	1.00	1.40	1.18	1.19	1.01	1.04
Bladder	188	0.88	0.92	0.86	0.91	0.95	1.03	1.02	0.94	0.98	0.92
Kidney *etc.*	189	1.02	0.96	0.93	0.98	0.91	0.95	0.88	0.93	0.94	0.98
Brain, nervous system	191–192	1.12	0.94	1.23	1.40	1.35	1.30	1.45	1.11	1.03	0.89
Thyroid	193	0.66	0.61	0.66	0.86	0.92	1.24	1.32	1.19	1.17	0.95
Lymphatic tissue	200–203	0.80	0.79	0.88	0.84	0.86	0.87	0.90	0.91	0.98	0.96
Non-Hodgkin's lymphoma	200, 202	0.71	0.71	0.81	0.80	0.83	0.79	0.81	0.86	0.92	0.96
Multiple myeloma	203	1.06	1.15	1.08	0.91	0.84	1.12	1.25	1.03	1.18	1.02
Leukemia	204–208	0.92	0.96	0.91	0.89	0.88	0.92	0.96	0.99	0.90	0.87
Lymphoid leukemia	204	0.92	0.97	0.86	0.83	0.90	0.93	0.85	0.79	0.74	0.59
Myeloid leukemia	205	0.85	0.94	0.96	0.98	0.94	0.93	1.02	1.17	1.04	1.04

TABLE XIII-2. Trends of Correction Coefficients Used for Correction of Estimated Incidence in Japan According to Sex and Primary Site (1975–1984), Female

Primary site	ICD, 9th	Year									
		1975	1976	1977	1978	1979	1980	1981	1982	1983	1984
All sites	140–208, 233	0.95	0.95	0.96	0.96	0.96	0.95	0.96	0.95	0.96	0.96
All sites	140–208	0.95	0.95	0.96	0.96	0.96	0.95	0.96	0.95	0.96	0.96
Mouth	140–145	0.91	0.85	0.92	0.96	0.91	1.26	0.85	0.88	0.75	0.99
Pharynx	146–149	0.81	0.84	1.01	0.99	0.91	0.91	0.79	1.13	0.94	0.97
Esophagus	150	0.84	0.91	0.93	1.00	0.96	0.99	0.92	0.95	1.08	1.01
Stomach	151	0.98	0.97	1.00	0.97	0.99	0.98	0.98	0.98	0.98	0.99
Colon	153	0.98	1.02	0.98	1.05	0.99	1.02	1.01	1.01	0.96	0.96
Rectum	154	1.00	1.00	1.05	0.97	0.95	0.87	0.96	0.94	0.96	0.91
Liver	155	0.97	0.97	0.96	0.93	0.96	0.88	0.89	0.84	0.84	0.85
Gallbladder *etc.*	156	0.92	0.87	0.89	0.91	0.96	0.96	0.99	1.01	1.01	0.98
Pancreas	157	0.91	0.88	0.86	0.87	0.92	0.98	0.99	0.93	0.98	0.96
Nose, sinuses	160	0.96	1.16	1.07	0.97	0.80	0.88	0.91	0.93	1.02	0.93
Larynx	161	1.00	1.32	1.48	0.96	0.81	1.01	0.81	0.92	1.01	1.71
Lung, trachea	162	0.88	0.88	0.83	0.86	0.85	0.92	0.90	0.91	0.92	0.97
Connective tissue	171	0.86	0.87	0.94	0.81	0.78	0.82	0.85	0.98	1.03	1.03
Skin	172, 173	1.01	0.93	1.45	1.60	1.40	1.48	1.34	1.18	0.88	0.88
Other skin	173	0.96	0.89	1.67	2.02	1.49	1.57	1.37	1.23	0.77	0.78
Breast	174–175, 2330	1.08	1.02	1.05	1.00	0.99	0.97	1.02	1.01	1.00	1.02
Uterus	179–182, 2331	1.02	1.01	1.01	1.01	1.00	0.95	0.94	0.94	0.96	1.00
Uterus	179–182	1.02	1.01	1.01	1.01	1.00	0.95	0.94	0.94	0.96	1.00
Cervix uteri	180	0.95	1.07	0.96	1.06	1.02	1.04	1.00	0.98	0.94	0.98
Corpus uteri	182	1.26	0.80	1.20	0.94	1.20	0.86	1.02	0.97	1.12	1.10
Uterus, unspecified	179	1.03	1.00	1.02	0.99	0.98	0.91	0.91	0.91	0.96	1.00
Ovary *etc.*	183	0.89	0.95	0.97	1.01	1.04	0.91	0.93	0.89	0.93	0.97
Bladder	188	1.01	1.04	0.88	0.86	0.76	0.95	0.91	0.97	0.98	0.83
Kidney *etc.*	189	0.89	0.96	0.96	1.17	1.04	0.94	1.00	1.05	0.93	0.80
Brain, nervous system	191–192	1.13	1.18	1.11	1.07	0.89	1.23	1.04	0.82	0.71	0.63
Thyroid	193	0.83	0.79	1.06	0.91	0.85	0.86	0.91	0.91	1.02	0.92
Lymphatic tissue	200–203	0.75	0.79	0.88	0.85	0.84	0.81	0.86	0.91	1.00	1.03
Non-Hodgkin's lymphoma	200, 202	0.70	0.78	0.89	0.84	0.78	0.77	0.84	0.92	0.98	1.02
Multiple myeloma	203	0.76	0.71	0.76	0.82	0.95	0.84	0.84	0.86	0.99	1.03
Leukemia	204–208	0.93	0.84	0.84	0.88	0.98	0.98	0.93	0.93	0.92	0.96
Lymphoid leukemia	204	0.85	0.81	0.67	0.57	0.76	0.92	0.71	0.72	0.66	0.73
Myeloid leukemia	205	0.88	0.82	0.84	0.95	1.08	1.04	1.04	1.04	1.05	1.11

TABLE XIV-1. Age-Specific Incidence Rates per 100,000 Population (Uncorrected Estimates[a]) in Japan According to Sex and Primary Site (1975), Male

Primary site	ICD, 9th	Age group 0–	5–	10–	15–	20–	25–	30–	35–	40–	45–	50–	55–	60–	65–	70–	75–	80–	85–	All ages
All sites	140–208, 233	17.9	9.6	9.2	12.6	12.2	22.0	36.2	64.7	114.6	229.6	362.2	575.2	893.5	1287.8	1783.5	2063.9	2173.5	1777.4	218.7
All sites	140–208	17.9	9.6	9.2	12.6	12.2	22.0	36.2	64.7	114.6	229.6	362.2	575.2	893.5	1287.8	1783.5	2063.9	2173.5	1777.4	218.7
Mouth	140–145	0.2	0.0	0.0	0.1	0.2	0.2	1.7	1.0	3.2	3.4	5.8	8.0	10.8	13.0	14.1	21.2	16.2	28.6	2.6
Pharynx	146–149	0.0	0.0	0.3	0.1	0.0	0.1	0.2	0.5	0.6	1.2	1.8	5.1	7.4	5.2	9.0	5.6	10.9	1.3	1.2
Esophagus	150	0.0	0.0	0.0	0.0	0.1	0.0	0.0	0.8	1.1	6.2	12.6	24.0	43.1	66.4	84.4	93.5	93.3	101.7	8.9
Stomach	151	0.0	0.0	0.0	0.3	2.9	4.9	11.3	26.7	51.6	107.2	162.7	246.0	366.7	540.0	706.0	767.8	756.0	566.7	88.9
Colon	153	0.0	0.1	0.0	0.2	0.3	1.2	2.3	3.4	6.6	9.3	14.9	15.4	37.1	43.5	73.4	96.0	95.2	59.0	8.6
Rectum	154	0.0	0.0	0.0	0.2	0.2	0.9	2.4	3.7	5.4	12.3	17.1	26.8	41.0	61.8	82.6	108.5	105.0	73.8	10.4
Liver	155	0.8	0.1	0.2	0.1	0.1	0.6	2.6	2.8	10.8	22.5	32.6	52.1	59.9	75.7	108.0	124.9	119.8	81.8	14.6
Gallbladder *etc.*	156	0.0	0.0	0.0	0.0	0.0	0.0	0.2	0.7	0.7	2.7	7.8	10.2	19.1	29.3	41.9	41.4	79.9	38.9	4.4
Pancreas	157	0.0	0.0	0.0	0.0	0.1	0.1	0.2	2.0	2.8	6.5	8.9	18.7	28.3	46.2	51.7	66.2	30.7	67.3	6.4
Nose, Sinuses	160	0.0	0.0	0.0	0.1	0.0	0.0	0.2	0.6	1.5	1.4	3.4	5.9	5.9	9.6	8.3	9.3	13.3	7.2	1.5
Larynx	161	0.0	0.0	0.0	0.0	0.0	0.0	0.1	0.0	0.5	1.0	4.2	9.5	16.6	18.1	27.9	22.2	45.8	26.7	2.7
Lung, trachea	162	0.0	0.0	0.0	0.4	0.3	0.6	0.9	3.1	7.1	20.4	30.8	55.2	113.5	191.5	292.2	323.4	298.9	265.2	26.3
Connective tissue	171	0.3	0.4	0.1	0.3	0.5	0.3	0.6	0.9	0.5	1.2	2.2	1.2	2.0	2.5	3.6	2.3	0.0	0.0	0.8
Skin	172, 173	0.0	0.3	0.1	0.1	0.2	0.7	0.3	1.2	1.3	2.1	2.9	7.5	8.9	14.1	17.7	41.6	36.0	37.4	2.6
Other skin	173	0.0	0.3	0.0	0.1	0.2	0.7	0.3	1.0	1.3	1.7	2.8	6.0	5.4	12.6	15.7	38.8	35.5	32.1	2.2
Prostate	185	0.0	0.0	0.0	0.1	0.0	0.0	0.2	0.1	0.0	0.6	0.9	4.4	16.5	28.2	65.1	109.8	160.7	185.0	5.3
Testis	186	1.9	0.0	0.0	1.1	0.9	1.5	1.4	1.8	1.0	0.9	1.0	0.1	0.1	0.1	0.4	0.0	5.1	0.0	1.0
Bladder	188	0.0	0.0	0.0	0.0	0.0	0.6	0.4	0.2	2.3	4.0	8.4	14.4	33.7	28.6	63.4	64.6	119.5	115.3	6.1
Kidney *etc.*	189	2.0	0.4	0.1	0.0	0.3	0.2	0.4	0.6	0.9	2.5	4.4	13.4	12.2	17.1	17.6	20.0	19.6	1.3	2.8
Brain, nervous system	191–192	2.1	1.6	1.6	1.6	1.0	0.8	1.8	2.3	1.7	2.0	3.4	3.9	2.5	5.8	3.2	4.2	2.7	1.3	2.0
Thyroid	193	0.0	0.0	0.0	0.3	0.2	0.3	0.3	0.4	1.7	2.1	1.3	2.3	2.5	5.7	9.6	9.6	7.9	1.3	1.1
Lymphatic tissue	200–203	0.5	0.9	1.7	1.9	1.6	2.6	3.2	4.2	5.6	7.5	12.6	23.5	28.9	38.8	35.3	36.5	56.2	20.1	7.2
Non-Hodgkin's lymphoma	200, 202	0.5	0.8	1.7	1.9	1.5	2.3	3.1	3.8	4.8	6.1	11.0	16.1	19.5	29.3	25.9	21.8	34.2	18.8	5.6
Multiple myeloma	203	0.0	0.0	0.0	0.0	0.0	0.0	0.0	0.1	0.4	1.3	1.1	5.0	3.6	5.4	4.2	9.9	13.5	0.0	0.9
Leukemia	204–208	6.7	4.8	2.9	3.0	1.4	3.8	4.1	5.0	3.0	5.6	9.9	11.3	11.6	11.6	17.1	19.2	31.0	28.6	5.6
Lymphoid leukemia	204	3.8	2.3	1.8	0.5	0.1	0.1	0.8	0.4	0.0	0.6	0.1	1.2	1.2	2.2	0.4	4.2	3.4	9.1	1.1
Myeloid leukemia	205	2.1	1.9	0.8	1.8	0.9	3.3	2.3	3.7	2.3	4.0	8.2	7.4	8.7	7.9	11.9	10.1	16.2	11.8	3.5

[a] See text.

TABLE XIV-2. Age-Specific Incidence Rates per 100,000 Population (Uncorrected Estimates[a]) in Japan According to Sex and Primary Site (1975), Female

Primary site	ICD, 9th	Age group																		All ages
		0–	5–	10–	15–	20–	25–	30–	35–	40–	45–	50–	55–	60–	65–	70–	75–	80–	85–	
All sites	140–208, 233	12.5	8.7	8.7	8.1	15.5	33.5	61.1	109.8	191.5	258.1	325.8	407.0	546.4	715.1	900.6	1107.2	1042.0	912.1	184.0
All sites	140–208	12.5	8.7	8.7	8.1	15.2	32.1	56.6	95.3	175.1	242.9	317.0	402.7	539.7	713.2	896.8	1106.9	1042.0	912.1	179.2
Mouth	140–145	0.0	0.0	0.0	0.0	0.5	0.1	0.6	1.0	0.8	1.0	1.8	3.7	6.6	4.5	8.5	8.3	10.4	4.9	1.4
Pharynx	146–149	0.0	0.0	0.0	0.0	0.0	0.0	0.0	0.1	0.4	1.4	1.0	0.7	1.2	0.5	1.3	3.7	0.5	0.6	0.4
Esophagus	150	0.0	0.0	0.0	0.0	0.0	0.0	0.0	0.1	0.5	0.6	3.6	4.1	9.5	11.6	17.8	36.3	27.2	41.0	2.7
Stomach	151	0.0	0.0	0.0	0.4	2.9	8.3	17.2	23.6	43.8	51.5	76.3	104.0	165.8	215.9	278.7	345.6	330.5	324.2	50.2
Colon	153	0.0	0.0	0.0	0.2	0.2	0.8	1.3	3.2	4.6	11.1	13.5	20.3	25.2	41.0	55.9	65.7	67.2	71.7	8.7
Rectum	154	0.0	0.0	0.0	0.0	0.2	1.0	2.0	3.8	4.6	5.6	13.7	19.8	22.2	27.5	46.1	58.4	68.6	39.8	7.6
Liver	155	0.7	0.0	0.3	0.0	0.2	0.4	1.1	1.1	2.2	5.2	7.0	15.2	17.9	32.4	48.5	63.7	68.3	65.3	6.6
Gallbladder *etc.*	156	0.0	0.4	0.0	0.0	0.0	0.0	0.5	0.7	1.7	4.9	7.9	11.3	17.3	32.6	50.4	57.2	56.4	28.5	6.0
Pancreas	157	0.0	0.0	0.0	0.1	0.0	0.2	0.3	1.3	2.8	4.6	6.2	12.5	20.1	27.4	27.8	45.0	28.4	35.9	5.1
Nose, sinuses	160	0.0	0.0	0.0	0.0	0.0	0.1	0.1	0.6	0.4	0.8	1.8	3.9	4.4	5.6	8.2	8.2	6.3	5.2	1.2
Larynx	161	0.0	0.0	0.0	0.0	0.0	0.0	0.0	0.0	0.0	0.1	0.6	0.4	1.9	3.2	2.5	1.9	2.0	1.7	0.3
Lung, trachea	162	0.2	0.0	0.0	0.0	0.1	0.2	0.9	2.8	4.6	6.5	12.8	21.8	30.2	50.2	69.1	90.5	97.6	55.2	9.6
Connective tissue	171	0.7	0.1	0.1	0.1	0.0	0.1	0.2	0.5	0.9	2.3	1.4	0.9	1.4	0.7	0.5	3.5	1.7	11.7	0.7
Skin	172, 173	0.4	0.0	0.1	0.2	0.2	0.3	0.1	0.9	0.5	0.5	2.4	3.0	5.9	8.5	15.9	19.5	21.1	33.0	2.0
Other skin	173	0.4	0.0	0.0	0.2	0.2	0.1	0.1	0.9	0.5	0.5	1.6	1.9	5.0	7.8	14.1	17.6	18.6	32.5	1.7
Breast	174–175, 2330	0.0	0.0	0.0	0.0	1.1	6.1	11.8	20.1	39.0	58.7	50.4	41.8	53.5	56.1	42.1	35.8	45.6	38.5	20.5
Uterus	179–182, 2331	0.0	0.0	0.0	0.2	1.6	5.8	11.3	34.0	57.3	64.6	73.8	84.2	86.7	85.6	97.3	113.1	67.0	27.7	30.9
Uterus	179–182	0.0	0.0	0.0	0.2	1.3	4.4	6.8	19.8	41.2	49.4	65.6	79.9	80.5	84.2	93.6	112.8	67.0	27.7	26.1
Cervix uteri	180	0.0	0.0	0.0	0.0	0.6	2.2	5.0	17.2	34.3	38.8	48.3	56.7	62.6	65.1	64.7	81.2	30.4	9.4	19.4
Corpus uteri	182	0.0	0.0	0.0	0.0	0.0	0.1	0.5	0.6	2.8	3.1	9.2	15.4	8.6	5.6	7.2	6.0	11.0	0.0	2.5
Uterus, unspecified	179	0.0	0.0	0.0	0.1	0.0	0.3	0.4	1.1	2.4	5.3	7.2	7.7	9.3	13.5	21.6	25.5	25.7	18.2	3.5
Ovary *etc.*	183	0.8	0.1	1.1	1.2	2.2	1.5	2.0	3.4	6.7	10.9	13.0	12.1	15.2	11.2	11.7	12.4	10.3	12.6	5.0
Bladder	188	0.0	0.0	0.0	0.0	0.0	0.0	0.0	0.2	0.4	0.4	2.3	4.3	5.1	11.8	16.5	24.2	16.0	23.7	2.0
Kidney *etc.*	189	0.5	0.0	0.0	0.0	0.3	0.1	0.2	0.1	0.0	1.0	1.9	3.0	6.0	5.1	7.2	8.9	10.5	10.1	1.3
Brain, nervous system	191–192	2.1	1.5	0.9	0.8	0.4	0.7	2.0	0.8	2.5	1.5	3.4	2.6	2.4	3.8	1.0	1.9	0.0	0.0	1.6
Thyroid	193	0.0	0.0	0.4	0.0	1.7	4.0	3.1	2.9	4.6	6.0	7.6	9.2	10.5	13.4	14.9	22.5	22.0	15.4	4.3
Lymphatic tissue	200–203	0.4	0.5	0.7	0.6	1.0	1.2	0.9	2.7	2.2	7.1	7.2	8.9	14.5	30.6	31.4	27.7	18.4	21.7	5.0
Non-Hodgkin's lymphoma	200, 202	0.4	0.5	0.7	0.6	0.7	1.1	0.9	2.5	1.6	5.8	5.2	6.4	9.0	17.4	16.2	20.5	12.0	16.9	3.4
Multiple myeloma	203	0.0	0.0	0.0	0.0	0.0	0.0	0.0	0.2	0.2	1.3	1.8	1.4	5.0	9.4	11.8	4.3	4.1	4.3	1.2
Leukemia	204–208	5.4	5.2	3.0	3.1	1.4	1.9	2.8	2.8	3.8	3.8	5.6	6.2	5.8	11.3	14.9	10.7	11.7	5.2	4.3
Lymphoid leukemia	204	1.8	2.6	1.2	0.1	0.0	0.2	0.2	0.5	0.0	0.4	0.8	0.4	0.3	0.2	1.7	1.4	0.0	0.0	0.7
Myeloid leukemia	205	1.5	1.9	1.5	2.7	1.2	1.2	2.1	1.7	3.3	3.0	3.5	4.4	4.4	8.8	11.3	6.9	7.0	3.7	2.8

[a] See text.

TABLE XV-1. Age-Specific Incidence Rates per 100,000 Population (Uncorrected Estimates[a]) in Japan According to Sex and Primary Site (1976), Male

Primary site	ICD, 9th	Age group																		All ages
		0–	5–	10–	15–	20–	25–	30–	35–	40–	45–	50–	55–	60–	65–	70–	75–	80–	85–	
All sites	140–208, 233	17.6	9.6	8.1	13.3	10.9	23.4	35.1	62.8	112.6	230.3	350.7	560.9	883.9	1301.5	1762.5	2102.7	2246.7	1737.8	221.5
All sites	140–208	17.6	9.6	8.1	13.3	10.9	23.4	35.1	62.8	112.6	230.3	350.7	560.9	883.9	1301.5	1762.5	2102.7	2246.7	1737.8	221.5
Mouth	140–145	0.2	0.0	0.0	0.1	0.2	0.2	1.2	1.3	2.6	3.3	5.5	8.1	10.8	15.9	15.2	17.9	17.4	9.1	2.6
Pharynx	146–149	0.0	0.0	0.3	0.1	0.0	0.4	0.1	0.2	0.6	1.4	3.2	5.4	7.8	4.7	9.5	5.9	10.4	6.1	1.3
Esophagus	150	0.0	0.0	0.0	0.0	0.1	0.0	0.1	0.4	0.9	5.3	12.4	22.7	40.3	63.4	81.5	107.3	100.5	99.1	9.0
Stomach	151	0.2	0.0	0.1	0.4	1.9	5.8	13.2	25.7	48.7	102.4	149.6	231.0	347.9	519.8	677.9	760.6	771.1	525.0	86.6
Colon	153	0.0	0.1	0.0	0.2	0.7	1.1	2.0	3.4	7.0	9.6	14.4	20.9	40.2	42.3	75.9	83.8	93.3	91.7	9.0
Rectum	154	0.0	0.0	0.0	0.2	0.1	0.8	1.9	3.0	4.8	12.2	17.3	29.8	36.8	52.5	81.3	100.2	99.9	78.8	10.0
Liver	155	1.1	0.1	0.2	0.0	0.2	0.2	3.0	2.5	13.5	25.6	33.7	57.0	66.4	87.4	120.1	116.3	118.0	63.1	16.2
Gallbladder *etc.*	156	0.0	0.0	0.0	0.0	0.0	0.1	0.2	1.2	0.6	2.1	8.5	10.0	16.3	23.7	43.1	58.1	79.1	42.5	4.5
Pancreas	157	0.0	0.0	0.0	0.1	0.1	0.2	0.1	2.6	2.9	6.6	8.4	20.7	27.8	57.9	53.5	60.3	43.5	58.3	6.9
Nose, sinuses	160	0.0	0.0	0.0	0.1	0.0	0.1	0.2	0.5	1.4	2.5	4.5	4.7	5.6	10.7	9.7	11.6	26.1	6.7	1.8
Larynx	161	0.0	0.0	0.0	0.0	0.0	0.0	0.1	0.2	0.5	1.8	4.6	9.3	16.2	21.4	29.6	24.2	31.7	28.7	2.9
Lung, trachea	162	0.0	0.0	0.0	0.6	0.2	0.7	1.0	2.9	7.4	18.5	30.5	57.6	119.0	199.9	274.1	323.7	339.1	267.8	27.1
Connective tissue	171	0.5	0.5	0.2	0.3	0.4	0.3	0.5	1.0	0.5	1.3	1.8	1.6	2.7	2.7	4.6	2.0	0.0	1.2	0.9
Skin	172,173	0.0	0.0	0.1	0.1	0.1	0.9	0.3	1.0	1.1	3.3	1.7	6.6	9.2	11.1	19.0	44.3	39.7	72.6	2.7
Other skin	173	0.0	0.0	0.0	0.1	0.1	0.9	0.1	1.0	0.8	3.1	1.5	5.2	7.4	10.4	17.8	39.3	38.0	67.8	2.4
Prostate	185	0.0	0.0	0.0	0.1	0.0	0.4	0.2	0.0	0.1	0.5	1.7	2.7	18.1	27.9	61.8	132.5	173.4	159.2	5.8
Testis	186	1.5	0.0	0.0	1.1	0.6	2.1	1.3	1.3	1.2	0.9	1.0	0.7	0.8	0.1	0.4	0.2	1.6	0.0	1.0
Bladder	188	0.0	0.0	0.0	0.2	0.2	0.9	0.6	0.7	2.0	3.6	7.5	11.4	25.1	31.4	59.8	75.9	111.8	100.5	6.0
Kidney *etc.*	189	1.6	0.2	0.1	0.1	0.0	0.4	0.6	0.6	1.2	3.0	5.4	11.2	14.6	19.9	19.9	27.5	19.9	20.1	3.2
Brain, nervous system	191–192	2.9	1.7	0.9	1.0	0.9	0.5	1.0	2.8	0.9	2.5	3.9	4.1	4.6	6.6	3.5	3.7	2.6	1.2	2.0
Thyroid	193	0.0	0.0	0.0	0.3	0.1	0.4	0.3	1.0	2.4	2.0	2.2	2.5	2.8	5.4	6.2	10.1	3.0	7.9	1.2
Lymphatic tissue	200–203	0.7	1.1	1.5	1.9	1.6	2.0	2.0	3.4	5.3	8.7	13.1	19.8	33.1	40.8	42.2	46.6	43.5	35.0	7.5
Non-Hodgkin's lymphoma	200, 202	0.7	1.1	1.4	1.4	1.6	1.9	1.9	2.9	4.5	7.1	11.5	14.4	24.0	32.1	29.1	16.4	26.5	35.0	5.7
Multiple myeloma	203	0.0	0.0	0.0	0.0	0.0	0.0	0.0	0.2	0.6	1.4	1.3	2.7	4.5	4.6	8.0	19.6	8.6	0.0	1.0
Leukemia	204–208	6.1	4.9	2.6	3.6	1.8	3.3	3.6	4.3	3.3	6.6	8.4	8.9	11.9	13.7	17.6	20.8	33.0	19.6	5.6
Lymphoid leukemia	204	3.4	2.4	1.3	0.7	0.5	0.3	0.5	0.9	0.1	0.2	0.1	1.0	1.4	2.0	1.0	3.1	3.3	8.6	1.1
Myeloid leukemia	205	1.8	2.0	0.9	2.4	0.9	2.6	2.2	3.1	2.5	5.0	7.5	5.9	8.2	9.7	12.5	10.7	12.0	11.0	3.4

[a] See text.

TABLE XV-2. Age-Specific Incidence Rates per 100,000 Population (Uncorrected Estimates[a]) in Japan According to Sex and Primary Site (1976), Female

Primary site	ICD, 9th	Age group 0–	5–	10–	15–	20–	25–	30–	35–	40–	45–	50–	55–	60–	65–	70–	75–	80–	85–	All ages
All sites	140–208, 233	12.9	7.4	9.2	7.6	13.6	35.8	56.8	107.6	186.6	249.4	334.9	404.9	526.5	705.4	888.3	1099.0	1110.0	977.5	185.5
All sites	140–208	12.9	7.4	9.2	7.6	13.1	34.3	53.1	96.4	172.0	234.9	324.7	400.5	519.6	703.9	884.9	1098.9	1108.0	977.5	180.9
Mouth	140–145	0.0	0.0	0.0	0.0	0.5	0.1	0.4	1.4	0.8	1.0	2.3	4.5	5.2	4.9	6.4	4.8	11.5	18.6	1.4
Pharynx	146–149	0.2	0.0	0.0	0.0	0.0	0.0	0.1	0.0	0.2	1.4	0.6	1.1	0.9	1.0	1.6	3.9	1.2	0.5	0.4
Esophagus	150	0.0	0.0	0.0	0.0	0.0	0.0	0.2	0.1	0.5	0.5	2.5	2.6	7.8	10.0	16.7	36.8	33.0	41.5	2.5
Stomach	151	0.0	0.0	0.0	0.5	1.9	8.6	15.0	25.9	44.5	51.9	73.6	99.3	148.4	211.0	277.6	345.4	342.5	333.8	50.0
Colon	153	0.0	0.0	0.0	0.3	0.3	0.9	1.3	3.1	3.9	8.7	15.3	23.6	26.9	37.1	47.6	72.8	84.7	81.4	9.0
Rectum	154	0.0	0.0	0.0	0.0	0.1	1.1	2.1	2.8	4.7	6.8	13.0	21.5	20.8	33.1	48.0	63.2	73.8	50.9	8.2
Liver	155	0.7	0.0	0.0	0.0	0.2	0.5	0.8	1.5	1.2	4.5	7.6	16.1	17.0	28.9	42.6	60.6	71.3	56.3	6.4
Gallbladder *etc.*	156	0.0	0.4	0.0	0.0	0.0	0.3	0.5	1.0	2.1	5.9	9.7	10.7	18.0	38.1	49.9	51.9	61.5	35.0	6.7
Pancreas	157	0.0	0.0	0.0	0.0	0.0	0.3	0.3	1.2	1.6	4.8	5.3	11.4	18.3	32.4	29.0	46.9	32.4	28.4	5.1
Nose, sinuses	160	0.0	0.0	0.0	0.0	0.0	0.3	0.1	0.2	0.4	0.6	1.4	4.2	4.4	4.3	8.9	6.7	6.9	4.4	1.1
Larynx	161	0.0	0.0	0.0	0.0	0.0	0.0	0.0	0.0	0.0	0.0	0.3	0.3	1.7	2.3	1.6	1.6	6.3	0.5	0.3
Lung, trachea	162	0.0	0.0	0.0	0.0	0.0	0.1	0.9	2.3	4.8	6.2	15.1	21.3	30.8	52.0	81.2	95.1	95.2	77.1	10.4
Connective tissue	171	0.6	0.1	0.0	0.1	0.5	0.1	0.2	0.2	0.4	1.5	1.5	1.4	2.0	1.1	1.0	0.1	1.9	10.4	0.6
Skin	172,173	0.0	0.0	0.4	0.6	0.2	0.3	0.2	0.5	0.8	1.1	3.6	1.4	5.0	6.9	15.1	20.3	21.7	37.5	2.0
Other skin	173	0.0	0.0	0.0	0.5	0.2	0.1	0.1	0.4	0.7	0.9	3.1	0.9	4.4	6.3	13.5	18.8	20.7	35.1	1.8
Breast	174–175, 2330	0.0	0.0	0.0	0.2	1.2	6.3	11.8	22.5	43.4	58.2	56.9	47.0	53.8	51.0	45.2	40.7	42.3	36.8	21.7
Uterus	179–182, 2331	0.0	0.0	0.0	0.1	1.1	6.0	11.0	28.6	50.2	58.5	77.0	78.9	83.0	86.3	90.2	92.6	87.0	35.5	29.4
Uterus	179–182	0.0	0.0	0.0	0.1	0.6	4.5	7.3	17.6	35.8	44.3	67.3	74.5	76.1	84.8	87.6	92.5	85.1	35.5	25.0
Cervix uteri	180	0.0	0.0	0.0	0.0	0.0	2.1	5.1	15.4	29.9	35.0	49.8	53.2	59.7	66.0	61.9	65.6	46.5	8.9	18.6
Corpus uteri	182	0.0	0.0	0.0	0.0	0.0	0.4	0.5	0.5	2.5	2.9	10.4	14.3	8.8	5.4	6.5	4.0	9.7	0.0	2.5
Uterus, unspecified	179	0.0	0.0	0.0	0.1	0.0	0.3	0.3	1.2	2.3	4.2	6.7	6.7	7.7	13.4	19.2	22.9	28.9	26.5	3.3
Ovary *etc.*	183	0.9	0.1	0.5	1.0	1.4	1.9	1.6	2.8	5.7	10.3	10.0	13.3	16.7	8.5	16.6	12.1	2.9	4.9	4.6
Bladder	188	0.0	0.0	0.0	0.0	0.2	0.0	0.0	0.3	0.6	0.5	1.8	4.0	5.1	11.6	11.9	26.4	20.6	34.6	2.0
Kidney *etc.*	189	0.8	0.4	0.0	0.0	0.4	0.3	0.3	0.6	0.6	1.2	1.8	2.8	3.8	4.4	8.0	8.6	10.3	10.7	1.3
Brain, nervous system	191–192	2.9	1.5	1.3	0.7	0.5	0.8	1.9	1.2	3.0	1.6	3.6	4.1	1.8	4.6	0.7	1.3	0.0	0.5	1.8
Thyroid	193	0.0	0.0	0.5	0.1	1.4	3.6	3.0	3.4	6.0	5.8	7.7	9.2	12.4	11.5	13.7	24.1	21.0	4.1	4.4
Lymphatic tissue	200–203	0.2	0.7	0.7	1.1	1.2	1.9	1.1	1.8	2.5	6.6	7.3	9.2	18.6	25.9	26.6	29.2	16.6	23.5	5.1
Non-Hodgkin's lymphoma	200, 202	0.2	0.6	0.7	1.1	0.9	1.9	1.1	1.6	1.4	5.3	3.8	7.2	11.9	14.3	14.2	19.1	9.8	18.9	3.3
Multiple myeloma	203	0.0	0.0	0.0	0.0	0.0	0.0	0.0	0.2	0.2	1.3	3.3	1.9	6.4	9.3	9.0	7.5	4.6	4.1	1.4
Leukemia	204–208	5.8	3.7	3.8	2.1	1.2	2.1	2.6	2.5	2.9	4.1	6.3	5.2	6.6	12.7	15.0	13.5	11.7	4.9	4.3
Lymphoid leukemia	204	2.5	2.2	1.6	0.2	0.1	0.3	0.2	0.1	0.0	0.2	0.8	0.3	0.5	0.9	1.6	1.5	0.0	0.0	0.7
Myeloid leukemia	205	1.7	1.0	1.9	1.7	1.0	1.4	2.1	1.6	2.4	3.5	3.9	4.0	4.9	9.4	10.8	8.5	5.6	3.5	2.7

[a] See text.

TABLE XVI-1. Age-Specific Incidence Rates per 100,000 Population (Uncorrected Estimates[a]) in Japan According to Sex and Primary Site (1977), Male

Primary site	ICD, 9th	Age group 0–	5–	10–	15–	20–	25–	30–	35–	40–	45–	50–	55–	60–	65–	70–	75–	80–	85–	All ages
All sites	140–208, 233	17.5	9.3	6.2	14.8	10.3	26.2	34.4	65.9	117.9	232.1	356.9	536.9	907.1	1320.4	1682.1	2060.3	2270.5	1864.1	225.8
All sites	140–208	17.5	9.3	6.2	14.8	10.3	26.2	34.4	65.9	117.9	232.1	356.9	536.9	907.1	1320.4	1682.1	2060.3	2270.5	1864.1	225.8
Mouth	140–145	0.2	0.0	0.0	0.4	0.3	0.3	1.4	1.2	1.3	2.7	6.6	9.3	9.4	13.3	18.3	18.7	25.0	10.1	2.7
Pharynx	146–149	0.0	0.0	0.1	0.0	0.0	0.4	0.0	0.3	0.4	1.9	2.7	4.6	9.5	4.2	8.2	3.8	10.2	5.6	1.3
Esophagus	150	0.0	0.0	0.0	0.0	0.0	0.0	0.2	0.6	0.8	5.3	13.1	21.1	41.9	63.5	79.6	108.8	94.4	104.9	9.3
Stomach	151	0.2	0.0	0.1	0.6	1.3	6.2	12.4	27.1	51.6	97.6	148.5	210.4	357.0	498.4	628.8	746.7	764.7	551.9	85.7
Colon	153	0.0	0.0	0.0	0.2	0.6	1.3	2.2	4.0	6.7	10.7	15.3	21.1	48.9	54.6	82.9	86.5	112.2	117.7	10.4
Rectum	154	0.0	0.0	0.0	0.2	0.0	0.6	1.9	4.2	5.9	10.1	18.5	28.1	33.4	54.4	75.1	86.4	88.3	98.9	9.9
Liver	155	1.0	0.1	0.1	0.0	0.1	0.2	2.4	1.9	14.4	30.1	36.2	54.0	70.3	89.2	108.0	104.3	102.0	73.6	16.4
Gallbladder *etc.*	156	0.0	0.0	0.0	0.0	0.0	0.1	0.3	1.5	0.7	3.9	7.6	13.2	22.7	27.2	43.6	53.4	88.3	41.5	5.2
Pancreas	157	0.0	0.0	0.0	0.1	0.1	0.2	0.4	2.6	3.6	7.8	8.7	19.8	27.9	56.1	53.7	56.7	57.4	52.7	7.2
Nose, sinuses	160	0.0	0.0	0.0	0.4	0.0	0.3	0.2	0.5	1.0	2.4	4.4	3.6	4.8	11.5	8.1	13.8	23.2	9.5	1.7
Larynx	161	0.0	0.0	0.0	0.0	0.0	0.0	0.2	0.2	0.5	2.1	4.8	9.5	13.5	29.6	27.2	29.7	20.6	19.2	3.1
Lung, trachea	162	0.0	0.0	0.0	1.0	0.2	0.6	1.0	2.1	8.1	18.1	33.1	53.4	117.2	202.8	260.9	319.2	338.0	281.5	27.3
Connective tissue	171	0.6	0.4	0.3	0.2	0.4	0.8	0.8	1.3	0.5	1.0	0.9	1.7	2.4	3.3	3.6	6.4	0.0	3.9	0.9
Skin	172, 173	0.0	0.0	0.1	0.1	0.1	1.1	0.5	1.3	1.6	3.6	2.7	6.0	7.3	10.3	19.0	40.6	51.3	92.6	2.8
Other skin	173	0.0	0.0	0.0	0.1	0.1	1.0	0.2	1.2	1.2	3.6	2.5	4.4	6.4	9.5	17.3	36.2	48.2	74.1	2.5
Prostate	185	0.0	0.0	0.0	0.0	0.0	0.4	0.2	0.0	0.1	0.4	1.5	4.7	17.3	33.7	57.5	130.0	183.4	172.6	6.1
Testis	186	1.2	0.0	0.0	1.3	0.8	2.2	1.4	1.2	1.7	1.2	1.2	0.8	0.9	0.1	0.9	0.2	1.9	4.5	1.1
Bladder	188	0.1	0.0	0.0	0.2	0.3	0.5	0.4	1.4	3.0	4.0	9.3	15.7	22.8	33.9	56.3	82.7	114.3	85.3	6.5
Kidney *etc.*	189	1.1	0.1	0.0	0.1	0.0	0.3	0.6	0.6	1.0	2.4	6.0	11.7	15.6	19.7	21.9	31.5	23.6	27.7	3.4
Brain, nervous system	191–192	2.9	2.5	1.1	1.2	1.0	1.3	1.8	2.2	1.0	2.9	4.6	4.5	4.9	5.4	2.8	4.7	2.4	0.0	2.3
Thyroid	193	0.0	0.0	0.0	0.2	0.1	0.4	0.5	1.5	2.8	3.1	2.9	3.2	3.9	5.2	8.9	8.9	3.9	7.3	1.5
Lymphatic tissue	200–203	0.9	0.9	1.5	1.7	0.9	2.4	1.1	2.6	3.4	9.0	10.7	19.7	37.2	44.3	40.4	48.4	40.6	32.6	7.5
Non-Hodgkin's lymphoma	200, 202	0.9	0.7	1.3	1.2	0.9	2.2	0.7	2.1	2.8	7.6	8.7	14.3	28.6	34.2	26.2	19.7	21.9	32.6	5.5
Multiple myeloma	203	0.0	0.0	0.0	0.0	0.0	0.0	0.2	0.2	0.4	1.0	1.8	3.0	5.1	7.5	12.0	18.7	12.0	0.0	1.3
Leukemia	204–208	6.6	4.3	1.7	4.5	2.1	4.2	3.1	4.7	4.1	6.1	6.3	7.5	11.1	14.7	17.5	14.6	32.9	18.6	5.5
Lymphoid leukemia	204	3.7	2.5	0.8	1.1	0.5	0.7	0.8	0.7	0.1	0.2	0.1	0.3	1.0	2.1	2.0	0.5	1.5	1.1	1.1
Myeloid leukemia	205	1.9	1.5	0.5	2.9	1.4	2.8	1.7	3.4	3.1	4.7	5.4	4.5	7.8	9.7	12.0	8.6	21.3	13.6	3.4

[a] See text.

TABLE XVI-2. Age-Specific Incidence Rates per 100,000 Population (Uncorrected Estimates[a]) in Japan According to Sex and Primary Site (1977), Female

Primary site	ICD, 9th	Age group 0–	5–	10–	15–	20–	25–	30–	35–	40–	45–	50–	55–	60–	65–	70–	75–	80–	85–	All ages
All sites	140–208, 233	14.3	7.0	9.7	9.7	13.1	35.4	58.0	113.9	180.4	247.0	322.6	399.3	517.1	715.1	862.6	1080.0	1093.8	915.1	187.3
All sites	140–208	14.3	7.0	9.7	9.7	12.9	33.9	54.4	102.0	166.4	233.1	314.0	394.1	510.0	713.6	859.8	1079.9	1092.0	915.1	182.9
Mouth	140–145	0.0	0.0	0.0	0.0	0.1	0.1	0.4	1.1	1.0	1.2	2.7	5.7	4.0	7.2	5.3	6.7	6.0	21.7	1.5
Pharynx	146–149	0.2	0.0	0.0	0.0	0.0	0.0	0.0	0.2	0.3	1.3	0.6	1.9	1.9	1.2	1.4	1.4	1.4	3.3	0.5
Esophagus	150	0.0	0.0	0.0	0.0	0.0	0.1	0.2	0.0	0.3	0.9	2.6	2.2	7.8	9.3	16.0	24.6	31.0	35.4	2.3
Stomach	151	0.0	0.0	0.0	0.5	1.2	8.3	17.0	28.6	44.6	48.3	69.5	98.1	137.3	203.4	274.3	340.1	335.0	303.5	49.8
Colon	153	0.0	0.0	0.0	0.3	0.2	0.8	0.9	2.7	4.2	8.6	16.2	25.4	29.6	42.1	49.1	70.2	76.5	84.2	9.6
Rectum	154	0.0	0.0	0.0	0.0	0.2	1.1	1.8	2.7	5.4	8.6	12.8	20.6	22.5	30.0	47.2	64.1	72.1	49.1	8.4
Liver	155	0.7	0.0	0.0	0.0	0.2	0.4	1.2	1.8	0.9	3.3	7.2	14.3	18.8	31.3	40.3	65.6	67.4	43.8	6.4
Gallbladder *etc.*	156	0.0	0.0	0.0	0.0	0.0	0.3	0.1	0.4	1.9	7.4	9.9	11.3	16.9	36.1	51.8	56.3	47.0	54.2	6.9
Pancreas	157	0.0	0.0	0.0	0.0	0.0	0.3	0.2	0.5	0.7	4.5	4.7	12.1	17.9	36.2	31.4	35.3	37.2	23.5	5.1
Nose, sinuses	160	0.0	0.0	0.0	0.0	0.0	0.2	0.1	0.1	0.3	0.6	1.9	3.6	4.1	4.3	8.5	7.4	3.9	3.3	1.1
Larynx	161	0.0	0.0	0.0	0.0	0.0	0.0	0.0	0.0	0.0	0.1	0.2	0.5	0.8	2.5	1.3	2.7	5.4	0.5	0.3
Lung, trachea	162	0.0	0.0	0.0	0.2	0.0	0.1	1.0	2.5	3.8	6.2	14.8	20.8	37.0	52.3	76.4	98.4	92.9	73.4	10.8
Connective tissue	171	0.9	0.0	0.3	0.2	1.0	0.1	0.2	0.0	0.8	1.5	1.7	1.3	1.3	1.7	0.9	0.2	0.7	0.5	0.7
Skin	172,173	0.0	0.0	0.4	0.5	0.1	0.6	0.3	0.4	1.2	2.3	2.6	2.2	4.7	7.7	10.8	21.5	27.2	49.5	2.2
Other skin	173	0.0	0.0	0.0	0.4	0.1	0.5	0.2	0.2	0.8	2.1	2.1	2.0	4.1	7.3	9.5	20.2	25.0	45.4	1.9
Breast	174–175, 2330	0.0	0.0	0.0	0.2	0.9	6.2	11.3	26.8	43.9	55.9	56.2	49.8	50.2	55.5	40.3	38.4	44.0	30.7	22.0
Uterus	179–182, 2331	0.0	0.0	0.0	0.0	0.8	5.9	11.1	28.0	42.7	58.4	70.8	71.5	79.4	86.4	88.5	82.3	96.4	32.6	28.3
Uterus	179–182	0.0	0.0	0.0	0.0	0.6	4.4	7.6	16.2	28.9	44.8	62.5	66.2	72.3	84.9	86.4	82.2	94.6	32.6	24.0
Cervix uteri	180	0.0	0.0	0.0	0.0	0.0	1.6	6.0	14.6	24.0	35.5	46.7	47.4	55.0	66.9	63.9	57.8	64.4	3.8	18.1
Corpus uteri	182	0.0	0.0	0.0	0.0	0.0	0.4	0.5	0.3	2.5	3.8	10.6	13.0	9.9	7.4	5.9	2.6	2.1	0.0	2.6
Uterus, unspecified	179	0.0	0.0	0.0	0.0	0.0	0.1	0.2	1.0	1.7	3.6	5.0	5.5	7.3	10.6	16.6	21.9	28.1	28.8	2.8
Ovary *etc.*	183	0.4	0.2	0.6	1.5	1.5	1.4	1.7	3.1	6.0	10.2	10.9	13.2	17.4	10.6	13.9	15.5	7.2	4.6	4.9
Bladder	188	0.0	0.0	0.0	0.0	0.2	0.1	0.1	0.3	0.6	0.8	2.7	4.0	5.7	11.2	14.5	25.1	26.8	28.8	2.2
Kidnay *etc.*	189	0.9	0.4	0.0	0.0	0.3	0.3	0.4	0.7	1.0	1.6	2.1	3.8	3.6	5.2	5.6	10.6	14.3	9.9	1.5
Brain, nervous system	191–192	2.9	1.8	1.6	0.7	0.5	0.8	1.2	1.6	3.2	3.5	3.3	4.2	2.0	6.5	0.7	0.6	0.9	1.0	2.1
Thyroid	193	0.0	0.0	0.4	0.4	2.2	3.1	5.1	4.5	7.2	6.2	6.4	7.4	9.6	14.0	17.2	21.1	21.5	7.1	4.7
Lymphatic tissue	200–203	0.9	0.6	0.7	1.8	0.9	2.0	1.0	1.0	2.8	4.3	6.4	10.6	20.2	18.7	22.8	34.3	19.4	12.7	4.9
Non-Hodgkin's lymphoma	200, 202	0.9	0.6	0.7	1.4	0.7	1.8	0.9	0.9	1.6	3.1	3.4	7.8	14.3	12.6	15.0	16.4	14.0	11.7	3.3
Multiple myeloma	203	0.0	0.0	0.0	0.0	0.0	0.0	0.0	0.1	0.2	1.2	2.8	2.5	5.5	5.3	5.3	16.5	3.2	1.0	1.3
Leukemia	204–208	6.0	3.4	3.6	2.5	2.1	2.5	1.6	2.6	2.9	4.3	5.7	4.3	8.3	10.0	13.0	13.6	11.0	1.8	4.2
Lymphoid leukemia	204	2.3	2.7	1.7	0.8	0.1	0.2	0.2	0.2	0.5	0.3	0.8	0.9	1.3	0.8	1.2	1.3	0.0	0.5	0.9
Myeloid leukemia	205	1.5	0.4	1.6	1.6	1.9	1.6	1.2	1.8	2.1	3.6	3.6	2.7	5.3	7.1	10.3	6.6	7.4	0.0	2.5

[a] See text.

TABLE XVII-1. Age-Specific Incidence Rates per 100,000 Population (Uncorrected Estimates[a]) in Japan According to Sex and Primary Site (1978), Male

Primary site	ICD, 9th	Age group 0–	5–	10–	15–	20–	25–	30–	35–	40–	45–	50–	55–	60–	65–	70–	75–	80–	85–	All ages
All sites	140–208,233	17.5	8.0	6.0	14.4	8.3	24.1	36.7	66.6	122.9	239.7	391.2	537.9	895.3	1331.3	1730.9	2132.5	2149.1	1929.7	235.0
All sites	140–208	17.5	8.0	6.0	14.4	8.3	24.1	36.7	66.6	122.9	239.7	391.2	537.9	895.3	1331.3	1730.9	2132.5	2149.1	1929.7	235.0
Mouth	140–145	0.0	0.0	0.0	0.3	0.1	0.3	1.0	0.7	1.0	3.7	5.7	9.3	10.6	15.0	21.6	20.2	26.4	12.6	2.8
Pharynx	146–149	0.0	0.0	0.1	0.3	0.0	0.4	0.0	0.4	0.9	2.6	2.8	4.2	7.3	5.7	9.7	5.2	9.3	10.5	1.4
Esophagus	150	0.0	0.0	0.0	0.0	0.0	0.0	0.2	1.0	1.8	5.4	13.6	23.0	40.9	64.7	83.7	98.1	103.5	107.2	9.8
Stomach	151	0.2	0.0	0.2	0.9	1.0	7.2	14.4	28.0	51.6	99.4	160.4	208.2	346.0	475.5	614.3	747.0	712.4	568.6	87.3
Colon	153	0.0	0.0	0.0	0.2	0.5	0.8	1.9	4.2	7.0	11.8	15.4	23.5	47.7	59.4	92.0	97.9	99.9	103.3	11.1
Rectum	154	0.0	0.0	0.0	0.2	0.1	0.3	1.8	4.5	9.2	9.4	18.8	27.6	35.5	59.3	60.4	86.3	93.7	105.3	10.2
Liver	155	0.8	0.0	0.2	0.0	0.2	0.3	2.1	1.5	13.0	34.3	45.3	55.7	76.5	95.4	109.3	103.8	106.2	103.8	17.9
Gallbladder *etc.*	156	0.0	0.0	0.0	0.0	0.0	0.1	0.2	1.5	1.1	4.2	6.7	11.4	24.2	28.8	57.0	58.0	56.6	46.7	5.5
Pancreas	157	0.0	0.1	0.0	0.1	0.0	0.3	0.6	3.3	3.3	8.7	10.5	20.0	29.6	56.3	56.0	72.5	55.0	45.5	7.8
Nose, sinuses	160	0.0	0.0	0.0	0.4	0.0	0.3	0.3	0.3	0.8	2.9	5.6	4.7	5.6	10.9	7.5	11.8	21.1	7.8	1.9
Larynx	161	0.0	0.0	0.0	0.0	0.0	0.0	0.2	0.5	0.7	1.9	6.2	10.0	11.7	30.9	24.3	30.9	13.5	13.5	3.2
Lung, trachea	162	0.0	0.0	0.0	0.7	0.3	0.5	1.4	2.0	8.0	15.4	37.2	54.0	117.0	210.8	281.1	346.5	348.6	240.1	29.1
Connective tissue	171	0.9	0.1	0.2	0.0	0.1	0.6	0.7	1.0	0.5	0.5	1.0	1.2	2.7	2.0	4.6	5.8	0.0	3.6	0.8
Skin	172,173	0.0	0.0	0.0	0.0	0.2	0.6	0.4	0.9	2.0	3.5	2.7	4.5	11.5	12.0	17.4	34.7	53.4	95.2	2.9
Other skin	173	0.0	0.0	0.0	0.0	0.2	0.5	0.1	0.9	1.6	3.4	2.1	4.0	10.7	9.4	14.5	26.8	49.0	82.4	2.4
Prostate	185	0.0	0.0	0.1	0.0	0.2	0.4	0.0	0.0	0.7	0.4	1.9	6.0	11.1	45.2	69.0	123.7	166.2	193.6	6.7
Testis	186	1.1	0.1	0.0	1.1	0.8	1.7	1.6	1.5	1.1	1.0	1.0	1.7	0.8	0.1	0.5	0.3	1.4	4.2	1.0
Bladder	188	0.1	0.0	0.0	0.2	0.3	0.9	0.9	1.5	2.6	5.1	11.3	16.6	23.4	35.8	66.1	99.7	109.7	125.5	7.5
Kidney *etc.*	189	0.6	0.2	0.0	0.1	0.0	0.3	0.1	1.0	1.2	2.4	5.6	9.8	16.7	15.6	20.3	32.8	20.6	30.9	3.2
Brain, nervous system	191–192	3.5	2.3	1.0	0.9	0.4	1.7	2.2	2.2	2.1	4.4	5.2	3.6	5.5	5.0	6.0	5.4	2.2	1.0	2.6
Thyroid	193	0.0	0.0	0.0	0.0	0.1	0.7	0.6	1.4	2.0	3.7	3.0	2.8	3.5	5.1	7.9	5.9	4.8	8.9	1.5
Lymphatic tissue	200–203	0.9	0.5	1.3	1.9	0.7	1.7	1.6	2.6	4.9	8.2	14.2	17.0	30.2	35.7	42.5	60.0	26.8	28.9	7.3
Non-Hodgkin's lymphoma	200, 202	0.9	0.4	1.2	1.5	0.7	1.6	1.1	2.1	3.6	7.2	11.2	13.1	22.0	25.9	24.0	27.5	16.9	28.9	5.2
Multiple myeloma	203	0.0	0.0	0.0	0.0	0.0	0.0	0.2	0.4	0.4	0.7	2.7	2.3	4.7	6.8	15.3	25.3	9.2	0.0	1.5
Leukemia	204–208	7.0	3.5	2.0	4.4	2.2	3.4	3.3	4.2	4.6	5.8	6.7	7.9	12.0	13.5	21.4	18.2	33.4	19.3	5.6
Lymphoid leukemia	204	4.5	2.5	1.2	1.3	0.5	0.6	0.7	0.7	0.3	0.3	0.1	0.8	1.2	0.4	2.9	0.5	1.5	2.0	1.2
Myeloid leukemia	205	1.3	0.7	0.3	2.7	1.3	2.1	2.1	2.8	3.7	4.5	6.1	4.6	8.4	9.8	13.0	11.3	23.7	12.6	3.3

[a] See text.

Table XVII-2. Age-Specific Incidence Rates per 100,000 Population (Uncorrected Estimates[a]) in Japan According to Sex and Primary Site (1978), Female

Primary site	ICD, 9th	Age group																		All ages
		0–	5–	10–	15–	20–	25–	30–	35–	40–	45–	50–	55–	60–	65–	70–	75–	80–	85–	
All sites	140–208, 233	14.2	7.8	7.5	9.8	15.4	29.6	58.2	115.2	174.4	243.2	319.2	404.2	532.5	747.6	852.6	1115.4	1126.1	1007.8	193.6
All sites	140–208	14.2	7.8	7.5	9.8	15.2	28.6	54.5	104.4	162.1	230.3	309.9	398.0	525.2	745.5	849.5	1114.2	1124.2	1007.8	189.3
Mouth	140–145	0.0	0.0	0.0	0.0	0.1	0.0	0.3	1.2	0.5	1.7	2.6	5.3	3.6	8.1	5.7	11.2	9.8	24.4	1.6
Pharynx	146–149	0.2	0.0	0.0	0.0	0.1	0.0	0.0	0.2	0.3	1.7	0.5	1.7	1.2	1.8	1.3	1.3	0.9	3.1	0.5
Esophagus	150	0.0	0.0	0.0	0.0	0.0	0.1	0.2	0.0	0.5	1.2	1.1	3.0	8.7	7.6	16.6	24.1	32.8	37.4	2.4
Stomach	151	0.2	0.0	0.0	0.2	1.9	7.1	16.1	26.2	38.0	45.7	69.6	99.2	135.1	208.8	256.9	329.6	336.5	310.7	49.7
Colon	153	0.0	0.0	0.0	0.0	0.6	0.8	1.2	3.5	3.9	7.5	16.5	25.3	35.2	47.6	52.8	77.8	87.7	97.7	10.7
Rectum	154	0.0	0.0	0.0	0.0	0.1	0.7	2.2	2.9	5.2	9.6	14.5	20.5	25.6	33.3	43.5	62.3	82.1	54.3	9.1
Liver	155	0.4	0.0	0.0	0.0	0.4	0.1	0.4	1.7	0.7	3.6	7.6	15.1	23.6	33.0	42.6	73.4	59.7	44.7	7.0
Gallbladder *etc.*	156	0.0	0.0	0.0	0.0	0.2	0.3	0.0	0.4	1.8	6.5	8.6	14.3	18.4	38.0	44.0	60.6	42.3	50.9	7.1
Pancreas	157	0.0	0.0	0.0	0.0	0.0	0.2	0.4	0.8	1.1	3.9	5.0	11.8	17.1	34.2	33.3	46.7	48.7	17.7	5.5
Nose, sinuses	160	0.0	0.0	0.0	0.0	0.2	0.2	0.1	0.2	0.3	0.6	1.3	3.8	3.0	2.6	6.5	7.6	6.1	1.9	1.0
Larynx	161	0.0	0.0	0.0	0.0	0.0	0.0	0.0	0.2	0.0	0.1	0.7	0.4	0.8	2.8	1.8	2.2	4.9	0.0	0.3
Lung, trachea	162	0.0	0.0	0.0	0.2	0.0	0.6	0.9	1.9	3.6	6.7	11.8	18.6	40.2	60.8	81.1	87.6	91.0	80.7	11.2
Connective tissue	171	0.9	0.8	0.3	0.2	1.0	0.1	0.0	0.2	0.9	1.1	1.3	2.0	0.9	2.6	1.5	0.8	2.2	2.2	0.8
Skin	172,173	0.0	0.0	0.4	0.6	0.2	0.5	0.5	0.2	1.6	2.7	3.5	3.1	5.0	8.4	10.5	17.9	22.9	54.8	2.4
Other skin	173	0.0	0.0	0.0	0.5	0.0	0.5	0.4	0.0	1.0	2.5	2.6	2.7	4.5	8.0	9.8	17.0	21.2	51.4	2.1
Breast	174–175,2330	0.0	0.0	0.0	0.2	0.5	3.8	10.2	28.5	49.3	59.0	60.3	54.8	52.4	57.2	39.4	40.9	34.8	38.7	23.3
Uterus	179–182,2331	0.0	0.0	0.0	0.0	0.7	5.0	12.0	27.7	40.2	56.6	72.1	66.4	81.4	88.1	82.6	89.0	106.2	45.4	28.6
Uterus	179–182	0.0	0.0	0.0	0.0	0.5	4.0	8.3	17.1	28.4	44.2	63.0	60.3	74.0	86.0	80.2	87.8	104.3	45.4	24.5
Cervix uteri	180	0.0	0.0	0.0	0.0	0.1	1.9	7.0	14.9	23.8	35.4	45.7	45.4	57.7	65.9	63.5	60.9	77.3	15.6	18.7
Corpus uteri	182	0.0	0.0	0.0	0.0	0.0	0.4	0.2	1.3	2.3	5.5	13.2	8.9	9.2	10.0	3.0	4.8	2.2	2.2	2.8
Uterus, unspecified	179	0.0	0.0	0.0	0.0	0.0	0.0	0.1	0.7	1.7	2.4	3.7	5.6	7.1	10.1	13.5	20.4	24.8	27.6	2.6
Ovary *etc.*	183	0.1	0.5	0.5	1.7	1.7	1.9	2.9	3.9	5.0	8.7	10.2	13.9	15.8	14.2	20.3	19.3	12.5	11.9	5.4
Bladder	188	0.0	0.0	0.0	0.0	0.2	0.2	0.1	0.5	0.4	1.0	1.7	2.7	6.3	12.8	20.3	22.8	35.3	36.0	2.5
Kidney *etc.*	189	1.5	0.4	0.0	0.0	0.2	0.1	0.3	0.7	1.0	1.1	1.9	3.6	2.8	7.6	8.8	10.9	11.7	13.6	1.7
Brain, nervous system	191–192	3.1	1.9	1.6	0.7	1.2	0.6	1.1	1.7	2.7	3.8	2.7	5.1	3.2	5.3	1.7	2.4	1.3	0.9	2.2
Thyroid	193	0.0	0.0	0.2	0.8	2.5	2.0	6.1	4.6	9.1	5.8	6.6	7.1	8.4	11.8	20.7	19.1	19.2	16.1	4.9
Lymphatic tissue	200–203	1.0	0.5	0.7	1.9	0.9	1.9	0.8	1.6	2.0	4.1	7.7	11.7	21.0	18.1	19.1	37.7	22.0	16.6	5.1
Non-Hodgkin's lymphoma	200, 202	1.0	0.4	0.7	1.3	0.8	1.7	0.7	1.5	1.1	2.6	4.7	8.5	14.0	11.9	12.3	16.7	15.6	12.6	3.4
Multiple myeloma	203	0.0	0.0	0.0	0.0	0.0	0.0	0.0	0.1	0.1	0.8	2.9	2.7	5.6	5.2	6.2	19.5	5.9	0.9	1.4
Leukemia	204–208	5.2	3.5	2.3	2.1	2.0	2.4	1.5	2.7	3.2	4.5	3.1	3.8	8.1	9.1	9.2	14.5	9.5	0.5	3.8
Lymphoid leukemia	204	2.5	2.6	0.9	0.8	0.1	0.3	0.2	0.2	0.6	0.4	0.2	0.9	1.8	0.8	1.0	2.5	0.7	0.5	0.9
Myeloid leukemia	205	0.8	0.5	1.2	1.1	1.7	1.5	1.2	2.2	1.9	3.0	2.3	1.8	4.9	5.8	6.3	7.8	5.4	0.0	2.1

[a] See text.

TABLE XVIII-1. Age-Specific Incidence Rates per 100,000 Population (Uncorrected Estimates[a]) in Japan According to Sex and Primary Site (1979), Male

Primary site	ICD, 9th	Age group																		All ages
		0–	5–	10–	15–	20–	25–	30–	35–	40–	45–	50–	55–	60–	65–	70–	75–	80–	85–	
All sites	140–208, 233	17.1	6.7	6.3	12.3	8.7	21.3	39.6	70.5	120.9	238.6	414.4	580.3	935.4	1319.6	1773.8	2167.6	2206.9	2026.3	245.6
All sites	140–208	17.1	6.7	6.3	12.3	8.7	21.3	39.6	70.5	120.9	238.6	414.4	580.3	935.4	1319.6	1773.8	2167.6	2206.9	2026.3	245.6
Mouth	140–145	0.0	0.0	0.0	0.3	0.1	0.2	1.4	0.7	1.0	3.6	7.7	10.4	9.9	15.1	21.1	19.8	32.5	13.7	3.1
Pharynx	146–149	0.0	0.0	0.0	0.3	0.1	0.0	0.1	0.7	1.3	2.9	1.9	4.3	10.4	6.9	12.4	5.6	8.8	5.8	1.6
Esophagus	150	0.0	0.0	0.0	0.0	0.0	0.0	0.1	0.8	2.2	6.4	14.1	24.7	41.4	60.4	82.4	91.8	98.6	113.8	9.9
Stomach	151	0.0	0.0	0.2	0.6	1.1	6.5	14.0	28.2	51.4	97.4	166.7	223.0	364.2	473.4	629.2	705.9	688.8	642.8	90.2
Colon	153	0.0	0.0	0.0	0.2	0.7	0.8	2.3	4.6	6.2	10.8	20.9	24.4	46.0	64.1	89.9	122.3	122.1	98.8	12.2
Rectum	154	0.0	0.0	0.0	0.2	0.1	0.4	2.5	5.9	9.1	11.8	20.5	27.6	41.2	62.8	64.5	88.2	85.5	98.1	11.2
Liver	155	0.5	0.0	0.1	0.0	0.1	0.2	1.2	2.2	11.7	34.2	49.1	64.2	88.8	91.3	111.4	110.9	115.0	144.8	19.1
Gallbladder *etc.*	156	0.0	0.0	0.0	0.0	0.0	0.0	0.2	1.1	1.1	4.3	5.8	11.5	22.3	29.3	57.2	61.6	57.6	43.9	5.6
Pancreas	157	0.0	0.2	0.0	0.0	0.0	0.2	0.9	2.4	3.0	9.3	10.6	22.3	34.6	47.8	62.1	84.4	60.8	44.0	8.3
Nose, sinuses	160	0.0	0.0	0.0	0.4	0.0	0.2	0.7	0.4	0.7	1.7	5.0	5.4	5.2	9.7	7.8	11.2	10.6	7.3	1.7
Larynx	161	0.0	0.0	0.0	0.0	0.0	0.0	0.2	0.4	0.9	2.2	7.9	10.7	13.3	27.8	21.5	32.6	17.1	8.5	3.4
Lung, trachea	162	0.0	0.0	0.0	0.4	0.2	0.3	1.6	3.3	6.6	14.8	40.3	59.6	115.7	212.6	296.8	391.8	367.5	267.7	31.3
Connective tissue	171	0.9	0.1	0.2	0.4	0.3	0.8	0.4	0.7	0.5	0.6	0.8	2.0	2.9	1.7	2.4	9.8	2.1	2.5	0.9
Skin	172,173	0.0	0.0	0.0	0.0	0.1	0.4	0.3	1.2	1.8	2.1	4.4	4.7	12.4	12.3	17.7	37.4	55.2	72.4	3.0
Other skin	173	0.0	0.0	0.0	0.0	0.1	0.2	0.1	1.0	1.7	2.0	3.7	3.6	11.6	9.8	14.7	32.9	51.4	58.1	2.6
Prostate	185	0.0	0.0	0.1	0.0	0.2	0.0	0.0	0.0	0.7	0.2	2.8	7.4	10.8	44.5	70.2	118.6	155.4	183.5	6.8
Testis	186	0.9	0.1	0.0	1.2	1.0	2.1	2.2	1.6	1.0	1.7	0.5	1.0	0.1	1.3	0.6	2.7	1.7	3.9	1.1
Bladder	188	0.1	0.4	0.0	0.4	0.4	0.6	1.1	2.4	2.9	4.9	10.8	18.7	30.2	40.8	63.4	94.9	132.1	119.2	8.1
Kidney *etc.*	189	0.5	0.2	0.0	0.0	0.0	0.0	0.0	1.7	1.3	2.5	4.1	9.6	15.4	17.2	20.8	30.3	27.2	13.7	3.2
Brain, nervous system	191–192	3.1	1.5	1.1	0.7	0.3	1.6	2.5	2.7	2.4	4.2	3.2	3.5	4.8	5.9	5.3	5.7	2.4	1.9	2.5
Thyroid	193	0.0	0.0	0.1	0.0	0.1	0.6	0.9	1.0	2.1	3.5	2.4	1.9	3.6	4.2	6.5	6.0	7.9	2.8	1.4
Lymphatic tissue	200–203	1.2	0.7	1.3	1.8	0.7	1.3	2.6	2.6	4.9	9.3	16.3	16.8	22.5	36.0	45.5	51.7	52.3	31.6	7.6
Non-Hodgkin's lymphoma	200, 202	1.2	0.4	1.1	1.7	0.6	1.1	2.1	2.2	3.6	8.6	11.9	12.7	15.0	23.1	27.5	32.4	38.5	18.9	5.4
Multiple myeloma	203	0.0	0.0	0.0	0.0	0.0	0.0	0.2	0.3	0.6	0.5	4.1	2.8	4.0	9.3	14.6	18.2	12.7	12.7	1.6
Leukemia	204–208	6.9	2.7	2.3	3.5	1.8	3.8	3.5	4.2	4.8	5.7	6.7	8.6	14.3	15.7	22.7	16.9	28.7	41.5	5.7
Lymphoid leukemia	204	4.8	2.0	1.2	1.1	0.1	0.9	0.8	0.4	0.4	1.1	0.1	0.8	1.0	2.4	3.4	0.5	4.4	1.9	1.3
Myeloid leukemia	205	1.4	0.3	0.6	2.1	1.3	2.3	2.4	2.7	3.6	3.8	6.2	5.0	11.3	10.1	12.4	10.1	21.2	35.3	3.4

[a] See text.

TABLE XVIII-2. Age-Specific Incidence Rates per 100,000 Population (Uncorrected Estimates[a]) in Japan According to Sex and Primary Site (1979), Female

Primary site	ICD, 9th	Age group																		All ages
		0–	5–	10–	15–	20–	25–	30–	35–	40–	45–	50–	55–	60–	65–	70–	75–	80–	85–	
All sites	140–208, 233	14.8	7.8	6.4	9.6	16.0	28.5	60.3	128.4	176.5	244.8	314.3	416.7	544.5	738.8	875.7	1131.0	1136.3	1003.0	200.1
All sites	140–208	14.8	7.8	6.4	9.6	16.0	27.7	55.3	116.4	164.7	234.1	306.6	410.2	539.4	736.8	872.8	1129.7	1136.1	1003.0	196.0
Mouth	140–145	0.0	0.1	0.0	0.0	0.0	0.0	0.6	1.4	0.9	1.9	3.1	4.3	5.4	7.2	7.7	14.4	10.1	9.0	1.8
Pharynx	146–149	0.0	0.0	0.0	0.0	0.1	0.0	0.0	0.3	0.1	1.5	0.7	1.6	1.4	1.3	2.0	1.7	1.6	4.6	0.5
Esophagus	150	0.0	0.0	0.0	0.0	0.0	0.1	0.0	0.0	1.0	1.4	1.4	4.1	9.9	9.4	17.2	23.9	24.3	29.3	2.5
Stomach	151	0.2	0.0	0.0	0.0	2.3	7.4	16.3	25.3	36.8	43.3	65.2	100.6	136.9	205.1	256.1	338.4	362.3	290.6	50.7
Colon	153	0.0	0.0	0.0	0.0	0.4	0.8	1.2	4.0	4.6	7.5	16.7	22.5	36.7	55.1	59.8	84.0	71.8	82.8	11.3
Rectum	154	0.0	0.0	0.0	0.1	0.2	0.2	1.7	4.3	5.9	10.5	16.3	20.5	27.3	34.7	39.2	59.3	74.9	58.6	9.4
Liver	155	0.3	0.0	0.0	0.0	0.4	0.2	0.4	1.7	1.2	3.7	5.8	16.3	22.8	35.5	47.4	68.4	55.7	44.7	7.1
Gallbladder *etc.*	156	0.0	0.0	0.0	0.0	0.2	0.0	0.0	0.1	1.4	5.4	7.1	16.0	21.6	28.7	45.3	66.8	43.4	58.0	7.1
Pancreas	157	0.0	0.0	0.0	0.0	0.0	0.0	0.5	1.1	1.1	3.0	4.5	13.1	18.5	31.4	40.0	40.8	56.7	29.0	5.9
Nose, sinuses	160	0.0	0.0	0.0	0.0	0.2	0.0	0.1	0.0	0.2	0.6	1.6	2.6	2.4	4.1	4.7	7.0	5.3	9.3	0.9
Larynx	161	0.0	0.0	0.0	0.0	0.0	0.0	0.0	0.2	0.1	0.1	0.8	0.5	0.5	2.3	2.6	1.9	3.3	0.9	0.3
Lung, trachea	162	0.0	0.0	0.0	0.2	0.0	0.7	0.7	2.3	4.0	7.7	11.9	20.9	41.8	61.4	78.2	94.3	101.8	83.8	11.9
Connective tissue	171	0.9	0.8	0.3	0.1	0.8	0.1	0.2	0.4	0.7	1.1	0.9	3.1	1.2	2.0	1.3	1.4	1.9	2.0	0.8
Skin	172, 173	0.0	0.0	0.0	0.4	0.2	0.9	0.4	0.3	2.2	3.1	3.0	5.1	5.7	7.6	9.2	21.4	32.2	61.3	2.7
Other skin	173	0.0	0.0	0.0	0.4	0.0	0.9	0.4	0.2	1.7	2.9	2.2	4.3	5.2	7.3	8.6	19.6	30.1	56.8	2.4
Breast	174–175, 2330	0.0	0.0	0.0	0.0	1.0	4.8	10.7	32.6	48.8	60.4	62.1	58.1	52.0	54.9	43.4	37.4	35.2	50.3	24.4
Uterus	179–182, 2331	0.0	0.0	0.0	0.0	0.8	4.4	13.6	32.6	40.5	54.2	69.1	65.7	74.1	78.7	82.6	92.4	98.1	41.3	28.5
Uterus	179–182	0.0	0.0	0.0	0.0	0.8	3.6	8.6	21.0	29.5	44.1	61.6	59.6	69.0	76.7	79.8	91.1	97.9	41.3	24.6
Cervix uteri	180	0.0	0.0	0.0	0.0	0.1	2.1	7.6	17.3	25.1	35.3	43.6	44.6	52.2	57.2	61.8	60.7	69.3	17.4	18.5
Corpus uteri	182	0.0	0.0	0.0	0.0	0.0	0.4	0.3	2.7	2.1	5.9	14.7	10.6	8.4	11.0	5.6	10.9	3.7	3.2	3.3
Uterus, unspecified	179	0.0	0.0	0.0	0.0	0.0	0.0	0.1	0.6	1.9	2.1	3.1	4.5	8.4	8.5	12.2	17.9	25.0	20.8	2.4
Ovary *etc.*	183	0.1	0.5	0.6	2.1	1.4	1.6	3.3	5.4	5.9	9.7	12.9	13.6	14.1	17.1	22.0	18.4	12.3	11.2	6.0
Bladder	188	0.0	0.0	0.0	0.0	0.0	0.2	0.2	0.6	0.4	1.3	2.2	3.2	7.8	11.9	23.9	21.6	34.0	24.8	2.7
Kidney *etc.*	189	1.4	0.2	0.0	0.0	0.2	0.0	0.2	0.4	0.7	1.9	2.4	4.0	4.4	7.6	10.7	7.4	13.2	12.0	1.8
Brain, nervous system	191–192	2.4	1.6	1.5	0.5	1.2	0.7	1.1	1.9	3.3	3.9	2.6	3.6	5.8	5.9	3.7	4.1	1.4	0.9	2.3
Thyroid	193	0.0	0.0	0.2	1.0	2.6	1.7	5.5	4.8	7.7	7.2	6.2	8.5	8.7	11.0	17.0	12.8	14.4	17.9	4.7
Lymphatic tissue	200–203	1.2	0.6	0.6	1.9	0.7	1.3	0.3	2.2	2.1	5.4	7.1	11.5	21.1	23.7	18.7	35.9	29.2	22.3	5.4
Non-Hodgkin's lymphoma	200, 202	1.2	0.4	0.6	1.4	0.7	1.0	0.2	2.1	1.6	3.2	5.0	7.4	13.8	14.7	10.5	15.4	16.6	18.5	3.5
Multiple myeloma	203	0.0	0.0	0.0	0.0	0.0	0.0	0.0	0.2	0.2	1.1	1.9	3.5	5.8	6.5	7.4	19.3	11.6	0.9	1.5
Leukemia	204–208	5.3	3.4	1.9	2.4	2.2	2.2	1.8	3.2	3.9	4.2	2.3	4.6	9.0	7.3	9.7	17.2	9.6	6.4	4.0
Lymphoid leukemia	204	3.0	2.4	0.7	1.2	0.0	0.4	0.3	0.7	0.9	0.6	0.4	1.1	2.2	1.2	1.7	1.4	1.4	0.4	1.0
Myeloid leukemia	205	0.4	0.8	1.0	1.1	1.9	1.2	1.3	2.4	2.4	2.7	1.3	2.5	5.8	4.0	6.2	9.3	6.0	5.9	2.2

[a] See text.

TABLE XIX-1. Age-Specific Incidence Rates per 100,000 Population (Uncorrected Estimates[a]) in Japan According to Sex and Primary Site (1980), Male

Primary site	ICD, 9th	Age group																		All ages
		0–	5–	10–	15–	20–	25–	30–	35–	40–	45–	50–	55–	60–	65–	70–	75–	80–	85–	
All sites	140–208, 233	16.2	7.7	8.0	10.7	9.9	19.2	36.3	64.9	109.0	221.8	393.1	590.4	895.7	1312.2	1820.5	2158.6	2297.2	2076.1	249.6
All sites	140–208	16.2	7.7	8.0	10.7	9.9	19.2	36.3	64.9	109.0	221.8	393.1	590.4	895.7	1312.2	1820.5	2158.6	2297.2	2076.1	249.6
Mouth	140–145	0.0	0.0	0.1	0.0	0.1	0.2	0.8	1.3	1.8	3.0	6.0	8.8	9.3	14.5	21.4	17.6	30.5	10.2	3.0
Pharynx	146–149	0.0	0.0	0.2	0.3	0.5	0.0	0.3	0.5	1.2	2.3	3.5	4.8	7.4	7.8	10.6	9.1	6.8	3.8	1.7
Esophagus	150	0.0	0.0	0.0	0.0	0.0	0.0	0.0	0.6	1.9	5.7	14.1	24.6	36.9	51.8	79.0	93.2	81.3	114.0	9.3
Stomach	151	0.0	0.2	0.1	0.3	1.4	6.5	12.7	25.5	45.0	89.8	151.4	227.5	337.0	473.9	646.0	700.8	666.3	649.9	90.0
Colon	153	0.0	0.0	0.0	0.2	0.5	0.8	2.5	4.2	6.3	11.4	18.9	25.4	41.1	57.9	83.2	116.7	137.4	117.0	11.9
Rectum	154	0.0	0.0	0.0	0.1	0.1	0.4	2.3	5.1	7.6	11.2	16.1	28.2	45.6	63.7	76.3	85.5	111.7	102.8	11.5
Liver	155	0.5	0.1	0.0	0.0	0.1	0.1	1.4	3.1	10.3	32.7	52.3	68.5	91.1	100.2	125.9	131.0	162.5	132.9	21.6
Gallbladder *etc.*	156	0.0	0.0	0.0	0.0	0.0	0.2	0.1	0.7	1.0	3.2	6.1	12.9	20.8	30.6	54.4	72.9	68.3	51.1	5.9
Pancreas	157	0.0	0.2	0.0	0.1	0.0	0.2	0.9	2.1	2.2	7.6	12.7	20.9	33.1	53.4	70.0	87.3	69.4	44.5	8.8
Nose, sinuses	160	0.0	0.0	0.0	0.0	0.0	0.0	0.4	0.2	1.0	2.2	4.9	4.2	5.5	10.0	7.2	7.9	8.2	6.4	1.6
Larynx	161	0.0	0.0	0.0	0.0	0.0	0.0	0.0	0.5	0.5	2.3	6.2	10.5	15.0	25.6	19.0	34.2	20.3	8.7	3.4
Lung, trachea	162	0.0	0.3	0.0	0.1	0.2	0.4	1.1	3.6	4.8	14.8	38.3	66.9	112.4	208.3	303.9	380.6	421.5	262.4	33.0
Connective tissue	171	0.9	0.2	0.2	0.8	0.4	0.5	0.6	0.5	0.4	1.2	1.1	1.6	3.1	3.2	2.8	5.1	3.9	0.0	0.9
Skin	172,173	0.0	0.0	0.0	0.0	0.1	0.3	0.2	1.0	1.6	1.8	3.9	5.0	11.5	11.8	18.6	35.9	45.0	45.8	2.9
Other skin	173	0.0	0.0	0.0	0.0	0.1	0.1	0.2	0.6	1.5	1.6	3.2	3.8	10.7	9.5	16.8	29.6	41.5	43.6	2.5
Prostate	185	0.0	0.0	0.1	0.0	0.1	0.0	0.0	0.0	0.6	0.1	1.9	5.1	8.5	35.6	72.8	126.9	165.3	201.4	6.7
Testis	186	0.9	0.2	0.0	0.7	1.0	2.3	1.8	2.0	0.8	1.4	0.8	1.3	0.0	0.9	0.1	1.9	1.1	0.0	1.0
Bladder	188	0.0	0.3	0.0	0.3	0.5	0.4	1.0	2.5	2.2	3.6	10.3	15.7	30.8	40.4	68.1	79.0	114.2	127.0	7.9
Kidney *etc.*	189	1.5	0.2	0.0	0.0	0.0	0.2	0.3	1.1	1.8	2.2	3.8	8.7	14.1	20.0	24.9	25.2	21.2	11.5	3.3
Brain, nervous system	191–192	2.3	1.1	1.3	1.2	0.4	0.6	2.2	2.1	1.9	3.7	2.1	2.5	5.7	6.6	5.5	8.2	2.9	3.8	2.2
Thyroid	193	0.0	0.0	0.1	0.0	0.0	0.5	1.1	1.2	1.7	2.1	1.4	2.2	2.7	3.7	4.5	4.8	8.7	3.5	1.1
Lymphatic tissue	200–203	1.1	0.7	1.5	1.5	0.7	1.2	2.0	2.5	5.1	8.0	16.8	17.5	20.7	35.4	43.3	55.1	53.2	61.3	7.8
Non-Hodgkin's lymphoma	200, 202	1.0	0.6	1.4	1.3	0.5	1.2	1.9	2.1	3.9	7.2	13.4	13.0	15.8	22.7	28.3	34.2	32.6	46.4	5.8
Multiple myeloma	203	0.0	0.0	0.1	0.0	0.0	0.0	0.0	0.3	0.7	0.7	3.0	3.9	3.1	8.7	12.5	19.7	19.3	12.4	1.5
Leukemia	204–208	6.3	3.7	3.4	3.4	2.1	2.8	3.3	3.3	6.1	5.0	7.5	12.5	15.9	16.1	24.1	16.6	20.6	36.7	6.0
Lymphoid leukemia	204	4.8	2.0	2.2	1.1	0.1	0.9	0.3	0.6	0.8	1.1	0.5	2.3	0.9	4.1	2.9	0.3	5.5	6.8	1.5
Myeloid leukemia	205	0.9	1.0	0.5	2.2	1.3	1.6	2.7	2.2	4.0	3.0	5.2	7.6	11.7	8.8	10.7	10.2	10.7	24.7	3.3

[a] See text.

TABLE XIX-2. Age-Specific Incidence Rates per 100,000 Population (Uncorrected Estimates[a]) in Japan According to Sex and Primary Site (1980), Female

Primary site	ICD, 9th	Age group																		All ages
		0–	5–	10–	15–	20–	25–	30–	35–	40–	45–	50–	55–	60–	65–	70–	75–	80–	85–	
All sites	140–208, 233	13.4	7.3	5.8	7.5	16.1	26.1	63.3	119.0	175.6	239.7	311.7	401.4	543.7	694.9	912.3	1085.9	1147.0	1058.0	201.5
All sites	140–208	13.4	7.3	5.8	7.5	15.7	24.8	56.4	106.3	160.2	229.8	301.5	395.0	538.3	690.8	910.3	1085.0	1146.9	1057.7	196.7
Mouth	140–145	0.0	0.1	0.0	0.0	0.4	0.0	0.5	1.1	0.9	2.4	2.5	4.1	6.5	4.9	4.8	13.0	8.2	14.4	1.7
Pharynx	146–149	0.0	0.0	0.0	0.2	0.2	0.2	0.3	0.2	0.1	1.3	0.5	1.0	1.6	1.4	2.5	1.8	2.2	2.2	0.5
Esophagus	150	0.0	0.0	0.0	0.0	0.0	0.0	0.0	0.0	0.8	1.0	1.6	4.5	9.4	10.7	15.9	26.9	18.3	28.6	2.6
Stomach	151	0.1	0.0	0.0	0.0	2.2	5.6	14.5	23.2	34.3	47.4	63.8	91.3	128.4	193.7	254.0	318.8	374.9	300.7	50.1
Colon	153	0.0	0.0	0.0	0.2	0.6	0.4	1.6	2.6	5.3	8.0	17.6	22.2	35.9	49.4	62.5	91.3	75.4	73.1	11.6
Rectum	154	0.0	0.0	0.0	0.1	0.1	0.4	1.6	4.3	5.4	9.0	13.5	19.7	27.4	36.2	40.2	54.4	74.8	68.3	9.3
Liver	155	0.2	0.0	0.0	0.2	0.1	0.3	0.3	0.9	1.9	4.6	7.7	15.8	25.1	38.2	50.7	59.1	86.2	74.1	8.3
Gallbladder *etc.*	156	0.0	0.1	0.0	0.0	0.1	0.5	0.1	0.5	1.7	4.2	5.9	16.8	24.7	30.3	56.6	66.5	59.5	50.0	7.9
Pancreas	157	0.0	0.0	0.0	0.0	0.0	0.3	0.6	0.9	1.2	2.6	5.5	12.1	17.4	27.4	41.3	45.6	53.0	36.1	6.1
Nose, sinuses	160	0.0	0.0	0.0	0.0	0.3	0.0	0.2	0.0	0.2	0.8	1.9	1.4	2.4	5.6	5.2	7.1	7.4	5.9	1.0
Larynx	161	0.0	0.0	0.0	0.0	0.0	0.0	0.0	0.1	0.1	0.1	0.9	0.5	0.4	1.5	2.2	2.9	2.8	4.5	0.3
Lung, trachea	162	0.0	0.0	0.0	0.0	0.0	0.9	0.9	1.8	4.8	9.5	11.0	20.2	40.0	58.0	84.7	85.8	100.1	96.3	12.3
Connective tissue	171	0.6	0.8	0.1	0.1	0.4	0.3	0.4	1.2	0.5	0.5	1.1	2.8	1.6	1.2	1.7	2.2	3.8	3.9	0.9
Skin	172,173	0.0	0.1	0.0	0.3	0.2	0.5	0.8	0.7	1.8	1.9	2.6	3.7	5.6	7.6	12.8	20.4	25.5	48.3	2.6
Other skin	173	0.0	0.1	0.0	0.2	0.1	0.4	0.7	0.4	1.4	1.6	2.1	2.9	4.6	7.3	11.4	17.4	24.3	44.9	2.2
Breast	174–175,2330	0.0	0.0	0.1	0.0	1.1	3.6	12.5	29.4	48.4	58.7	61.7	58.1	57.4	44.9	49.0	42.3	36.5	52.3	24.4
Uterus	179–182,2331	0.0	0.0	0.0	0.0	1.4	4.3	15.6	33.1	42.2	51.7	66.3	67.7	78.4	72.7	81.5	81.0	87.3	50.6	28.9
Uterus	179–182	0.0	0.0	0.0	0.0	1.0	3.0	8.9	21.0	27.8	42.2	56.5	61.9	73.0	68.6	79.6	80.1	87.2	50.3	24.3
Cervix uteri	180	0.0	0.0	0.0	0.0	0.2	2.3	8.1	17.6	23.2	33.2	39.9	44.1	56.2	50.0	58.3	53.3	54.5	21.3	17.9
Corpus uteri	182	0.0	0.0	0.0	0.0	0.0	0.3	0.4	2.8	3.0	6.3	13.2	12.1	9.3	8.8	6.3	12.0	5.2	2.7	3.4
Uterus, unspecified	179	0.0	0.0	0.0	0.0	0.0	0.0	0.2	0.3	1.1	1.8	3.0	5.4	7.5	9.7	14.9	13.7	27.5	26.3	2.6
Ovary *etc.*	183	0.1	0.7	0.8	1.8	1.9	1.8	3.5	5.7	7.3	9.7	13.9	13.2	15.3	14.9	21.0	16.6	13.1	14.1	6.2
Bladder	188	0.0	0.0	0.0	0.0	0.0	0.1	0.4	0.7	0.5	0.7	2.5	1.9	6.8	13.5	24.0	26.0	24.4	27.6	2.7
Kidney *etc.*	189	1.3	0.2	0.0	0.0	0.1	0.0	0.4	0.2	0.6	1.2	1.3	3.7	6.0	6.5	14.3	9.7	6.5	3.6	1.7
Brain, nervous system	191–192	2.1	1.1	1.2	0.6	1.1	0.8	1.2	1.5	2.0	2.2	2.8	2.9	5.1	6.2	4.2	2.8	0.8	0.6	2.0
Thyroid	193	0.2	0.0	0.3	1.0	2.1	1.5	3.7	3.2	5.3	6.8	7.1	6.9	9.2	10.9	15.2	10.0	12.7	15.6	4.2
Lymphatic tissue	200–203	0.7	0.5	0.2	0.8	0.8	0.9	0.4	2.7	2.1	5.6	8.7	11.8	16.5	23.6	24.3	31.3	25.1	17.9	5.4
Non-Hodgkin's lymphoma	200, 202	0.7	0.4	0.2	0.6	0.8	0.8	0.4	2.5	1.7	3.9	6.2	8.5	10.0	12.6	15.0	16.2	15.0	13.6	3.6
Multiple myeloma	203	0.0	0.0	0.0	0.0	0.0	0.0	0.0	0.1	0.1	0.8	2.3	2.7	5.4	9.0	8.4	14.2	8.9	2.3	1.5
Leukemia	204–208	5.4	3.1	2.2	1.6	1.8	2.7	2.2	3.4	4.3	4.6	2.7	5.3	7.4	8.5	8.0	14.0	6.9	12.8	4.0
Lymphoid leukemia	204	3.9	2.3	1.2	0.3	0.5	0.4	0.5	0.7	0.5	1.6	0.7	0.9	1.7	1.8	2.3	3.0	1.5	0.0	1.2
Myeloid leukemia	205	0.5	0.7	0.9	1.2	1.1	1.8	1.5	2.3	2.6	2.0	1.5	3.6	4.2	4.4	3.7	7.7	3.9	8.4	2.0

[a] See text.

TABLE XX-1. Age-Specific Incidence Rates per 100,000 Population (Uncorrected Estimates[a]) in Japan According to Sex and Primary Site (1981), Male

Primary site	ICD, 9th	Age group																		All ages
		0–	5–	10–	15–	20–	25–	30–	35–	40–	45–	50–	55–	60–	65–	70–	75–	80–	85–	
All sites	140–208, 233	14.6	9.7	8.4	9.9	9.7	19.3	36.8	60.4	109.6	227.2	397.0	629.9	922.2	1359.3	1857.8	2227.4	2438.9	2084.3	263.0
All sites	140–208	14.6	9.7	8.4	9.9	9.7	19.3	36.8	60.4	109.6	227.2	397.0	629.9	922.2	1359.3	1857.8	2227.4	2438.9	2084.3	263.0
Mouth	140–145	0.0	0.0	0.3	0.0	0.1	0.5	1.2	1.1	2.4	2.7	6.1	11.4	10.4	12.5	22.2	15.5	22.3	13.3	3.2
Pharynx	146–149	0.0	0.0	0.3	0.2	0.5	0.0	0.3	0.3	0.7	2.5	3.7	5.9	7.7	7.6	11.6	10.4	9.6	4.8	1.8
Esophagus	150	0.0	0.0	0.0	0.0	0.0	0.0	0.0	0.2	1.6	6.1	15.5	26.6	38.2	54.3	81.9	95.9	72.4	90.2	9.8
Stomach	151	0.0	0.2	0.0	0.1	1.2	5.3	11.6	22.4	46.0	87.2	146.5	233.3	338.8	480.5	641.5	717.8	692.7	653.2	92.2
Colon	153	0.0	0.0	0.0	0.0	0.8	1.1	2.3	4.4	6.5	13.8	21.9	31.5	47.1	65.4	98.2	123.7	159.5	130.3	13.9
Rectun	154	0.0	0.0	0.3	0.0	0.0	0.4	2.9	4.1	6.0	14.5	16.5	28.2	46.9	63.8	86.8	97.5	119.4	106.0	12.5
Liver	155	0.2	0.0	0.0	0.0	0.1	0.2	1.7	4.0	11.1	32.7	56.2	81.9	97.1	115.9	138.9	131.3	166.9	131.1	23.9
Gallbladder *etc.*	156	0.0	0.0	0.0	0.0	0.0	0.2	0.1	0.5	1.2	3.3	6.7	12.8	19.7	34.7	52.0	79.8	77.2	56.0	6.3
Pancreas	157	0.0	0.1	0.0	0.1	0.0	0.1	0.9	1.5	2.4	6.5	13.7	20.4	31.1	49.9	66.0	85.9	86.6	44.4	8.9
Nose, sinuses	160	0.0	0.0	0.0	0.1	0.0	0.0	0.4	0.1	0.7	2.1	4.0	3.9	4.9	11.2	8.7	6.4	10.3	3.9	1.6
Larynx	161	0.0	0.0	0.0	0.0	0.0	0.0	0.0	0.1	0.7	2.5	6.2	10.8	17.5	25.5	22.1	37.0	19.5	8.7	3.6
Lung, trachea	162	0.0	0.3	0.0	0.0	0.1	0.4	0.9	3.5	4.7	17.6	37.0	68.7	117.9	216.9	306.0	408.4	439.9	274.7	35.1
Connective tissue	171	0.7	0.2	1.0	0.7	0.4	0.4	0.4	0.6	0.4	1.7	0.9	3.4	3.9	1.9	5.0	4.4	6.9	3.7	1.1
Skin	172, 173	0.0	0.0	0.0	0.0	0.0	0.4	0.4	1.1	1.8	2.0	5.0	7.6	8.8	14.8	20.5	33.2	51.6	54.3	3.3
Other skin	173	0.0	0.0	0.0	0.0	0.0	0.4	0.4	0.6	1.4	1.3	4.2	6.5	8.2	13.0	20.0	27.7	46.5	52.2	2.9
Prostate	185	0.0	0.1	0.0	0.3	0.0	0.0	0.0	0.0	0.0	0.1	2.3	3.9	14.3	32.0	73.0	130.3	169.6	177.9	7.0
Testis	186	1.0	0.2	0.0	0.6	1.2	2.9	2.1	1.8	0.7	1.9	1.2	0.4	0.4	1.0	0.2	1.8	0.4	0.0	1.1
Bladder	188	0.0	0.3	0.1	0.3	0.6	0.5	0.9	2.8	2.5	4.1	10.0	20.6	27.6	45.4	63.1	76.5	118.5	95.7	8.2
Kidney *etc.*	189	1.4	0.1	0.0	0.0	0.0	0.2	0.5	0.7	2.3	2.6	4.5	8.4	15.3	21.4	28.2	25.0	21.4	16.5	3.5
Brain, nervous system	191–192	1.5	1.8	1.3	1.1	0.4	0.9	2.5	2.2	1.7	3.6	2.2	3.9	5.9	7.1	4.6	9.0	3.4	3.5	2.3
Thyroid	193	0.0	0.0	0.1	0.0	0.1	0.3	1.5	1.3	2.0	0.9	1.5	3.4	3.1	3.9	5.0	3.6	8.2	8.7	1.2
Lymphatic tissue	200–203	1.3	1.3	1.3	1.5	0.9	1.3	2.6	3.1	4.1	8.5	15.5	16.0	22.7	38.8	47.5	55.7	65.4	69.8	8.3
Non-Hodgkin's lymphoma	200, 202	1.3	1.2	1.2	1.3	0.7	1.3	2.5	3.0	3.4	7.2	12.2	11.2	16.6	24.6	32.8	40.2	43.8	51.9	6.2
Multiple myeloma	203	0.0	0.0	0.1	0.0	0.0	0.0	0.0	0.1	0.5	1.1	2.8	3.9	4.4	11.6	13.1	13.9	20.3	15.0	1.7
Leukemia	204–208	5.6	4.5	2.8	3.6	1.8	3.0	2.4	3.4	6.2	4.7	7.5	11.4	16.9	18.7	23.0	19.6	28.2	37.6	6.2
Lymphoid leukemia	204	3.5	2.7	2.0	1.1	0.2	1.3	0.3	0.7	1.4	1.2	0.7	1.8	1.8	5.8	3.0	1.6	8.6	5.6	1.7
Myeloid leukemia	205	0.9	1.1	0.4	2.2	1.1	1.5	1.9	2.3	4.0	2.7	5.5	7.3	11.0	9.4	12.0	12.4	9.9	19.9	3.3

[a] See text.

TABLE XX-2. Age-Specific Incidence Rates per 100,000 Population (Uncorrected Estimates[a]) in Japan According to Sex and Primary Site (1981), Female

Primary site	ICD, 9th	Age group																		All ages
		0–	5–	10–	15–	20–	25–	30–	35–	40–	45–	50–	55–	60–	65–	70–	75–	80–	85–	
All sites	140–208, 233	14.1	6.9	6.7	8.5	16.3	26.5	69.4	121.4	181.7	243.1	305.4	399.0	532.1	694.9	930.1	1058.3	1185.7	1097.5	207.3
All sites	140–208	14.1	6.9	6.7	8.5	15.9	24.8	61.9	108.6	166.0	232.6	295.9	392.9	527.5	689.6	928.5	1056.2	1185.5	1097.2	202.3
Mouth	140–145	0.0	0.1	0.0	0.0	0.4	0.1	0.8	1.9	0.9	2.3	3.1	3.6	5.3	5.6	5.5	11.7	9.5	19.8	1.9
Pharynx	146–149	0.1	0.0	0.0	0.1	0.2	0.2	0.3	0.4	0.3	0.7	0.7	0.8	2.4	1.8	1.5	2.0	2.2	2.8	0.5
Esophagus	150	0.0	0.0	0.0	0.0	0.0	0.0	0.0	0.0	0.8	0.9	1.9	4.0	8.7	10.3	13.9	23.7	23.5	22.2	2.5
Stomach	151	0.0	0.0	0.0	0.0	2.3	5.4	14.4	23.4	36.2	48.1	63.6	88.9	124.6	185.0	253.0	305.4	377.2	311.2	50.7
Colon	153	0.0	0.0	0.0	0.1	0.6	0.5	1.9	2.1	7.2	8.4	17.9	24.8	37.3	46.7	73.1	98.4	87.7	80.2	12.9
Rectum	154	0.0	0.0	0.0	0.1	0.2	0.4	1.3	4.1	6.5	10.4	13.1	19.7	28.4	41.2	41.8	49.5	66.4	68.5	9.7
Liver	155	0.3	0.0	0.0	0.2	0.0	0.2	0.7	1.1	3.0	4.7	7.7	16.6	23.7	39.6	54.3	51.8	85.1	76.4	8.6
Gallbladder *etc.*	156	0.0	0.1	0.0	0.0	0.0	0.4	0.1	1.0	1.5	3.8	6.6	14.4	24.2	33.8	61.2	72.5	72.0	55.0	8.5
Pancreas	157	0.0	0.0	0.1	0.0	0.0	0.3	0.3	0.7	1.3	2.2	6.6	11.4	18.7	28.9	42.4	45.5	56.2	37.3	6.4
Nose, sinuses	160	0.0	0.0	0.0	0.0	0.2	0.0	0.2	0.2	0.2	0.9	1.6	1.6	2.8	6.9	6.2	5.7	5.9	5.1	1.0
Larynx	161	0.0	0.0	0.0	0.0	0.0	0.0	0.1	0.0	0.1	0.0	0.5	0.5	0.3	1.7	2.2	4.1	3.9	4.1	0.3
Lung, trachea	162	0.0	0.0	0.0	0.0	0.0	0.7	1.7	2.5	5.3	10.1	13.1	19.9	41.1	58.3	88.7	100.2	103.4	114.2	13.5
Connective tissue	171	0.5	0.3	0.2	0.1	0.6	0.3	0.5	0.9	0.7	0.9	0.9	2.4	2.0	1.1	0.9	2.1	2.9	2.6	0.8
Skin	172,173	0.2	0.1	0.0	0.4	0.1	0.3	1.0	0.8	2.2	2.3	1.9	4.6	4.7	8.4	14.0	23.4	36.3	49.2	3.0
Other skin	173	0.1	0.1	0.0	0.2	0.1	0.3	0.8	0.5	1.7	1.6	1.7	3.7	4.0	8.2	12.3	21.2	35.2	45.9	2.6
Breast	174–175, 2330	0.0	0.0	0.1	0.1	1.5	3.3	15.1	31.0	48.3	60.5	55.6	55.7	58.7	44.2	51.4	41.9	43.9	47.3	25.0
Uterus	179–182, 2331	0.0	0.0	0.0	0.2	1.2	4.9	17.8	32.8	41.2	48.5	58.9	69.0	68.7	68.0	78.5	69.0	69.3	52.5	27.8
Uterus	179–182	0.0	0.0	0.0	0.2	0.8	3.2	10.5	20.6	26.5	38.4	49.7	63.8	64.2	63.5	77.0	66.8	69.2	52.3	23.1
Cervix uteri	180	0.0	0.0	0.0	0.0	0.2	2.2	9.8	17.3	21.1	30.4	34.5	45.3	48.7	45.9	54.4	44.6	42.8	20.1	16.9
Corpus uteri	182	0.0	0.0	0.0	0.2	0.0	0.4	0.4	2.4	3.8	5.8	12.4	13.5	9.8	8.9	9.0	9.7	5.6	2.2	3.6
Uterus, unspecified.	179	0.0	0.0	0.0	0.0	0.0	0.1	0.2	0.6	1.2	1.5	2.5	4.6	5.6	8.7	13.6	12.5	20.8	29.9	2.4
Ovary *etc.*	183	0.0	0.3	0.9	1.9	1.4	2.1	2.6	4.5	7.4	11.8	15.3	13.8	15.9	17.9	20.7	14.1	12.0	14.5	6.4
Bladder	188	0.0	0.0	0.0	0.0	0.0	0.0	0.3	0.4	0.5	0.6	2.5	2.6	5.5	12.9	20.2	22.9	24.3	27.8	2.6
Kidney *etc.*	189	1.2	0.2	0.0	0.0	0.2	0.1	0.3	0.6	0.7	1.5	2.1	5.1	5.3	6.4	14.6	10.8	5.2	2.8	1.9
Brain, nervous system	191–192	2.8	1.4	1.3	0.8	1.1	1.2	1.0	1.9	2.2	2.5	2.9	2.2	5.6	7.4	5.2	2.4	1.4	0.8	2.2
Thyroid	193	0.1	0.0	0.1	0.8	2.2	2.0	3.6	3.4	4.6	6.3	7.4	7.3	8.8	12.5	14.2	12.0	12.8	8.9	4.2
Lymphatic tissue	200–203	0.7	0.5	0.4	0.7	0.7	0.6	0.8	2.3	2.6	5.8	8.4	12.2	16.6	24.0	23.4	27.6	29.3	18.4	5.5
Non-Hodgkin's lymphoma	200, 202	0.7	0.5	0.4	0.6	0.7	0.5	0.7	2.1	2.4	4.3	6.1	9.1	10.4	14.0	15.1	15.0	19.8	11.7	3.8
Multiple myeloma	203	0.0	0.0	0.0	0.0	0.0	0.0	0.0	0.1	0.1	1.1	2.2	2.6	4.6	8.7	8.0	11.7	9.0	6.7	1.5
Leukemia	204–208	5.7	3.1	2.5	1.8	1.5	2.6	2.7	3.5	4.1	4.8	4.4	6.0	7.4	8.3	9.2	14.1	9.5	14.2	4.4
Lymphoid leukemia	204	3.9	2.3	1.3	0.6	0.6	0.4	0.5	1.2	0.8	2.2	1.6	1.1	2.2	3.1	2.3	3.2	1.1	0.0	1.5
Myeloid leukemia	205	0.8	0.7	1.0	1.2	0.8	1.7	1.7	2.0	2.1	2.1	1.8	3.9	3.7	2.9	4.7	7.1	5.7	12.3	2.1

[a] See text.

TABLE XXI-1. Age-Specific Incidence Rates per 100,000 Population (Uncorrected Estimates[a]) in Japan According to Sex and Primary Site (1982), Male

Primary site	ICD, 9th	Age group																		All ages
		0–	5–	10–	15–	20–	25–	30–	35–	40–	45–	50–	55–	60–	65–	70–	75–	80–	85–	
All sites	140–208, 233	13.6	10.3	8.3	8.6	11.1	20.4	36.4	57.6	116.4	229.6	415.7	656.5	918.6	1388.5	1883.0	2264.2	2610.2	2294.8	276.9
All sites	140–208	13.6	10.3	8.3	8.6	11.1	20.4	36.4	57.6	116.4	229.6	415.7	656.5	918.6	1388.5	1883.0	2264.2	2610.2	2294.8	276.9
Mouth	140–145	0.0	0.0	0.3	0.0	0.1	0.5	1.1	0.9	3.2	3.4	5.3	10.7	9.6	14.6	23.6	19.6	19.9	15.3	3.4
Pharynx	146–149	0.0	0.0	0.3	0.1	0.2	0.0	0.3	0.4	0.8	2.0	4.3	6.4	7.9	7.1	9.5	11.8	15.5	4.9	1.9
Esophagus	150	0.0	0.0	0.0	0.0	0.0	0.0	0.0	0.5	1.8	6.1	16.7	30.4	36.6	56.1	84.6	96.1	87.7	70.2	10.5
Stomach	151	0.0	0.1	0.0	0.2	1.8	5.6	12.0	22.1	48.3	86.4	148.6	233.8	323.2	469.5	610.3	716.3	738.6	660.1	93.8
Colon	153	0.0	0.0	0.0	0.0	0.8	1.1	2.3	4.8	7.9	14.7	24.3	39.1	51.5	74.5	103.8	124.2	186.2	172.4	16.0
Rectum	154	0.0	0.0	0.3	0.0	0.0	0.3	1.8	3.6	7.7	15.5	20.8	29.4	45.5	66.4	93.3	99.9	129.3	129.8	13.6
Liver	155	0.2	0.0	0.0	0.0	0.1	0.4	1.8	3.9	10.6	32.8	65.6	91.6	103.8	120.8	143.1	144.2	183.4	114.4	26.3
Gallbladder *etc.*	156	0.0	0.0	0.0	0.0	0.0	0.0	0.2	0.4	1.7	4.1	6.9	13.0	21.3	37.0	59.5	76.5	98.6	83.7	7.1
Pancreas	157	0.0	0.0	0.0	0.0	0.0	0.1	1.1	1.5	2.1	6.7	13.1	19.1	32.5	53.4	63.3	83.2	84.3	69.6	9.1
Nose, sinuses	160	0.0	0.0	0.0	0.2	0.0	0.0	0.3	0.1	0.5	1.9	4.3	3.1	6.1	8.8	9.1	6.9	7.6	12.4	1.6
Larynx	161	0.0	0.0	0.0	0.0	0.0	0.0	0.1	0.3	0.6	1.8	5.8	11.9	19.6	25.9	23.8	41.8	24.0	15.4	4.0
Lung, trachea	162	0.0	0.3	0.0	0.0	0.1	0.5	1.0	2.8	4.7	19.3	36.9	72.2	122.2	223.1	318.3	397.0	474.1	327.6	37.4
Connective tissue	171	0.5	0.2	1.3	0.6	0.3	0.3	0.7	0.4	0.4	1.6	0.7	2.3	2.6	1.7	6.7	4.4	7.5	3.9	1.1
Skin	172, 173	0.0	0.0	0.0	0.0	0.0	0.4	0.5	1.1	1.7	2.8	4.9	8.8	7.2	17.2	20.5	27.6	52.2	55.4	3.5
Other skin	173	0.0	0.0	0.0	0.0	0.0	0.4	0.5	0.9	1.2	2.1	4.3	8.1	6.5	15.7	19.4	21.4	49.7	53.0	3.1
Prostate	185	0.0	0.1	0.0	0.3	0.0	0.0	0.0	0.0	0.0	0.1	1.5	4.4	13.4	35.8	79.9	141.8	189.6	185.4	7.7
Testis	186	1.1	0.2	0.0	0.4	2.0	2.4	2.5	1.8	1.3	1.7	1.7	0.4	0.6	0.6	0.8	0.4	1.0	4.7	1.2
Bladder	188	0.0	0.0	0.2	0.1	0.4	0.9	0.7	2.1	2.3	5.5	11.9	22.2	27.0	48.7	65.3	81.9	116.4	98.4	8.9
Kidney *etc.*	189	1.3	0.1	0.0	0.0	0.0	0.1	0.5	0.3	2.0	3.1	5.6	8.5	15.8	19.8	32.2	24.0	14.7	26.2	3.7
Brain, nervous system	191–192	1.9	2.5	1.3	0.8	0.5	1.4	2.2	2.1	2.0	2.8	2.2	5.1	4.7	6.9	5.0	9.4	5.6	3.2	2.5
Thyroid	193	0.0	0.0	0.0	0.0	0.1	0.5	1.1	1.4	2.2	0.9	1.3	3.4	3.0	3.3	6.6	5.6	11.1	8.0	1.2
Lymphatic tissue	200–203	1.2	1.2	1.0	1.1	1.3	1.1	2.4	2.9	4.2	5.4	12.6	15.2	26.2	39.1	46.6	59.3	59.6	77.6	8.0
Non-Hodgkin's lymphoma	200, 202	1.2	1.1	0.9	1.0	1.0	0.9	2.0	2.7	3.8	4.5	10.2	10.1	20.1	23.1	32.7	43.4	41.8	58.7	6.0
Multiple myeloma	203	0.0	0.0	0.1	0.0	0.0	0.0	0.0	0.2	0.3	0.9	2.0	3.6	4.5	13.0	12.7	14.4	16.8	18.4	1.6
Leukemia	204–208	4.8	5.0	2.5	3.5	1.6	2.9	1.9	2.8	6.0	4.9	10.1	11.9	14.0	20.6	25.1	26.5	24.4	38.8	6.4
Lymphoid leukemia	204	3.0	3.3	1.8	1.2	0.4	1.5	0.1	0.5	1.8	1.7	2.4	2.9	2.9	6.1	5.1	3.0	7.2	5.6	2.0
Myeloid leukemia	205	0.6	1.0	0.2	1.9	0.7	1.2	1.6	1.7	3.5	2.5	5.7	6.8	7.1	8.0	13.1	16.2	8.4	22.0	3.0

[a] See text.

TABLE XXI-2. Age-Specific Incidence Rates per 100,000 Population (Uncorrected Estimates[a]) in Japan According to Sex and Primary Site (1982), Female

Primary site	ICD, 9th	Age group																		All ages
		0–	5–	10–	15–	20–	25–	30–	35–	40–	45–	50–	55–	60–	65–	70–	75–	80–	85–	
All sites	140–208, 233	14.5	8.2	7.0	9.1	16.5	27.2	75.7	114.4	184.0	238.7	312.0	397.5	523.2	708.9	937.1	1061.8	1241.7	1188.0	214.6
All sites	140–208	14.5	8.2	7.0	9.1	16.1	25.7	66.6	100.3	166.7	225.4	302.9	391.1	517.7	703.3	935.2	1059.2	1241.6	1186.8	209.0
Mouth	140–145	0.0	0.1	0.0	0.2	0.3	0.3	1.1	1.4	0.8	2.0	2.9	3.6	5.2	6.5	6.1	8.0	11.3	29.7	2.0
Pharynx	146–149	0.1	0.0	0.0	0.1	0.2	0.2	0.3	0.3	0.2	0.8	0.9	1.2	2.7	3.4	1.9	2.8	1.4	1.6	0.7
Esophagus	150	0.0	0.0	0.0	0.0	0.0	0.0	0.0	0.0	0.5	0.8	1.6	3.0	6.2	11.5	13.8	21.4	28.2	31.4	2.4
Stomach	151	0.0	0.0	0.0	0.0	2.3	6.6	14.4	21.3	35.1	44.6	66.1	88.8	120.8	182.7	251.5	301.1	362.5	322.7	51.4
Colon	153	0.0	0.0	0.0	0.3	0.8	0.6	2.0	2.8	7.1	10.5	18.2	28.9	41.3	49.0	83.7	97.0	110.6	99.0	14.7
Rectum	154	0.0	0.0	0.0	0.0	0.2	0.4	1.4	3.1	6.7	10.9	13.2	21.2	30.8	39.2	47.9	48.3	68.4	59.0	10.1
Liver	155	0.4	0.0	0.1	0.1	0.0	0.4	1.0	0.8	3.3	4.4	9.0	18.2	29.2	40.8	55.2	59.8	94.9	82.2	9.7
Gallbladder *etc.*	156	0.0	0.0	0.0	0.0	0.0	0.5	0.3	1.1	1.7	3.8	7.9	13.5	20.9	36.8	58.6	69.6	86.0	54.0	8.8
Pancreas	157	0.0	0.0	0.1	0.0	0.0	0.4	0.3	0.5	1.9	2.8	7.2	10.7	17.5	32.2	43.8	55.5	59.4	46.1	7.1
Nose, sinuses	160	0.0	0.0	0.0	0.0	0.1	0.1	0.1	0.2	0.5	0.7	1.3	1.7	3.1	5.8	6.6	4.1	7.6	4.4	1.0
Larynx	161	0.0	0.0	0.0	0.0	0.0	0.0	0.1	0.0	0.0	0.0	0.6	1.7	0.8	2.1	1.8	3.9	1.9	3.3	0.4
Lung, trachea	162	0.0	0.0	0.0	0.1	0.0	0.5	1.6	2.6	5.0	8.9	13.8	20.1	39.4	57.6	89.4	102.6	113.9	115.1	13.9
Connective tissue	171	0.6	0.4	0.2	0.1	0.6	0.3	0.4	0.9	1.2	1.3	1.2	1.2	1.6	1.4	0.8	1.4	2.2	4.2	0.8
Skin	172,173	0.2	0.1	0.2	0.2	0.1	0.1	1.1	1.0	2.1	3.2	3.2	3.7	5.3	11.4	16.2	23.0	37.2	65.3	3.5
Other skin	173	0.2	0.1	0.0	0.0	0.1	0.0	0.9	0.6	1.5	2.7	2.6	3.1	4.8	10.7	13.9	21.4	36.1	63.9	3.1
Breast	174–175,2330	0.0	0.0	0.1	0.1	1.6	3.1	16.7	31.2	48.7	60.0	54.8	56.2	64.5	52.0	50.1	47.7	43.0	36.6	26.0
Uterus	179–182,2331	0.0	0.0	0.0	0.2	1.1	4.2	19.1	30.2	41.7	46.3	55.7	65.5	58.9	61.3	67.2	64.3	65.5	59.5	26.6
Uterus	179–182	0.0	0.0	0.0	0.2	0.7	2.7	10.3	16.8	25.5	33.9	47.0	59.5	53.7	57.3	65.7	62.3	65.3	58.4	21.3
Cervix uteri	180	0.0	0.0	0.0	0.0	0.2	2.0	9.4	13.9	20.5	24.9	32.2	40.3	40.8	42.3	46.6	39.3	41.4	23.2	15.3
Corpus uteri	182	0.0	0.0	0.0	0.1	0.0	0.2	0.7	2.2	3.6	6.9	12.3	15.2	8.5	7.2	7.1	7.3	4.9	4.9	3.6
Uterus, unspecified	179	0.0	0.0	0.0	0.0	0.0	0.2	0.2	0.6	0.9	1.9	2.2	3.6	4.5	7.7	12.0	15.7	19.1	30.4	2.3
Ovary *etc.*	183	0.2	0.3	0.9	2.0	1.5	2.2	3.1	4.1	6.5	11.9	15.0	13.1	14.6	18.5	19.7	17.5	14.0	18.7	6.5
Bladder	188	0.0	0.0	0.0	0.0	0.0	0.2	0.3	0.3	0.4	0.4	2.5	2.9	4.7	15.6	18.6	22.9	23.9	38.6	2.8
Kidney *etc.*	189	0.9	0.1	0.0	0.0	0.0	0.2	0.3	0.5	1.9	0.8	2.6	5.0	5.4	8.8	16.2	11.6	4.8	5.9	2.1
Brain, nervous system	191–192	3.1	1.5	1.2	0.9	1.1	1.1	1.1	1.8	1.5	1.9	2.9	3.1	5.2	6.8	4.6	2.1	1.9	1.0	2.1
Thyroid	193	0.1	0.0	0.0	0.8	2.0	1.9	4.8	4.0	6.4	5.8	10.3	7.4	7.7	11.8	12.5	12.9	15.4	7.0	4.6
Lymphatic tissue	200–203	0.8	0.5	0.6	0.3	1.4	1.1	1.2	1.6	3.1	5.9	7.5	11.4	15.0	23.2	26.4	26.5	26.9	16.9	5.6
Non-Hodgkin's lymphoma	200, 202	0.8	0.4	0.6	0.3	1.4	0.9	1.0	1.4	3.0	4.7	5.5	9.0	8.6	14.6	18.0	16.6	19.0	10.6	4.0
Multiple myeloma	203	0.0	0.0	0.0	0.0	0.0	0.0	0.0	0.1	0.1	1.0	1.8	2.1	4.8	8.2	8.2	9.1	7.9	6.3	1.4
Leukemia	204–208	5.1	4.0	2.7	1.9	1.4	2.3	3.2	2.4	3.2	5.9	5.2	6.3	7.0	9.2	8.6	11.7	7.0	19.6	4.4
Lymphoid leukemia	204	3.7	3.2	1.2	0.4	0.7	0.2	0.4	1.0	0.4	2.3	1.9	1.2	2.4	4.3	1.9	4.4	1.2	3.0	1.6
Myeloid leukemia	205	0.6	0.4	1.3	1.3	0.6	1.4	2.1	1.0	1.8	3.0	2.1	3.9	3.4	3.1	4.8	5.5	4.3	11.5	2.0

[a] See text.

TABLE XXII-1. Age-Specific Incidence Rates per 100,000 Population (Uncorrected Estimates[a]) in Japan According to Sex and Primary Site (1983), Male

Primary site	ICD, 9th	Age group																		All ages
		0–	5–	10–	15–	20–	25–	30–	35–	40–	45–	50–	55–	60–	65–	70–	75–	80–	85–	
All sites	140–208, 233	11.6	10.5	8.1	8.8	12.5	19.6	38.4	57.8	122.5	230.4	430.3	674.1	941.0	1390.9	1889.1	2278.9	2598.8	2412.5	287.7
All sites	140–208	11.6	10.5	8.1	8.8	12.5	19.6	38.4	57.8	122.5	230.4	430.3	674.1	941.0	1390.9	1889.1	2278.9	2598.8	2412.5	287.7
Mouth	140–145	0.0	0.0	0.2	0.0	0.1	0.4	2.0	0.7	2.8	4.1	7.4	11.7	8.9	13.6	19.1	19.3	20.1	29.6	3.6
Pharynx	146–149	0.0	0.0	0.1	0.1	0.0	0.1	0.1	1.1	1.1	2.1	4.1	6.0	7.4	7.7	10.4	12.0	14.0	6.5	2.0
Esophagus	150	0.0	0.0	0.0	0.0	0.0	0.0	0.0	0.4	2.2	6.7	15.5	28.9	41.2	57.8	75.2	92.9	87.9	70.8	10.7
Stomach	151	0.0	0.0	0.0	0.1	1.5	4.4	12.6	21.8	47.6	82.1	155.0	233.4	322.3	462.1	599.0	699.9	773.2	726.2	95.5
Colon	153	0.0	0.0	0.1	0.0	0.9	0.8	2.4	5.1	8.6	15.5	28.0	46.7	55.8	78.6	117.8	149.7	181.8	151.3	18.1
Rectum	154	0.0	0.0	0.3	0.1	0.2	0.2	1.7	2.6	8.9	15.4	22.3	31.6	44.5	66.3	87.9	101.8	126.2	128.1	13.9
Liver	155	0.0	0.0	0.0	0.0	0.2	0.3	1.8	5.3	11.6	32.3	71.2	101.1	113.3	127.3	151.5	143.5	176.5	142.6	28.8
Gallbladder *etc.*	156	0.0	0.0	0.0	0.0	0.0	0.0	0.2	0.4	2.0	5.0	5.9	10.8	18.7	43.8	60.3	71.7	89.2	95.3	7.2
Pancreas	157	0.0	0.0	0.0	0.0	0.0	0.0	1.0	1.3	2.1	5.5	13.7	21.0	31.7	50.2	61.9	79.6	95.3	72.9	9.2
Nose, sinuses	160	0.0	0.0	0.0	0.2	0.0	0.1	0.3	0.1	0.6	1.6	3.7	3.2	5.2	9.5	10.2	6.3	6.8	8.3	1.5
Larynx	161	0.0	0.0	0.0	0.0	0.0	0.0	0.2	0.1	1.0	2.2	5.8	10.3	19.4	23.1	30.8	37.4	21.6	23.6	4.1
Lung, trachea	162	0.0	0.0	0.0	0.0	0.0	0.5	1.7	3.1	7.3	20.9	38.8	72.9	127.6	220.7	319.4	411.4	461.6	368.3	39.3
Connective tissue	171	0.5	0.3	1.3	0.7	0.4	0.4	0.6	0.4	0.5	1.2	0.9	3.3	3.1	1.7	7.0	5.7	11.5	4.5	1.2
Skin	172, 173	0.0	0.0	0.0	0.1	0.0	0.4	0.6	1.0	1.6	2.4	4.0	7.7	8.1	18.4	21.2	21.8	51.8	57.2	3.5
Other skin	173	0.0	0.0	0.0	0.1	0.0	0.4	0.6	0.8	1.3	1.9	3.7	6.8	7.6	16.3	19.9	17.2	49.2	55.4	3.1
Prostate	185	0.0	0.1	0.0	0.3	0.0	0.0	0.1	0.0	0.1	0.2	1.7	6.2	15.3	39.5	88.5	138.6	174.1	182.0	8.3
Testis	186	0.7	0.0	0.0	0.7	2.3	2.3	3.3	1.4	1.4	1.5	1.3	0.5	1.2	0.8	1.1	0.4	0.8	4.3	1.3
Bladder	188	0.0	0.0	0.2	0.2	0.2	0.8	0.6	1.3	2.1	5.7	10.0	21.2	29.8	49.1	60.8	90.8	110.3	104.2	9.0
Kidney *etc.*	189	0.6	0.2	0.0	0.0	0.1	0.2	0.4	0.6	1.4	4.1	6.5	10.5	16.5	21.5	30.3	27.6	17.4	27.0	4.1
Brain, nervous system	191–192	1.6	2.5	1.6	0.8	0.9	1.6	1.5	2.9	1.9	3.0	3.3	5.7	3.9	8.2	5.3	7.0	6.2	1.4	2.6
Thyroid	193	0.0	0.1	0.1	0.0	0.0	0.7	1.0	0.9	1.8	1.1	1.8	2.5	3.6	3.1	7.0	5.9	9.1	6.0	1.3
Lymphatic tissue	200–203	0.9	1.6	1.0	1.3	1.5	1.0	2.5	3.7	4.9	5.6	10.3	15.0	26.3	36.3	44.1	58.6	57.7	81.1	8.0
Non-Hodgkin's lymphoma	200, 202	0.9	1.3	1.0	1.3	1.2	0.8	2.1	2.9	4.2	4.8	8.6	10.2	17.7	23.6	30.8	43.1	40.8	58.8	5.9
Multiple myeloma	203	0.0	0.1	0.0	0.0	0.0	0.0	0.0	0.1	0.5	0.7	1.5	3.0	6.9	10.6	11.1	14.5	16.3	19.8	1.6
Leukemia	204–208	3.8	4.9	2.0	2.4	1.9	3.7	2.5	2.2	5.9	6.3	9.3	9.8	16.0	19.6	27.0	31.2	24.1	30.7	6.4
Lymphoid leukemia	204	2.3	3.9	1.2	1.0	0.5	1.4	0.5	0.4	2.0	2.4	2.8	2.3	5.0	5.6	5.4	7.6	5.3	0.9	2.1
Myeloid leukemia	205	0.5	0.5	0.4	1.1	1.2	2.1	1.7	1.3	3.3	3.1	5.0	5.5	7.5	7.7	14.7	16.2	9.9	22.0	3.0

[a] See text.

TABLE XXII-2. Age-Specific Incidence Rates per 100,000 Population (Uncorrected Estimates[a]) in Japan According to Sex and Primary Site (1983), Female

Primary site	ICD, 9th	Age group 0–	5–	10–	15–	20–	25–	30–	35–	40–	45–	50–	55–	60–	65–	70–	75–	80–	85–	All ages
All sites	140–208,233	13.4	8.1	7.1	8.6	15.9	27.9	73.4	110.7	185.9	240.3	320.7	407.3	530.0	702.7	921.7	1074.2	1316.2	1215.2	221.5
All sites	140–208	13.4	8.1	7.1	8.6	15.3	26.2	64.8	97.2	170.4	225.9	312.8	400.4	525.0	697.4	919.4	1071.5	1314.5	1212.9	216.0
Mouth	140–145	0.2	0.1	0.1	0.2	0.1	0.5	1.5	1.6	1.0	1.2	3.2	3.7	4.8	6.4	7.5	10.7	11.8	24.6	2.2
Pharynx	146–149	0.1	0.0	0.0	0.0	0.2	0.0	0.0	0.3	0.2	1.2	1.1	1.6	2.5	3.0	2.2	1.9	0.8	3.0	0.7
Esophagus	150	0.0	0.0	0.0	0.0	0.0	0.0	0.1	0.0	0.5	0.6	1.7	2.9	5.3	10.7	14.6	18.7	31.7	36.3	2.5
Stomach	151	0.0	0.0	0.0	0.0	3.1	7.4	14.6	20.8	35.7	44.0	67.3	89.5	120.7	178.0	252.2	291.9	359.3	322.7	52.7
Colon	153	0.0	0.0	0.0	0.2	0.5	0.5	1.8	3.1	6.4	12.3	19.5	28.2	47.2	54.1	86.8	97.3	126.2	110.0	16.1
Rectum	154	0.0	0.0	0.0	0.0	0.3	0.1	1.0	2.2	6.6	10.4	15.9	20.3	29.2	40.1	44.4	57.1	77.3	59.9	10.6
Liver	155	0.4	0.1	0.1	0.0	0.0	0.3	0.9	1.0	3.5	4.3	9.6	20.0	30.3	39.0	55.0	66.3	84.9	79.7	10.2
Gallbladder *etc.*	156	0.0	0.0	0.0	0.0	0.0	0.1	0.3	0.9	2.5	4.3	9.3	13.5	22.9	40.6	61.1	67.8	96.7	64.4	9.8
Pancreas	157	0.0	0.0	0.1	0.0	0.0	0.1	0.4	0.6	1.8	2.7	6.5	10.7	18.1	30.4	43.0	54.8	65.9	53.6	7.2
Nose, sinuses	160	0.0	0.3	0.0	0.0	0.0	0.2	0.2	0.4	0.5	0.7	1.5	1.8	2.9	4.1	5.1	4.1	7.5	4.1	1.0
Larynx	161	0.0	0.0	0.0	0.0	0.0	0.0	0.1	0.1	0.0	0.0	0.5	1.7	1.1	1.2	1.2	3.5	1.9	0.9	0.4
Lung, trachea	162	0.0	0.0	0.0	0.2	0.0	0.3	2.1	1.9	5.5	7.7	14.2	21.0	39.5	58.2	86.1	115.1	141.6	107.4	14.9
Connective tissue	171	0.6	0.2	0.2	0.0	0.6	0.2	0.6	0.2	1.1	1.3	0.7	1.0	1.0	2.8	1.0	1.2	1.6	4.2	0.7
Skin	172, 173	0.2	0.0	0.4	0.1	0.2	0.3	0.7	0.5	2.1	3.6	4.4	4.2	6.1	10.4	15.1	20.8	39.9	61.9	3.7
Other skin	173	0.2	0.0	0.0	0.0	0.2	0.2	0.5	0.3	1.3	3.0	3.7	3.5	5.6	9.1	13.1	19.7	38.9	59.0	3.2
Breast	174–175,2330	0.0	0.0	0.1	0.1	1.5	3.7	16.6	31.0	51.3	64.4	56.5	59.7	64.0	54.9	47.5	49.2	40.9	37.9	27.2
Uterus	179–182,2331	0.0	0.0	0.1	0.2	0.9	4.4	17.6	28.4	38.5	45.2	52.7	64.4	56.3	57.8	60.4	66.0	62.3	47.2	25.6
Uterus	179–182	0.0	0.0	0.1	0.2	0.4	2.8	9.2	15.7	24.0	32.3	45.3	58.0	51.7	54.4	58.6	64.1	60.6	46.4	20.6
Cervix uteri	180	0.0	0.0	0.0	0.0	0.3	1.6	8.3	12.8	19.1	23.5	31.1	38.8	39.7	41.6	40.2	40.8	37.8	20.1	14.7
Corpus uteri	182	0.0	0.0	0.1	0.2	0.0	0.5	0.7	1.8	3.0	6.7	12.1	15.8	8.2	6.6	7.7	6.7	5.2	5.2	3.6
Uterus, unspecified	179	0.0	0.0	0.0	0.0	0.0	0.2	0.0	0.8	1.3	1.6	2.1	3.4	3.9	6.2	10.7	16.7	17.7	21.1	2.1
Ovary *etc.*	183	0.2	0.2	0.3	1.7	1.8	2.2	2.7	3.9	6.9	11.4	14.3	15.0	15.0	18.0	19.7	18.0	13.5	23.4	6.5
Bladder	188	0.0	0.0	0.0	0.0	0.0	0.2	0.4	0.1	1.0	0.7	2.8	3.7	6.0	13.9	16.6	22.9	29.1	35.8	3.0
Kidney *etc.*	189	0.7	0.0	0.0	0.0	0.1	0.2	0.2	0.7	1.6	1.1	3.4	4.4	5.4	8.5	13.6	12.1	6.7	8.4	2.2
Brain, nervous system	191–192	2.5	1.7	1.4	0.8	1.2	1.3	1.5	1.6	1.6	2.3	3.7	3.9	5.6	6.3	4.0	3.5	2.9	1.1	2.4
Thyroid	193	0.0	0.0	0.1	0.6	1.8	2.4	4.5	5.6	6.9	5.9	11.2	9.0	8.6	10.5	10.2	13.3	13.4	9.6	4.8
Lymphatic tissue	200–203	0.9	0.6	0.9	0.7	1.3	1.3	1.3	0.8	3.8	5.1	7.0	9.5	15.7	19.9	28.2	24.1	28.8	24.7	5.5
Non-Hodgkin's lymphoma	200,202	0.9	0.5	0.9	0.6	1.2	1.1	1.1	0.7	3.5	4.3	5.3	6.8	8.6	13.7	19.5	15.7	16.9	17.8	3.9
Multiple myeloma	203	0.0	0.0	0.0	0.0	0.0	0.0	0.0	0.0	0.2	0.8	1.3	2.5	5.5	5.4	8.2	8.2	11.9	6.7	1.4
Leukemia	204–208	4.9	3.7	2.2	1.7	0.7	1.8	2.4	2.1	2.8	4.4	5.5	7.5	6.9	10.7	11.3	13.1	12.0	20.9	4.4
Lymphoid leukemia	204	3.3	2.6	0.9	0.5	0.3	0.3	0.1	1.0	0.4	1.2	1.9	1.7	2.3	4.3	2.5	4.8	5.3	2.8	1.5
Myeloid leukemia	205	0.6	0.6	1.1	1.0	0.4	0.8	1.6	1.0	1.8	2.7	2.6	4.0	3.2	5.0	6.2	5.8	4.6	12.3	2.0

[a] See text.

TABLE XXIII-1. Age-Specific Incidence Rates per 100,000 Population (Uncorrected Estimates[a]) in Japan According to Sex and Primary Site (1984), Male

Primary site	ICD, 9th	Age group 0–	5–	10–	15–	20–	25–	30–	35–	40–	45–	50–	55–	60–	65–	70–	75–	80–	85–	All ages
All sites	140–208, 233	12.6	8.6	8.9	9.3	13.1	21.2	38.3	62.4	126.8	222.8	433.0	692.3	963.2	1391.4	1897.5	2352.9	2689.7	2606.0	299.6
All sites	140–208	12.6	8.6	8.9	9.3	13.1	21.2	38.3	62.4	126.8	222.8	433.0	692.3	963.2	1391.4	1897.5	2352.9	2689.7	2606.0	299.6
Mouth	140–145	0.0	0.0	0.0	0.0	0.1	0.1	1.7	1.0	2.2	4.1	7.1	9.5	8.0	16.8	19.4	26.7	19.1	28.6	3.6
Pharynx	146–149	0.2	0.0	0.0	0.3	0.1	0.1	0.2	1.2	1.6	1.8	4.0	5.6	8.2	7.5	10.1	15.9	26.1	6.5	2.1
Esophagus	150	0.0	0.0	0.0	0.0	0.0	0.0	0.0	0.7	2.7	6.8	14.0	29.5	40.0	57.5	63.4	93.4	84.4	72.4	10.5
Stomach	151	0.0	0.0	0.0	0.2	1.1	5.5	12.3	22.0	49.2	78.3	151.0	232.0	316.3	442.3	582.5	678.8	757.3	779.0	96.0
Colon	153	0.0	0.0	0.1	0.0	1.0	0.6	2.1	5.8	8.5	14.5	31.0	46.0	59.6	86.7	122.7	162.8	195.2	183.0	19.6
Rectum	154	0.0	0.0	0.0	0.1	0.2	0.3	1.7	2.8	10.2	13.8	22.8	35.8	49.7	74.1	82.8	99.6	134.2	127.9	14.9
Liver	155	0.1	0.1	0.1	0.0	0.2	0.3	1.8	5.0	11.2	30.0	81.8	111.8	123.4	131.9	163.2	168.1	212.3	149.9	32.1
Gallbladder *etc.*	156	0.0	0.0	0.0	0.0	0.1	0.0	0.6	0.7	2.0	5.2	6.3	12.9	19.4	44.3	55.9	79.2	100.9	99.2	7.8
Pancreas	157	0.0	0.0	0.0	0.0	0.0	0.1	1.1	1.2	3.1	6.0	11.5	21.7	33.3	52.2	69.0	86.1	97.8	104.3	9.9
Nose, sinuses	160	0.0	0.0	0.0	0.2	0.0	0.2	0.3	0.2	0.7	1.5	3.1	2.7	4.6	7.3	10.1	11.2	5.6	12.1	1.5
Larynx	161	0.0	0.0	0.0	0.0	0.0	0.0	0.2	0.1	0.9	1.8	5.9	10.3	20.0	21.6	34.4	30.9	30.6	20.7	4.2
Lung, trachea	162	0.0	0.0	0.0	0.0	0.2	0.1	1.8	4.1	6.8	18.8	37.0	81.1	136.2	218.2	316.8	414.1	473.0	390.0	40.9
Connective tissue	171	0.5	0.3	0.6	0.9	0.4	0.4	0.6	0.4	0.7	0.8	1.0	2.0	2.4	2.0	5.0	5.8	9.9	1.7	1.0
Skin	172, 173	0.0	0.0	0.2	0.1	0.0	0.6	0.6	1.6	2.5	2.8	4.1	6.9	9.4	15.4	25.4	27.1	44.4	64.9	3.8
Other skin	173	0.0	0.0	0.2	0.1	0.0	0.5	0.6	1.5	2.0	2.5	3.9	6.0	8.5	14.0	23.5	21.8	42.6	60.9	3.4
Prostate	185	0.0	0.0	0.0	0.0	0.0	0.0	0.1	0.0	0.1	0.2	1.0	6.8	14.7	43.9	91.3	153.2	191.1	213.3	9.2
Testis	186	1.3	0.0	0.0	0.5	2.4	2.2	3.2	1.9	1.7	1.6	1.1	0.2	0.9	1.2	2.6	0.4	0.8	4.1	1.4
Bladder	188	0.0	0.0	0.1	0.2	0.2	0.8	0.6	2.1	2.8	6.1	8.4	18.1	35.1	49.6	69.6	100.1	109.4	109.7	9.6
Kidney *etc.*	189	0.9	0.1	0.0	0.1	0.1	0.3	0.3	1.0	1.9	4.6	7.8	11.1	18.4	25.4	31.6	27.5	26.9	38.4	4.8
Brain, nervous system	191–192	1.5	2.6	1.9	1.5	1.2	1.3	1.7	2.4	2.2	2.5	3.5	5.6	3.4	6.8	6.6	9.7	4.8	1.3	2.7
Thyroid	193	0.0	0.1	0.3	0.0	0.3	1.4	0.9	1.0	1.8	1.7	1.4	3.3	3.4	4.5	6.8	6.7	9.6	6.7	1.5
Lymphatic tissue	200–203	0.6	1.2	1.2	1.1	1.3	1.0	2.1	3.5	4.6	5.7	9.6	14.3	24.3	31.8	42.4	53.0	56.6	69.0	7.6
Non-Hodgkin's lymphoma	200, 202	0.5	0.9	1.2	0.9	1.0	0.8	1.5	2.3	3.9	4.7	7.2	9.7	16.1	20.9	26.2	35.2	33.8	49.0	5.3
Multiple myeloma	203	0.0	0.1	0.0	0.0	0.0	0.0	0.0	0.4	0.5	0.7	2.1	3.2	7.0	8.4	12.9	17.6	21.1	16.9	1.8
Leukemia	204–208	4.7	3.5	2.6	2.4	1.7	4.2	2.9	2.3	6.0	7.1	9.7	11.4	14.4	21.2	27.0	30.4	19.1	32.5	6.7
Lymphoid leukemia	204	3.6	2.9	1.6	1.3	0.3	1.4	0.8	0.6	2.7	3.0	4.0	4.1	5.3	5.9	6.2	7.2	3.7	0.9	2.5
Myeloid leukemia	205	0.8	0.3	0.6	0.7	1.3	2.6	1.9	1.3	2.6	3.3	4.2	5.1	7.1	9.3	12.6	14.6	10.7	25.8	3.0

[a] See text.

TABLE XXIII-2. Age-Specific Incidence Rates per 100,000 Population (Uncorrected Estimates[a]) in Japan According to Sex and Primary Site (1984), Female

Primary site	ICD, 9th	Age group																		All ages
		0–	5–	10–	15–	20–	25–	30–	35–	40–	45–	50–	55–	60–	65–	70–	75–	80–	85–	
All sites	140–208, 233	13.7	8.5	7.6	10.0	15.4	31.3	73.7	113.4	190.8	243.4	316.3	407.2	534.8	688.3	909.7	1121.7	1327.7	1292.6	228.7
All sites	140–208	13.7	8.5	7.6	9.9	14.7	29.0	63.4	98.3	174.4	227.5	307.6	398.8	530.1	683.9	905.9	1120.9	1325.6	1287.9	222.6
Mouth	140–145	0.2	0.1	0.1	0.2	0.1	0.5	1.4	0.8	1.0	1.8	3.1	3.9	5.1	6.8	6.6	9.7	7.4	19.3	2.0
Pharynx	146–149	0.2	0.0	0.0	0.0	0.3	0.0	0.3	0.2	0.1	1.7	0.9	1.9	2.4	2.7	2.0	2.6	0.6	3.9	0.7
Esophagus	150	0.0	0.0	0.0	0.0	0.0	0.0	0.1	0.0	0.9	0.5	1.6	3.0	4.6	10.1	14.6	20.9	29.1	39.2	2.6
Stomach	151	0.0	0.0	0.0	0.4	2.2	8.6	15.5	19.7	33.3	46.9	64.8	85.7	119.8	170.7	246.7	292.7	343.5	334.8	53.0
Colon	153	0.0	0.0	0.0	0.2	0.3	0.7	1.7	3.7	7.2	11.9	22.1	27.4	47.6	57.4	85.4	98.7	133.6	108.6	17.0
Rectum	154	0.0	0.0	0.0	0.0	0.1	0.1	1.1	1.8	8.1	10.8	14.4	20.9	29.8	38.0	44.1	64.8	72.7	58.7	10.9
Liver	155	0.3	0.1	0.1	0.1	0.0	0.3	0.6	1.1	2.2	4.3	9.8	19.2	33.4	42.8	49.6	70.4	90.3	74.5	10.7
Gallbladder *etc.*	156	0.0	0.0	0.0	0.0	0.0	0.2	0.3	0.7	3.2	3.5	9.9	14.9	22.4	41.6	58.2	69.6	99.9	82.7	10.4
Pancreas	157	0.0	0.0	0.0	0.0	0.0	0.1	0.4	0.5	1.8	2.6	5.6	9.9	18.4	27.5	43.8	55.6	74.8	66.0	7.5
Nose, sinuses	160	0.0	0.3	0.0	0.1	0.0	0.2	0.2	0.5	0.6	0.5	1.2	1.4	2.0	2.6	3.3	5.4	7.1	3.9	0.9
Larynx	161	0.0	0.0	0.0	0.0	0.0	0.0	0.0	0.1	0.0	0.0	0.7	1.8	1.0	1.0	1.1	3.3	0.8	1.1	0.4
Lung, trachea	162	0.0	0.0	0.0	0.2	0.0	0.3	1.2	2.4	6.9	6.0	12.5	20.5	36.7	56.6	86.9	118.0	144.2	113.9	15.2
Connective tissue	171	0.8	0.2	0.4	0.2	0.5	0.3	0.4	0.5	0.7	1.0	0.6	0.5	0.9	3.3	1.5	1.8	1.7	9.0	0.8
Skin	172,173	0.0	0.0	0.4	0.1	0.2	0.6	0.3	0.7	2.0	3.5	5.0	4.1	7.0	10.4	15.8	21.1	36.5	55.5	3.8
Other skin	173	0.0	0.0	0.0	0.1	0.2	0.5	0.2	0.5	1.3	2.9	4.2	3.2	6.9	9.2	13.7	20.5	35.2	53.7	3.3
Breast	174–175,2330	0.0	0.0	0.0	0.2	1.1	4.7	14.8	32.1	53.5	66.9	60.9	64.6	65.3	56.7	51.3	52.5	40.9	34.9	28.7
Uterus	179–182,2331	0.0	0.0	0.1	0.1	1.3	5.2	20.3	30.4	41.2	45.7	50.1	62.2	57.4	54.2	56.3	69.1	63.3	61.5	26.3
Uterus	179–182	0.0	0.0	0.1	0.0	0.8	3.0	10.3	16.4	26.1	31.8	42.6	54.7	53.2	50.9	53.4	69.0	61.3	58.2	20.8
Cervix uteri	180	0.0	0.0	0.0	0.0	0.7	2.2	8.4	13.4	21.6	22.7	28.6	34.7	40.0	39.3	36.6	46.3	39.3	31.5	14.8
Corpus uteri	182	0.0	0.0	0.1	0.0	0.0	0.4	1.2	2.0	3.0	6.6	11.8	18.0	9.3	6.9	8.0	6.7	3.3	6.8	3.9
Uterus, unspecified	179	0.0	0.0	0.0	0.0	0.0	0.0	0.4	0.8	1.1	2.0	1.9	2.1	3.9	4.8	8.9	16.0	18.8	19.9	2.0
Ovary *etc.*	183	0.2	0.2	0.4	1.9	2.7	3.1	3.3	4.9	6.7	11.4	13.5	14.3	16.9	16.5	18.6	20.0	19.1	18.5	7.0
Bladder	188	0.2	0.0	0.0	0.0	0.0	0.2	0.6	0.0	1.0	0.9	3.4	3.0	7.2	12.8	15.5	27.2	30.2	46.1	3.3
Kidney *etc.*	189	0.5	0.2	0.0	0.0	0.2	0.1	0.2	0.6	1.6	1.3	2.7	4.5	7.4	8.5	15.6	12.0	11.4	10.9	2.4
Brain, nervous system	191–192	2.0	1.6	1.4	1.0	1.1	1.1	1.8	2.1	1.1	2.5	3.6	4.3	5.7	6.2	5.4	6.6	4.2	2.2	2.5
Thyroid	193	0.0	0.0	0.2	0.8	1.7	2.1	4.3	5.6	7.4	7.3	10.6	10.4	9.6	10.4	11.2	13.3	12.3	12.3	5.1
Lymphatic tissue	200–203	1.0	0.6	0.8	0.8	1.7	1.2	1.3	0.9	3.7	4.6	5.8	9.5	12.8	20.8	27.8	26.2	30.5	31.0	5.7
Non-Hodgkin's lymphoma	200, 202	1.0	0.6	0.8	0.5	1.6	1.0	1.1	0.6	3.4	3.9	3.9	6.2	6.8	14.2	17.5	17.4	13.1	19.3	3.8
Multiple myeloma	203	0.0	0.0	0.0	0.1	0.0	0.0	0.0	0.2	0.3	0.7	1.5	3.0	5.7	5.8	9.3	8.8	16.3	11.5	1.7
Leukemia	204–208	4.6	3.8	2.6	1.8	1.1	1.4	2.3	1.6	2.8	3.7	5.4	9.2	8.7	9.7	11.5	15.4	16.6	23.5	4.7
Lymphoid leukemia	204	3.5	2.5	1.2	0.5	0.6	0.3	0.0	0.5	0.7	0.7	2.1	2.8	3.7	4.0	3.5	6.7	7.8	4.4	1.8
Myeloid leukemia	205	0.2	0.8	1.2	1.2	0.5	0.8	1.8	0.9	1.9	2.6	2.6	4.7	3.7	4.3	5.3	5.5	6.8	11.4	2.1

[a] See text.

CANCER SURVIVAL IN OSAKA

Aya HANAI, Hideaki TSUKUMA,
Tomohiko HIYAMA, and Isaburo FUJIMOTO

*Department of Field Research, Center for Adult Diseases, Osaka**

Survival rates for cancer patients from population-based cancer registries is one of the important indices for evaluating comprehensive cancer medical care in registration areas.

The Osaka Cancer Registry has provided and published five-year survival rates for cancer patients since 1975 by collecting their prognosis through combined passive and active follow up. Three to five percent of the cases were lost during the observation period.

Time trends of five-year relative survival rates for both sexes were prepared according to primary site and 3-year period from 1975 to 1983, as well as according to extent of disease for 1981–1983. Survival rate for all sites of cancer during the most recent period from 1981–1983 was 36.9% for all incident cases and 75.5% for localized cases for both sexes in Osaka.

The cancer patient data bank for specific cancer sites in Japan, managed by organ-specific cancer medical associations, has released reports on patient survival rates (*7*). However, cases in these reports do not constitute a representative sample of all cancer patients from the population, but rather those admitted to a limited number of university hospitals or large hospitals scattered throughout the country. It is therefore difficult to estimate survival rates from these results for cancer patients in a population.

Cancer patient survivals from population-based cancer registries enable evaluation of cancer prevention and cancer medical care activities in the community (*3, 4*). To provide survival, follow-up survey of every cancer patient not known to be dead is necessary. Difficulties in follow-up procedures limit the availability of population-based survival data, except that from Osaka, Yamagata, and Fukui Cancer Registries (*1*). Of these, the Osaka Cancer Registry, having the largest population and a large number of incident cases, has been analyzing and presenting statistically stable data (*2, 5*). This report summarizes patient survival data based on patients diagnosed from 1975 through 1983 in Osaka.

Methods

The first step in the follow-up of registered cases in the Osaka Cancer Registry is a passive one: matching registered patient files with the files of all deaths of Osaka Prefecture residents. The second step is an individual patient survey on those cases surviving 5 years after their first diagnosis; this is done by inquiry to the citizen

* 3-3, Nakamichi 1-chome, Higashinari-ku, Osaka 537, Japan (花井　彩，津熊秀明，日山興彦，藤本伊三郎)

register with the support of health center personnel.

The subjects of this report were 69,432 reported cases diagnosed during 1975–1983 in Osaka Prefecture (excluding those living in Osaka City). Of these, 4.4% were lost in the follow-up (*5*).

Relative survival rates (RSR) were calculated by the actuarial method (*6*). Cumulative survival rates were calculated first, and these were then divided by the expected survival rates of the patient groups based on mortality in the general population of Japan. Expected survival rates used in calculating relative rates were obtained from the National Cancer Center.

Results

Table I shows 5-year RSR for both sexes together with the number of cases observed and the standard error according to primary site and 3-year period during the period from 1975–1983. Trends of 5-year RSR for major sites are illustrated in Fig. 1. The breast, uterus, and bladder showed survival rates higher than 60%, while all sites and the stomach, colon, and rectum showed rates of around 40%. Rates for the lung, liver, esophagus, pancreas, and gallbladder were below 12%.

Table II shows 5-year RSR of reported cases diagnosed in 1981–1983 according to the extent of disease: localized, regional lymph node metastasis, direct extension to the adjacent organs or tissues, and distant metastasis. The curves of RSR after diagnosis are illustrated in Fig. 2. Two classes of regional spread in Table II appeared in total in these charts under the category designated "regional". Localized patients showed high rates of survival in most sites.

Acknowledgments

Authors would like to acknowledge the Osaka Prefectural Government, the Osaka Medical Association, all medical institutions and health centers in Osaka Prefecture, and the City Health Departments of both Sakai City and Higashi-Osaka City. This study was supported partly by a grant-in-aid (2-5 & 5-3) from the Ministry of Health and Welfare, Japan.

REFERENCES

1. Fujimoto, I., Hanai, A., Kitagawa, T., Morinaga, K., and Ominato, S. Regional cancer registry. *Taisya*, **27**, 361–369 (1990) (in Japanese).
2. Hanai, A. and Fujimoto, I. Five-year survival rates for cancer patients in Osaka. *Jpn. J. Cancer Clin.*, **27**, 589–601 (1981) (in Japanese).
3. Hanai, A. and Fujimoto, I. Survival rate as an index in evaluating cancer control. *In* "The Role of the Registry in Cancer Control," IARC Scientific Publications No. 66, eds. D.M. Parkin, G. Wagner, and C.S. Muir, pp.87–107 (1985). IARC, Lyon.
4. Hanai, A. and Fujimoto, I. Evaluation of cancer care by the measure of survival for cancer patients. *In* "Clinical Epidemiology on Cancer," Progress in Cancer Clinics No. 36, eds. K. Suemasu and A. Oshima, pp.83–92 (1992). Medical View, Tokyo (in Japanese).
5. Osaka Prefectural Department of Health, Osaka Medical Association and Center for Adult Diseases, Osaka. Cancer in Osaka No 49,—Five-Year Relative Survival Rates for

Cancer Patients in Osaka and the Trends, 1975–1983. (1991). Osaka Prefectural Government, Osaka (in Japanese).
6. Parkin, D.M. and Hakulinen, T. Analysis of survival. *In* "Cancer Registration Principles and Methods," IARC Scientific Publication No. 95, eds. O.M. Jensen, D.M. Parkin, R. Maclennan, C.S. Muir, and R.G. Skeet, pp.159–176 (1991). IARC, Lyon.
7. Segi, M., Suemasu, K., Tominaga, S., Fujimoto, I., Fukushima, N., Aoki, K., and Hirayama, T. (eds.). Prognosis of cancer patients by site: oesophagus, stomach, lung, bone, breast, uterus, brain, and haematopoietic tissue. *Jpn. J. Cancer Clin.*, **27**, 537–588 (1981) (in Japanese).

TABLE I. Five-Year Observed and Relative Survival Rates by Primary Site and Period of Diagnosis in Osaka, Both Sexes

Site	ICD, 9th	1975–77			1978–80			1981–83		
		Number of cases	Observed rate (%)	Relative rate (%)	Number of cases	Observed rate (%)	Relative rate (%)	Number of cases	Observed rate (%)	Relative rate (%)
All sites	140–208	17,807	28.9	32.6	22,424	30.9	34.8	26,888	32.6	36.9
Esophagus	150	405	5.1	6.2	486	9.0	10.7	595	10.5	12.6
Stomach	151	5,860	25.4	29.1	6,785	30.1	34.3	7,395	34.1	39.0
Colon	153	768	31.8	36.5	1,088	32.0	36.5	1,477	35.1	40.4
Rectum	154	699	25.6	29.5	1,017	33.6	38.1	1,223	37.5	42.9
Liver	155	990	1.4	1.6	1,440	2.5	2.8	2,354	2.8	3.2
Gallbladder *etc.*	156	226	2.4	2.8	405	6.5	7.5	614	5.9	6.9
Pancreas	157	378	3.0	3.5	543	1.9	2.2	760	2.3	2.7
Lung, trachea	162	1,731	5.8	6.9	2,330	8.3	10.0	2,712	8.6	10.3
Breast	174–175	1,195	65.9	69.0	1,577	67.3	69.9	1,966	75.6	78.7
Uterus	179–182	1,640	59.6	63.0	1,718	60.1	63.7	1,755	64.4	67.9
Ovary	1830	187	22.5	23.4	317	31.6	33.1	402	28.7	30.2
Prostate	185	169	35.5	49.1[a]	240	34.0	47.0	311	37.8	51.0
Bladder	188	358	45.7	54.4	529	49.3	59.9	591	55.6	67.1
Thyroid	193	209	77.3	82.3	270	69.8	76.1	344	74.7	79.7
Lymphatic tissue	200–203	471	18.0	19.6	565	24.8	27.1	801	24.6	27.4
Leukemia	204–208	449	12.1	12.6	529	17.7	18.5	635	19.3	20.3

[a] The standard error of the survival rate is between 5 and 10 percentage points.

TABLE II. Five-Year Relative Survival Rates in Osaka According to Primary Site and Clinical Stage (1981–1983), Both Sexes

Site	All reported cases		Localized		Regional				Distant		Stage unknown	
					Lymphnodes		Direct extension					
	Number of cases	5-Year R.S.R. (SE) %	Number of cases	5-Year R.S.R. (SE) %	Number of cases	5-Year R.S.R. (SE) %	Number of cases	5-Year R.S.R. (SE) %	Number of cases	5-Year R.S.R. (SE) %	Number of cases	5-Year R.S.R. (SE) %
All sites	26,888	36.9 (0.3)	7,555	75.5 (0.6)	4,484	47.0 (0.8)	3,919	13.0 (0.6)	5,451	6.6 (0.3)	5,479	21.8 (0.6)
Stomach	595	12.6 (1.6)	116	25.5 (4.7)	125	15.7 (3.5)	105	6.9 (2.7)	85	1.4 (1.4)	164	10.4 (2.8)
Colon	7,395	39.0 (0.7)	1,913	85.1 (1.1)	1,695	46.3 (1.3)	1,244	10.9 (0.9)	1,282	1.9 (0.5)	1,261	21.4 (1.3)
Rectum	1,477	40.4 (1.5)	341	85.2 (2.7)	344	57.4 (3.1)	225	18.9 (2.9)	324	4.0 (1.1)	243	21.9 (3.0)
Liver	2,354	3.2 (0.3)	465	8.5 (1.3)	81	0.0 (0.0)	356	0.7 (0.5)	442	0.6 (0.4)	1,010	3.0 (0.6)
Lung	2,712	10.3 (0.6)	379	39.3 (2.9)	474	13.1 (1.7)	497	5.4 (1.1)	870	1.3 (0.5)	492	7.7 (1.4)
Breast	1,966	78.7 (1.0)	929	95.8 (0.9)	712	73.3 (1.8)	53	56.2 (7.4)	86	13.9 (3.9)	186	50.1 (3.9)
Uterus	1,755	67.9 (1.3)	1,060	88.0 (1.1)	177	46.1 (4.0)	245	32.0 (3.3)	70	3.2 (2.2)	203	45.6 (3.8)
Bladder	591	67.1 (2.5)	361	87.2 (2.7)	16	45.1 (14.6)	43	28.9 (8.4)	40	0.0 (0.0)	131	42.7 (5.3)
Lymphatic tissue	801	27.4 (1.7)	80	59.7 (6.4)	87	36.5 (5.7)	44	21.0 (6.7)	364	14.3 (2.0)	226	35.0 (3.4)
Leukemia	635	20.3 (1.7)	—	— (—)	—	— (—)	—	— (—)	—	— (—)	—	— (—)

R.S.R.: relative survival rate.
SE: standard error.

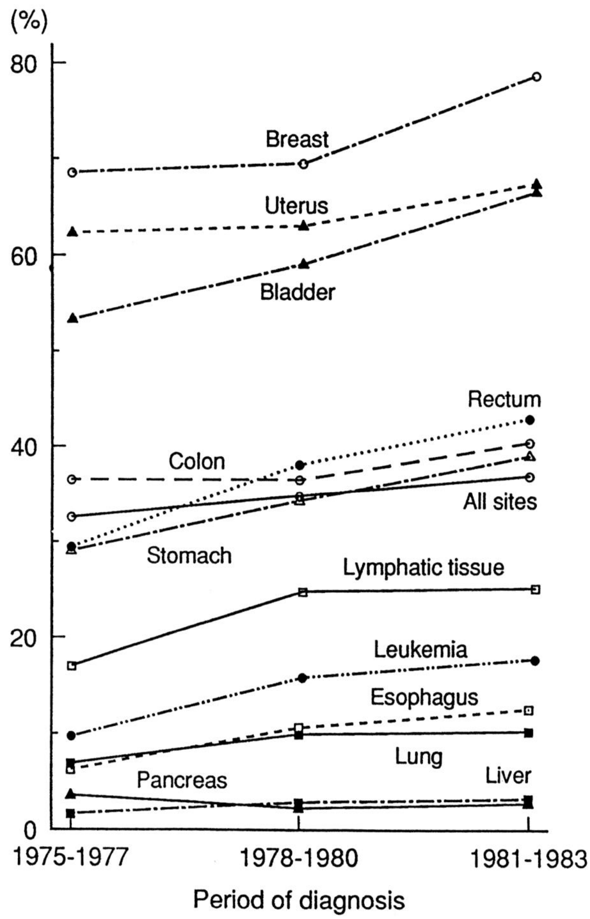

FIG. 1. Trends of 5-year relative survival rates according to primary site in Osaka for 1975–1983

Primary sites can be classified by their survival rates into three classes: the first group including sites with survival rates higher than 60%, the second group including sites with survival rates between 59 and 20%, and the third group made up of the remaining sites with unfavorable survival rates under 19%. Survival rates were improved in most sites during the 9-year period, except those for the liver and pancreas which showed the lowest rates and remained unchanged during the period.

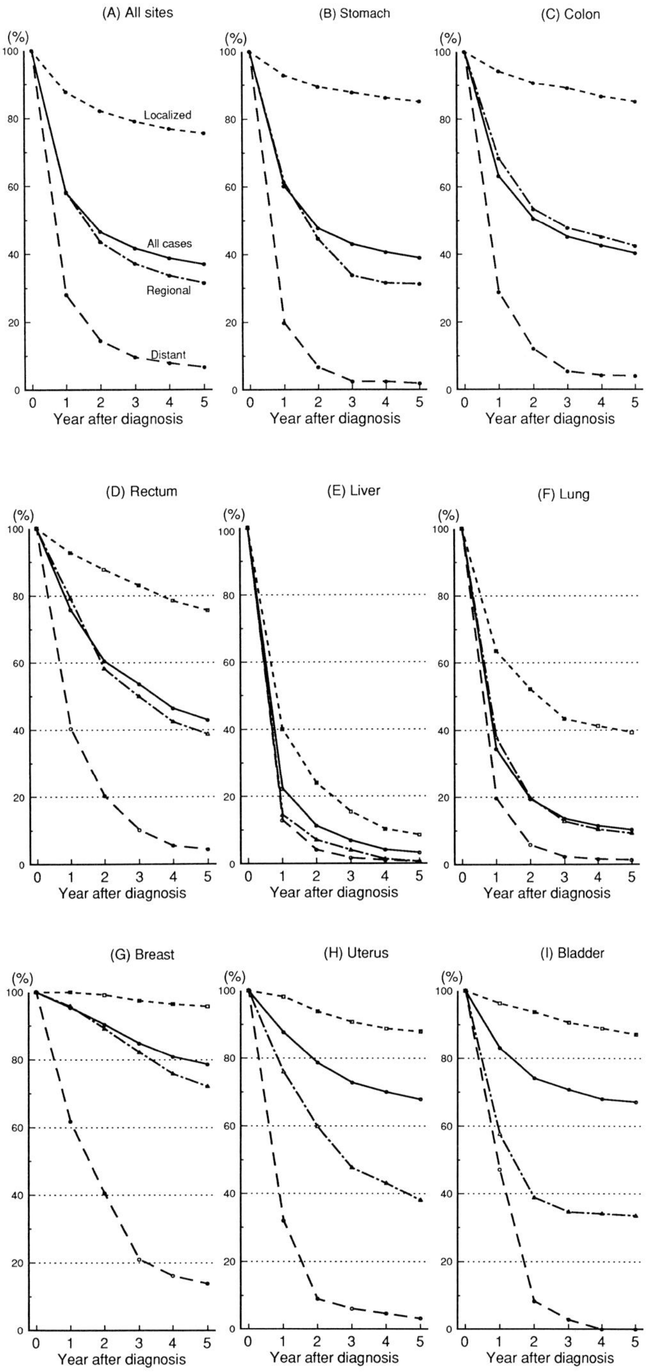

FIG. 2. Relative survival curves according to primary site, extent of disease, and year after diagnosis

Cancer cases were divided into three groups according to extent of disease: "localized", "regional spread", and "remote metastasis", as reported by in cancer notifications. Localized cases had survival rates higher than 70% in every site shown in this figure except the liver and the lung.

CANCER MORTALITY IN 33 COUNTRIES OF THE WORLD (1953–1987)

Tetsuo KUROISHI,*[1] Norihiko HAYAKAWA,*[2] Minoru KURIHARA,*[2] and Kunio AOKI*[3]

*Division of Epidemiology, Aichi Cancer Center Research Institute,**[1] *Department of Epidemiology and Social Medicine, Research Institute for Nuclear Medicine and Biology, Hiroshima University,**[2] *and Aichi Cancer Center**[3]

Cancer mortality statistics in 33 countries of the world were compiled and calculated from data edited from a magnetic tape copy of the WHO data base of cancer mortality.

This report includes the following cancer mortality statistics:

1) Age-adjusted death rates of cancer by site and year for 33 countries of the world (1953–1957 to 1983–1987).
2) Bar graphs of the age-adjusted death rates of cancer by site for 33 countries (1963–1967 and 1983–1987).
3) Line graphs for trends in the age-adjusted death rate of cancer by site for 33 countries (1953–1957 to 1983–1987).

The report entitled "World Cancer Mortality" was published as one chapter in *"Cancer Mortality and Morbidity Statistics—Japan and the World"* in 1981 by some of the authors (*2,5*). Since then, two monographs of "Cancer Mortality Statistics in the World" were issued as UICC publications in 1984 (*4*) and in 1989 (*3*). The first one contained cancer mortality statistics from 24 countries for 2 year periods from 1950–1979, with age-specific death rates for 1978–1979 (*4*). The second one was a revised edition of the first updating the data from 1980 to 1985 (*3*); this, however, did not include any age-specific death rates of cancer by site. A monograph entitled "Death Rates for Malignant Neoplasms for Selected Sites by Sex and Five-Year Age Group in 33 Countries 1953–1957 to 1983–1987" was recently compiled for use in time trend or cohort studies on cancer mortality and had/but offered limited graphic illustrations (*1*).

The aim of this paper is to show graphically an international comparison of cancer mortality rates and also secular trends of cancer mortality by site in each country; this may be useful not only to cancer researchers and clinicians, but also to public health workers working with cancer control programs. Nineteen sites of malignant neoplasms were selected considering frequency of disease and common interest. Original data on cancer mortality and population in each country were courteously supplied by the World Health Organization (WHO) in the form of a magnetic tape copy of the WHO data base of cancer mortality in the world. The International Classification of Diseases (ICD) corresponding to each type of malignant neoplasm in the 6th to 9th revisions are listed as follows:

[1],[3] 1-1 Kanokoden, Chikusa-ku, Nagoya 464, Japan (黒石哲生, 青木國雄).
*[2] 1-2-3 Kasumi, Minami-ku, Hiroshima 734, Japan (早川式彦, 栗原　登).

Site of malignant neoplasm	ICD			
	6th revision	7th revision	8th revision	9th revision
All sites	140–205	140–205	140–209	140–208
Lip, oral cavity, and pharynx	140–148	140–148	140–149	140–149
Esophagus	150	150	150	150
Stomach	151	151	151	151
Intestine, except rectum	152, 153	152, 153	152, 153	152, 153
Rectum, rectosigmoid junction, and anus	154	154	154	154
Liver and intrahepatic bile ducts			155, 197.8	155
Gallbladder and extrahepatic bile ducts		155.1	156	156
Pancreas	157	157	157	157
Larynx	161	161	161	161
Trachea, bronchus, and lung	162, 163	162, 163	162	162
Skin	190, 191	190, 191	172, 173	172, 173
Female breast	170	170	174	174
Uterus (all parts)	171–174	171–174	180–182	179–182
Ovary and other uterine adnexa	175	175	183	183
Prostate	177	177	185	185
Bladder	181	181	188	188
Thyroid gland	194	194	193	193
Leukaemia	204	204	204–207	204–208

Age-Adjusted Death Rates from Malignant Neoplasms by Site in 33 Countries (1953–1957 to 1983–1987)

The age-adjusted death rates for 19 selected sites of malignant neoplasms including all sites in 33 countries from 1953–1957 to 1983–1987 were calculated based on cancer mortality data and population data provided by WHO, and these rates are given in Tables I-1 to I-19. The age-adjusted death rates were standardized on the age distribution of Segi-Doll's World Population (see p. 2 of this monograph). The age-adjusted death rates for 1983–1987 as the latest 5-year period are illustrated by sex and site in Fig. 1-1 (below) to Fig. 1-19 as a bar graph in descending rate order. For the sake of comparison, the age-adjusted death rates for 1963-1967 as the data of 20 years ago are also illustrated in Figs. 1-1 (above) to 1-19. Trends in the age-adjusted death rate for countries are illustrated by sex and site in Figs. 2-1 to 2-19. To avoid complexity in this latter group of figures, the trend in the United Kingdom is represented by that of England and Wales, and the trend of the United States by U.S. White.

The contents of these tables and figures are as follows:

			Site of malignant neoplasm	ICD
				(9th revision)
Table I-1	Fig. 1-1	Fig. 2-1	All sites	140–208
Table I-2	Fig. 1-2	Fig. 2-2	Lip, oral cavity, and pharynx	140–149
Table I-3	Fig. 1-3	Fig. 2-3	Esophagus	150
Table I-4	Fig. 1-4	Fig. 2-4	Stomach	151
Table I-5	Fig. 1-5	Fig. 2-5	Intestine, except rectum	152, 153
Table I-6	Fig. 1-6	Fig. 2-6	Rectum	154
Table I-7	Fig. 1-7	Fig. 2-7	Liver	155
Table I-8	Fig. 1-8	Fig. 2-8	Biliary passages	156

			Site of malignant neoplasm	ICD (9th revision)
Table I-9	Fig. 1-9	Fig. 2-9	Pancreas	157
Table I-10	Fig. 1-10	Fig. 2-10	Larynx	161
Table I-11	Fig. 1-11	Fig. 2-11	Trachea, bronchus, and lung	162
Table I-12	Fig. 1-12	Fig. 2-12	Skin	172, 173
Table I-13	Fig. 1-13	Fig. 2-13	Female breast	174
Table I-14	Fig. 1-14	Fig. 2-14	Uterus (all parts)	179–182
Table I-15	Fig. 1-15	Fig. 2-15	Ovary and other uterine adnexa	183
Table I-16	Fig. 1-16	Fig. 2-16	Prostate	185
Table I-17	Fig. 1-17	Fig. 2-17	Urinary Bladder	188
Table I-18	Fig. 1-18	Fig. 2-18	Thyroid gland	193
Table I-19	Fig. 1-19	Fig. 2-19	Leukaemia	204–208

Acknowledgments

We would like to express our thanks to Dr. A. D. Lopez, Global Epidemiological Surveillance and Health Situation Assessment and Projections, WHO, for providing us the magnetic tape copy of the WHO data base of cancer mortality in the world from 1950 onward; Dr. J. Stjernswärd, Chief, Cancer Unit, WHO, and Mr. A. J. Turnbull, Executive Director of the UICC also helped us to whom we express deep thanks. We also thank Miss E. Nakamura for her excellent technical assistance in illustrating the figures and making the tables by personal computer.

REFERENCES

1. Aoki, K., Kurihara, M., Hayakawa, N., and Suzuki, S. (eds.). Death Rates for Malignant Neoplasms for Selected Sites by Sex and Five-Year Age Group in 33 Countries 1953–57 to 1983–87 (1992). International Union against Cancer, The University of Nagoya Press, Nagoya.
2. Aoki, K., Tominaga, S., and Kuroishi, T. Age-adjusted death rates for cancer by site (ICD, 8th revision) in 50 countries in 1975. *In* "Cancer Mortality and Morbidity—Japan and the World," Gann Monograph on Cancer Research, No. 26, eds. M. Segi, S. Tominaga, K. Aoki, and I. Fujimoto, pp.251–274 (1981). Japan Scientific Societies Press, Tokyo.
3. Kurihara, M., Aoki, K., and Hisamichi, S. (eds.). Cancer Mortality Statistics in the World 1950–1985 (1989). The University of Nagoya Press, Nagoya.
4. Kurihara, M., Aoki, K., and Tominaga, S. (eds.). Cancer Mortality Statistics in the World 1950–1979 (1984). The University of Nagoya Press, Nagoya.
5. Segi, M., Aoki, K., and Kurihara, M. World cancer mortality. *In* "Cancer Mortality and Morbidity—Japan and the World," Gann Monograph on Cancer Research, No. 26, eds. M. Segi, S. Tominaga, K. Aoki, and I. Fujimoto, pp.121–250 (1981). Japan Scientific Societies Press, Tokyo.

TABLE I-1. Age-Adjusted Death Rates of Cancer

All sites (male)

	Country	1953–1957	1958–1962	1963–1967	1968–1972	1973–1977	1978–1982	1983–1987
1.	Australia	130.4	135.7	143.6	156.9	161.6	163.5	164.0
2.	Austria		193.5	195.0	193.4	187.8	184.6	176.9
3.	Belgium	154.0[a)]	169.0	183.5	193.8	202.1	213.3	209.5[b)]
4.	Canada	134.3	139.3	145.4	155.2	160.5	164.7	167.5
5.	Chile		150.9	155.9	163.0	153.7	145.4	141.9
6.	Costa Rica			147.8	135.5	129.5	136.4	147.2
7.	Czechoslovakia	162.1	179.7	198.1	202.5	210.8	213.0	223.3
8.	Denmark	152.4	161.3	165.2	165.6	167.9	178.3	184.1
9.	Finland	188.5	192.5	189.0	192.6	184.5	178.5	165.9
10.	France	151.7	166.2	180.2	183.6	193.7	199.8	203.6
11.	Germany, Fed. Repub.	156.0	164.9	175.1	179.1	181.5	181.6	180.7
12.	Greece			123.3	125.4	137.7	142.9	144.3
13.	Hong Kong		130.7	156.1	169.9	180.2	184.3	178.4
14.	Hungary		151.9	163.5	178.1	193.0	211.0	227.5
15.	Ireland	130.2	135.7	142.0	155.4	164.3	164.2	171.3
16.	Israel	115.4	117.8	120.4	125.5	128.6	124.7	117.5
17.	Italy	124.2	138.9	154.4	169.0	173.7	183.2	192.7
18.	Japan	124.6	136.1	141.6	143.1	142.9	146.3	149.8
19.	Mexico		48.3	55.6	54.3	60.0	66.7[c)]	75.9[d)]
20.	Netherlands	149.7	161.2	176.0	187.2	195.1	199.6	199.7
21.	New Zealand	138.5	141.8	149.3	163.7	173.5	171.7	173.2
22.	Norway	125.7	125.7	127.5	135.3	136.9	143.2	147.1
23.	Poland		114.8[e)]	142.2	154.8	164.2	177.2	194.6
24.	Portugal		103.8	116.1	125.2	131.2	137.1	136.9
25.	Singapore			168.5	165.7	189.8	189.4	187.0
26.	Spain	104.0	121.0	132.7	135.0	146.4	150.8	157.1[f)]
27.	Sweden	118.8	128.8	128.8	136.1	147.0	139.5	129.4
28.	Switzerland	170.8	170.4	171.1	176.5	179.0	176.0	177.7
29.	U.K., England & Wales	171.5	178.4	184.5	189.5	188.6	184.9	184.0
30.	U.K., Northern Ireland	143.6	150.4	151.8	164.2	172.6	167.2	174.2
31.	U.K., Scotland	184.8	194.1	205.0	207.0	206.1	205.8	200.6
32.	U.S., White	139.5	142.1	147.3	153.7	157.8	160.0	158.9
33.	U.S., Nonwhite	146.5	157.7	174.6	190.3	198.8	206.5	204.9
34.	Yugoslavia			101.3	114.0	126.9	142.1	148.0

[a)] 1954–57, [b)] 1983, 84, 86, [c)] 1978, 81, 82, [d)] 1983, 85, 86, [e)] 1959–62, [f)] 1983–86.

by Site and Year (1953–57 to 1983–87)
All sites (female)

Country	1953–1957	1958–1962	1963–1967	1968–1972	1973–1977	1978–1982	1983–1987
1. Australia	102.6	98.1	98.5	101.6	101.5	98.9	102.5
2. Austria		133.3	132.3	127.9	121.8	115.2	112.0
3. Belgium	124.4[a]	125.0	122.7	118.9	114.3	114.8	111.6[b]
4. Canada	116.7	113.9	111.6	110.3	108.1	108.0	109.7
5. Chile		137.3	143.8	142.2	125.2	115.3	112.9
6. Costa Rica			132.0	119.0	104.3	106.4	109.1
7. Czechoslovakia	118.2	117.8	119.6	118.8	116.8	117.1	118.8
8. Denmark	144.1	142.3	138.7	134.1	130.9	134.2	138.1
9. Finland	117.9	111.5	107.1	102.9	97.6	94.9	93.0
10. France	106.5	105.5	103.9	98.7	96.3	92.6	90.6
11. Germany, Fed. Repub.	129.3	127.9	128.6	124.7	120.4	115.6	111.8
12. Greece			75.2	75.4	79.1	81.3	79.4
13. Hong Kong		88.0	96.3	98.4	99.5	97.8	96.6
14. Hungary		119.5	120.5	123.5	128.1	127.8	127.9
15. Ireland	111.3	111.9	115.2	122.9	127.5	122.9	124.1
16. Israel	119.9	120.3	118.1	121.0	115.1	108.6	100.3
17. Italy	97.5	99.7	102.0	102.7	100.7	98.8	100.0
18. Japan	93.8	97.2	95.9	92.8	88.0	84.3	79.9
19. Mexico		72.5	76.8	71.7	74.4	73.3[c]	79.1[d]
20. Netherlands	125.3	121.0	121.7	119.2	113.1	109.8	109.1
21. New Zealand	111.4	111.5	112.0	114.0	121.3	121.8	123.3
22. Norway	109.9	104.4	100.5	102.0	100.0	100.6	101.0
23. Poland		88.3[e]	104.5	103.9	101.7	103.6	106.6
24. Portugal		80.1	85.5	88.8	86.4	85.1	83.3
25. Singapore			99.7	96.5	102.0	110.1	109.0
26. Spain	77.7	86.3	90.1	87.0	87.6	82.1	79.7[f]
27. Sweden	111.8	111.6	107.3	109.1	110.6	105.6	98.7
28. Switzerland	122.2	117.0	112.3	110.5	104.7	103.0	101.4
29. U.K., England & Wales	115.7	115.3	115.9	119.5	121.6	123.0	126.3
30. U.K., Northern Ireland	118.1	111.4	109.6	117.0	120.1	119.7	119.3
31. U.K., Scotland	129.4	127.0	126.0	129.7	129.5	135.0	136.3
32. U.S.,White	113.8	108.3	106.1	105.7	105.7	106.4	108.2
33. U.S., Nonwhite	126.5	123.6	123.0	121.8	119.4	117.6	117.0
34. Yugoslavia			73.2	76.4	80.5	84.8	86.6

[a] 1954–57, [b] 1983, 84, 86, [c] 1978, 81, 82, [d] 1983, 85, 86, [e] 1959–62, [f] 1983–86.

TABLE I-2. Age-Adjusted Death Rates of Cancer

Lip, oral cavity, and pharynx (male)

Country	1953–1957	1958–1962	1963–1967	1968–1972	1973–1977	1978–1982	1983–1987
1. Australia	4.0	3.3	3.5	3.9	4.2	4.4	4.8
2. Austria		2.8	2.9	3.7	4.1	4.6	5.5
3. Belgium	2.7[a]	2.9	2.7	2.8	3.0	3.5	3.8[b]
4. Canada	4.7	4.2	4.2	4.4	4.4	4.4	4.5
5. Chile		2.1	2.3	2.3	2.8	2.7	2.4
6. Costa Rica			3.7	3.6	3.0	3.0	3.6
7. Czechoslovakia	3.5	3.4	3.3	3.3	4.0	5.3	7.2
8. Denmark	2.5	2.2	2.0	2.2	2.1	3.1	3.4
9. Finland	4.3	3.2	3.0	2.6	2.3	2.5	2.0
10. France	6.7	8.3	9.9	12.2	14.9	15.6	15.0
11. Germany, Fed. Repub.	1.6	1.7	1.8	2.1	2.6	3.9	5.4
12. Greece			1.4	1.5	1.5	1.7	1.8
13. Hong Kong		15.2	17.9	18.8	19.6	17.7	15.6
14. Hungary		4.1	4.1	4.5	5.5	7.9	11.1
15. Ireland	7.6	6.1	4.6	4.5	4.2	4.0	4.4
16. Israel	1.5	1.5	1.7	1.4	1.6	1.3	1.5
17. Italy	5.1	5.4	5.6	6.0	5.9	6.2	6.6
18. Japan	1.3	1.3	1.4	1.6	1.7	1.9	2.1
19. Mexico		1.3	1.6	1.3	1.5	1.7[c]	1.7[d]
20. Netherlands	1.9	1.8	1.8	1.9	1.9	2.0	2.4
21. New Zealand	3.6	3.4	2.6	3.3	3.3	4.0	3.9
22. Norway	3.2	2.9	2.7	3.1	2.8	2.5	3.0
23. Poland		2.5[e]	3.5	4.3	4.8	4.8	5.5
24. Portugal		4.5	4.9	4.9	5.0	5.0	5.0
25. Singapore			12.7	13.9	15.9	14.8	14.5
26. Spain	2.5	2.8	3.0	2.9	3.8	4.2	5.2[f]
27. Sweden	2.2	2.3	2.3	2.3	2.5	2.7	2.7
28. Switzerland	6.4	6.9	6.8	6.0	6.6	6.5	6.8
29. U.K., England & Wales	4.8	3.9	3.1	3.0	2.7	2.8	2.9
30. U.K., Northern Ireland	5.1	4.4	3.8	3.5	2.6	2.4	3.1
31. U.K., Scotland	6.0	4.3	3.9	3.1	3.0	3.2	3.7
32. U.S., White	4.8	4.7	4.6	4.7	4.5	4.1	3.6
33. U.S., Nonwhite	4.5	4.8	5.8	6.3	7.0	7.8	7.1
34. Yugoslavia			1.9	2.8	3.4	4.5	5.6

[a] 1954–57, [b] 1983,84,86, [c] 1978,81,82, [d] 1983,85,86, [e] 1959–62, [f] 1983–86.

by Site and Year (1953–57 to 1983–87)
Lip, oral cavity, and pharynx (female)

Country	1953–1957	1958–1962	1963–1967	1968–1972	1973–1977	1978–1982	1983–1987
1. Australia	1.1	1.1	1.2	1.2	1.2	1.3	1.4
2. Austria		0.8	0.8	0.8	0.7	0.6	0.9
3. Belgium	0.7[a]	0.7	0.7	0.6	0.7	0.8	1.0[b]
4. Canada	1.2	1.2	1.1	1.3	1.3	1.3	1.4
5. Chile		0.9	0.8	0.9	0.8	0.6	0.6
6. Costa Rica			1.2	1.1	0.9	0.8	1.3
7. Czechoslovakia	0.9	1.0	0.9	0.8	0.8	0.9	1.0
8. Denmark	0.9	1.0	1.0	1.0	1.0	1.4	1.4
9. Finland	1.8	1.6	1.1	1.1	1.1	1.2	0.9
10. France	0.7	0.8	0.8	1.0	1.1	1.2	1.3
11. Germany, Fed. Repub.	0.7	0.6	0.6	0.6	0.7	0.8	0.9
12. Greece			0.6	0.5	0.6	0.6	0.6
13. Hong Kong		6.7	7.1	7.1	6.8	6.1	4.8
14. Hungary		0.9	0.8	0.9	1.0	1.2	1.5
15. Ireland	2.5	2.1	1.9	1.9	1.8	1.4	1.5
16. Israel	0.6	1.0	0.8	0.8	1.1	0.7	0.8
17. Italy	0.9	0.9	0.9	0.9	0.9	0.9	1.0
18. Japan	0.6	0.6	0.6	0.6	0.7	0.7	0.6
19. Mexico		0.6	0.7	0.6	0.7	0.6[c]	0.7[d]
20. Netherlands	0.9	0.9	0.8	0.6	0.7	0.8	0.8
21. New Zealand	1.5	1.5	1.2	1.0	1.3	1.3	1.3
22. Norway	1.5	1.4	1.4	1.0	0.9	0.9	1.0
23. Poland		0.8[e]	1.0	1.0	1.0	1.0	1.0
24. Portugal		1.1	1.1	1.1	0.9	0.9	0.8
25. Singapore			5.2	4.8	5.5	5.3	5.2
26. Spain	0.5	0.5	0.6	0.6	0.6	0.6	0.7[f]
27. Sweden	1.7	1.6	1.4	1.1	1.1	0.9	1.0
28. Switzerland	1.0	1.0	0.9	1.0	1.0	1.1	1.2
29. U.K., England & Wales	1.7	1.6	1.4	1.4	1.3	1.3	1.3
30. U.K., Northern Ireland	2.3	2.0	2.2	2.0	1.4	1.4	1.2
31. U.K., Scotland	2.0	1.8	1.7	1.5	1.3	1.5	1.4
32. U.S., White	1.1	1.2	1.3	1.5	1.5	1.5	1.4
33. U.S., Nonwhite	1.4	1.5	1.7	1.8	1.9	2.0	1.8
34. Yugoslavia			0.5	0.6	0.7	0.8	0.9

[a] 1954–57, [b] 1983,84,86, [c] 1978,81,82, [d] 1983,85,86, [e] 1959–62, [f] 1983–86.

TABLE I-3. Age-Adjusted Death Rates of Cancer

Esophagus (male)

	Country	1953–1957	1958–1962	1963–1967	1968–1972	1973–1977	1978–1982	1983–1987
1.	Australia	3.4	3.3	3.5	3.8	4.4	4.2	4.4
2.	Austria		4.4	4.3	4.3	3.8	3.9	3.7
3.	Belgium	3.8[a)]	3.7	3.9	3.7	3.8	4.3	4.6[b)]
4.	Canada	3.0	3.1	3.3	3.4	3.7	3.7	4.2
5.	Chile		8.6	10.4	10.9	10.0	9.3	8.3
6.	Costa Rica			5.7	4.3	4.6	2.9	4.1
7.	Czechoslovakia	3.4	2.7	2.6	2.5	2.7	3.1	3.7
8.	Denmark	3.6	3.1	2.8	2.7	3.2	3.5	4.5
9.	Finland	8.5	6.8	5.6	4.7	3.7	3.6	2.9
10.	France	10.8	12.6	14.3	14.2	14.3	13.3	12.4
11.	Germany, Fed. Repub.	4.0	3.9	3.7	3.6	3.6	4.0	4.7
12.	Greece			1.7	1.8	2.0	1.9	1.8
13.	Hong Kong		8.5	11.1	10.9	11.5	12.3	11.2
14.	Hungary		2.4	2.7	2.5	2.9	4.1	5.7
15.	Ireland	4.3	5.1	4.9	5.2	5.8	6.1	6.4
16.	Israel	4.5	3.8	2.8	2.4	2.2	1.8	1.6
17.	Italy	3.8	4.3	4.4	4.7	4.6	4.8	4.7
18.	Japan	6.9	6.9	7.3	7.8	7.3	7.0	6.9
19.	Mexico		1.3	1.5	1.5	1.6	1.6[c)]	1.9[d)]
20.	Netherlands	3.7	3.2	3.0	2.9	3.1	3.4	4.2
21.	New Zealand	3.7	3.5	4.0	3.8	5.1	4.7	4.7
22.	Norway	3.2	3.0	2.5	2.5	2.6	2.6	2.4
23.	Poland		4.4[e)]	5.0	4.7	4.2	4.2	4.9
24.	Portugal		4.7	5.5	5.5	6.0	5.8	5.8
25.	Singapore			13.9	14.6	13.9	10.6	8.8
26.	Spain	2.5	3.3	3.8	4.5	5.2	5.4	5.4[f)]
27.	Sweden	2.8	2.5	2.5	2.8	2.9	2.9	2.9
28.	Switzerland	12.8	11.2	9.5	8.6	7.4	6.6	5.8
29.	U.K., England & Wales	4.6	4.5	4.5	5.0	5.4	5.9	6.7
30.	U.K., Northern Ireland	4.0	3.4	4.1	4.1	4.3	5.2	5.6
31.	U.K., Scotland	5.7	5.5	5.5	6.1	6.6	8.1	8.9
32.	U.S., White	3.4	3.4	3.3	3.3	3.4	3.5	3.7
33.	U.S., Nonwhite	7.1	8.4	9.7	10.2	11.4	12.0	10.7
34.	Yugoslavia			2.0	2.3	2.8	3.6	3.9

[a)] 1954–57, [b)] 1983, 84, 86, [c)] 1978, 81, 82, [d)] 1983, 85, 86, [e)] 1959–62, [f)] 1983–86.

by Site and Year (1953–57 to 1983–87)
Esophagus (female)

Country	1953–1957	1958–1962	1963–1967	1968–1972	1973–1977	1978–1982	1983–1987
1. Australia	1.2	1.3	1.4	1.6	1.7	1.7	1.7
2. Austria		0.8	0.8	0.6	0.6	0.5	0.5
3. Belgium	1.3[a]	1.1	1.0	1.0	0.9	1.1	1.0[b]
4. Canada	1.2	1.2	1.2	1.2	1.1	1.2	1.1
5. Chile		5.0	5.6	5.1	4.6	4.1	3.7
6. Costa Rica			2.1	2.8	1.6	1.6	1.6
7. Czechoslovakia	0.8	0.5	0.5	0.5	0.5	0.4	0.5
8. Denmark	1.7	1.4	1.2	1.2	1.1	1.2	1.3
9. Finland	5.8	5.2	4.3	3.4	2.6	2.2	1.9
10. France	1.1	1.1	1.1	1.1	1.1	1.0	1.0
11. Germany, Fed. Repub.	1.2	1.1	1.0	0.9	0.8	0.7	0.8
12. Greece			0.6	0.7	0.7	0.6	0.5
13. Hong Kong		2.3	2.4	3.5	2.9	2.3	2.0
14. Hungary		0.5	0.5	0.5	0.5	0.6	0.6
15. Ireland	3.3	3.3	4.0	4.2	4.0	3.9	3.7
16. Israel	2.5	2.4	2.1	1.6	1.5	1.2	0.9
17. Italy	0.9	0.8	0.8	0.8	0.8	0.8	0.8
18. Japan	2.3	2.2	2.2	2.0	1.7	1.4	1.1
19. Mexico		0.6	0.7	0.7	0.7	0.7[c]	0.8[d]
20. Netherlands	1.5	1.4	1.2	1.2	1.1	1.2	1.4
21. New Zealand	1.9	1.7	1.8	1.9	2.1	2.0	1.9
22. Norway	1.0	0.6	0.8	0.7	0.7	0.6	0.6
23. Poland		1.3[e]	1.3	1.1	0.9	0.8	0.8
24. Portugal		1.7	1.9	2.0	1.8	1.6	1.4
25. Singapore			4.0	5.3	3.7	3.0	2.5
26. Spain	0.7	1.0	1.1	1.1	1.0	0.8	0.7[f]
27. Sweden	1.4	1.1	1.0	0.9	0.9	0.8	0.8
28. Switzerland	1.5	1.4	1.1	1.1	0.9	0.9	1.0
29. U.K., England & Wales	2.3	2.3	2.4	2.6	2.8	2.8	3.0
30. U.K., Northern Ireland	3.1	2.2	3.3	2.5	2.5	2.4	2.9
31. U.K., Scotland	3.4	3.2	3.0	3.5	3.6	4.0	4.0
32. U.S., White	0.8	0.8	0.8	0.9	0.9	1.0	0.9
33. U.S., Nonwhite	1.7	1.9	2.3	2.6	3.0	3.0	2.8
34. Yugoslavia			0.5	0.5	0.7	0.7	0.8

[a] 1954–57, [b] 1983, 84, 86, [c] 1978, 81, 82, [d] 1983, 85, 86, [e] 1959–62, [f] 1983–86.

TABLE I-4. Age-Adjusted Death Rates of Cancer

Stomach (male)

	Country	1953–1957	1958–1962	1963–1967	1968–1972	1973–1977	1978–1982	1983–1987
1.	Australia	22.5	19.1	16.1	14.9	12.5	10.7	9.1
2.	Austria		46.2	41.8	36.4	29.9	25.5	20.5
3.	Belgium	33.2[a)]	31.0	27.6	23.4	19.0	16.4	13.5[b)]
4.	Canada	23.5	20.2	17.5	15.0	12.6	10.5	8.7
5.	Chile		67.9	62.1	62.2	52.0	42.8	35.3
6.	Costa Rica			60.9	52.9	48.3	45.7	46.0
7.	Czechoslovakia	46.5	44.8	42.2	37.1	31.7	25.7	21.5
8.	Denmark	31.2	26.8	21.6	17.2	14.7	12.2	9.9
9.	Finland	59.6	49.1	38.8	31.3	24.7	20.2	16.0
10.	France	27.6	25.2	22.0	18.0	15.2	12.5	10.6
11.	Germany, Fed. Repub.	44.0	40.2	36.6	31.6	26.4	21.2	17.0
12.	Greece			16.0	14.4	13.6	12.0	10.5
13.	Hong Kong		19.9	19.3	18.0	16.4	13.9	11.5
14.	Hungary		47.2	42.6	40.6	35.9	31.6	25.9
15.	Ireland	28.7	25.2	24.3	22.6	19.6	16.2	14.1
16.	Israel	23.4	22.3	18.2	16.8	14.3	11.1	9.9
17.	Italy	36.0	34.6	34.0	30.9	25.8	22.6	20.4
18.	Japan	69.5	70.3	68.3	63.6	55.8	47.8	40.8
19.	Mexico		8.6	10.4	10.2	9.6	9.5[c)]	9.8[d)]
20.	Netherlands	36.0	31.4	28.1	24.1	21.1	17.5	15.0
21.	New Zealand	21.6	19.5	16.9	14.9	14.3	12.3	10.7
22.	Norway	37.5	30.2	26.2	22.5	17.5	14.6	12.9
23.	Poland		40.1[e)]	43.7	39.7	35.0	30.4	26.8
24.	Portugal		31.4	34.2	34.9	33.9	29.8	25.8
25.	Singapore			39.0	31.7	33.5	26.4	24.0
26.	Spain	28.3	30.0	31.2	27.4	24.7	19.2	16.2[f)]
27.	Sweden	30.5	26.8	21.8	17.9	16.0	12.8	10.1
28.	Switzerland	38.3	31.9	27.0	22.6	18.3	14.3	11.5
29.	U.K., England & Wales	27.7	26.0	23.8	21.5	19.4	16.8	14.8
30.	U.K. Northern Ireland	28.0	28.6	22.9	21.4	19.9	17.5	14.8
31.	U.K., Scotland	30.2	28.0	25.9	22.2	19.6	17.4	14.3
32.	U.S., White	14.7	11.8	9.2	7.6	6.5	5.6	5.0
33.	U.S., Nonwhite	23.7	20.7	18.4	15.3	12.7	11.0	9.8
34.	Yugoslavia			21.9	23.2	22.8	21.1	18.5

[a)] 1954–57, [b)] 1983, 84, 86, [c)] 1978, 81, 82, [d)] 1983, 85, 86, [e)] 1959–62, [f)] 1983–86.

by Site and Year (1953–57 to 1983–87)
Stomach (female)

Country	1953–1957	1958–1962	1963–1967	1968–1972	1973–1977	1978–1982	1983–1987
1. Australia	12.2	9.7	8.1	7.6	6.2	4.7	4.0
2. Austria		25.7	23.2	19.4	15.5	12.3	9.9
3. Belgium	19.9[a]	18.4	15.3	11.9	9.9	7.8	6.5[b]
4. Canada	12.1	9.9	8.1	6.9	5.6	4.6	3.9
5. Chile		42.4	39.2	35.0	25.3	18.9	14.7
6. Costa Rica			32.7	31.8	22.2	21.5	22.5
7. Czechoslovakia	26.0	24.3	22.1	18.6	15.2	12.1	10.1
8. Denmark	20.5	16.3	12.7	9.4	7.6	6.2	5.0
9. Finland	34.9	27.3	20.0	15.8	12.3	10.5	8.9
10. France	14.6	12.9	10.7	8.4	6.8	5.4	4.3
11. Germany, Fed. Repub.	27.2	23.6	20.5	16.8	13.7	11.0	8.9
12. Greece			9.5	8.3	7.7	6.7	5.4
13. Hong Kong		11.5	11.2	8.9	7.7	6.8	6.5
14. Hungary		25.7	22.7	20.3	17.1	14.0	11.3
15. Ireland	19.2	17.0	16.1	14.8	11.9	8.8	7.0
16. Israel	17.2	14.9	12.2	9.7	8.2	7.0	5.0
17. Italy	20.7	18.7	17.5	15.2	12.6	10.7	9.5
18. Japan	37.0	37.0	35.3	33.2	28.5	23.6	19.0
19. Mexico		8.7	9.4	9.0	8.6	7.8[c]	7.8[d]
20. Netherlands	22.5	17.1	15.1	11.9	9.6	7.4	6.1
21. New Zealand	12.8	9.9	8.2	6.9	6.3	5.5	4.8
22. Norway	21.6	17.5	14.4	11.8	9.0	7.4	6.3
23. Poland		19.6[e]	20.9	17.4	14.0	11.6	9.8
24. Portugal		17.8	19.5	19.2	17.4	14.5	12.7
25. Singapore			17.1	14.8	15.0	13.1	11.3
26. Spain	17.1	17.7	17.5	15.0	12.8	9.6	7.7[f]
27. Sweden	19.3	14.8	11.8	9.8	8.1	6.7	5.3
28. Switzerland	23.4	19.0	14.9	11.6	9.0	7.0	5.3
29. U.K., England & Wales	15.0	13.5	11.6	10.1	8.7	7.4	6.0
30. U.K., Northern Ireland	19.4	16.7	13.4	11.3	11.1	9.0	6.3
31. U.K., Scotland	19.6	16.7	13.9	11.8	10.2	8.2	7.3
32. U.S.,White	7.6	6.0	4.7	3.8	3.1	2.6	2.2
33. U.S., Nonwhite	10.8	9.2	8.2	6.5	5.8	5.0	4.5
34. Yugoslavia			12.0	11.8	10.9	10.2	8.7

[a] 1954–57, [b] 1983, 84, 86, [c] 1978, 81, 82, [d] 1983, 85, 86, [e] 1959–62, [f] 1983–86.

TABLE I-5. Age-Adjusted Death Rates of Cancer

Intestine, except rectum (male)

	Country	1953–1957	1958–1962	1963–1967	1968–1972	1973–1977	1978–1982	1983–1987
1.	Australia	13.2	12.6	12.7	13.6	14.9	15.1	15.7
2.	Austria		9.7	10.6	12.7	13.8	14.0	13.4
3.	Belgium	11.1[a)]	12.2	12.8	13.4	13.2	14.2	13.3[b)]
4.	Canada	13.7	13.9	14.1	14.8	14.9	13.9	13.3
5.	Chile		3.2	3.7	4.6	4.5	4.5	4.2
6.	Costa Rica			3.6	2.7	3.6	3.6	4.3
7.	Czechoslovakia	6.6	6.6	7.5	8.7	10.8	12.0	14.0
8.	Denmark	12.4	13.4	13.5	11.8	12.9	13.9	14.2
9.	Finland	4.9	5.0	5.7	5.9	6.1	6.3	7.0
10.	France	11.1	11.7	12.2	12.7	13.3	12.2	12.4
11.	Germany, Fed. Repub.	6.8	8.0	10.2	12.6	13.6	13.7	14.2
12.	Greece			4.6	4.8	5.6	5.0	4.9
13.	Hong Kong		7.9	7.5	8.3	8.4	8.3	9.4
14.	Hungary		6.6	7.8	9.6	11.8	12.8	14.1
15.	Ireland	12.9	12.1	12.4	14.2	15.5	14.8	15.7
16.	Israel	5.3	6.5	7.2	8.8	10.5	11.3	11.5
17.	Italy	5.8	7.4	8.6	10.2	11.0	9.0	9.8
18.	Japan	2.4	2.8	3.3	4.1	5.2	6.3	7.8
19.	Mexico		1.7	1.9	1.9	2.0	1.7[c)]	2.2[d)]
20.	Netherlands	9.5	9.7	10.9	11.4	12.4	12.7	13.8
21.	New Zealand	13.0	12.7	13.3	15.9	16.3	15.8	15.8
22.	Norway	7.3	8.0	8.3	9.7	8.8	10.0	11.0
23.	Poland		2.8[e)]	4.1	4.8	5.2	5.1	5.7
24.	Portugal		6.5	7.9	8.4	8.8	8.6	8.5
25.	Singapore			6.3	7.2	9.4	9.9	11.2
26.	Spain	4.4	5.7	6.2	6.4	6.9	6.1	7.1[f)]
27.	Sweden	9.6	9.8	10.0	10.9	11.8	10.4	10.0
28.	Switzerland	11.5	11.2	11.8	12.5	12.4	12.3	12.7
29.	U.K., England & Wales	14.1	12.5	12.1	12.7	12.6	12.0	12.5
30.	U.K., Northern Ireland	13.0	12.5	12.9	14.6	16.2	13.7	15.6
31.	U.K., Scotland	19.0	16.6	15.9	15.5	15.2	14.1	13.4
32.	U.S., White	13.2	13.4	13.8	14.3	15.1	15.3	15.1
33.	U.S., Nonwhite	9.6	10.3	11.6	12.7	13.7	14.7	15.4
34.	Yugoslavia			2.3	3.4	4.1	4.9	5.4

[a)] 1954–57, [b)] 1983,84,86, [c)] 1978,81,82, [d)] 1983,85,86, [e)] 1959–62, [f)] 1983–86.

by Site and Year (1953–57 to 1983–87)
Intestine, except rectum (female)

Country	1953–1957	1958–1962	1963–1967	1968–1972	1973–1977	1978–1982	1983–1987
1. Australia	14.2	13.6	13.3	13.6	13.5	12.7	12.5
2. Austria		8.3	9.2	10.3	11.0	10.2	10.0
3. Belgium	12.1[a]	13.1	12.8	13.0	12.4	11.8	11.1[b]
4. Canada	16.0	15.9	15.1	14.6	13.9	11.9	10.6
5. Chile		4.3	4.6	5.3	5.1	4.4	4.6
6. Costa Rica			4.6	2.7	4.3	4.3	4.2
7. Czechoslovakia	5.7	5.1	5.7	6.5	7.5	8.1	9.1
8. Denmark	13.5	13.8	13.3	12.7	12.2	12.7	12.4
9. Finland	5.4	5.6	5.7	6.3	6.1	6.0	5.9
10. France	11.3	11.0	10.5	10.0	9.9	8.3	8.0
11. Germany, Fed. Repub.	5.8	7.1	9.1	11.3	12.0	11.7	11.7
12. Greece			4.7	4.8	5.7	4.6	4.5
13. Hong Kong		5.7	4.9	5.5	6.0	6.3	6.9
14. Hungary		7.3	8.2	9.2	10.5	10.8	10.9
15. Ireland	13.1	13.2	13.5	15.1	15.3	13.2	13.4
16. Israel	5.8	6.9	7.8	7.9	9.5	9.6	9.7
17. Italy	5.9	6.7	7.5	8.3	9.0	6.8	6.9
18. Japan	2.5	2.9	3.3	3.8	4.5	5.2	5.9
19. Mexico		2.6	2.8	2.5	2.5	2.1[c]	2.3[d]
20. Netherlands	11.2	11.4	11.9	12.1	11.6	11.4	11.4
21. New Zealand	15.1	14.3	14.5	14.9	17.0	15.6	15.5
22. Norway	7.2	7.6	8.1	8.8	8.6	9.7	9.7
23. Poland		2.6[e]	3.9	4.1	4.3	4.1	4.6
24. Portugal		7.6	8.8	8.5	8.2	7.1	6.5
25. Singapore			5.3	6.0	7.7	9.9	10.9
26. Spain	5.3	6.6	7.0	6.6	6.6	5.2	5.4[f]
27. Sweden	8.9	9.7	9.1	9.4	9.7	9.1	8.0
28. Switzerland	9.5	9.2	9.2	8.8	8.8	8.6	8.6
29. U.K., England & Wales	13.7	12.6	11.9	12.0	11.6	10.5	10.4
30. U.K., Northern Ireland	14.3	13.4	12.3	15.0	14.8	13.6	12.5
31. U.K., Scotland	18.1	16.1	15.2	15.2	14.1	12.5	11.2
32. U.S., White	14.0	13.5	13.0	12.6	12.4	11.6	10.8
33. U.S., Nonwhite	10.4	11.4	11.9	12.5	12.7	12.5	12.4
34. Yugoslavia			2.2	3.0	3.6	3.8	4.2

[a] 1954–57, [b] 1983,84,86, [c] 1978,81,82, [d] 1983,85,86, [e] 1959–62, [f] 1983–86.

TABLE I-6. Age-Adjusted Death Rates of Cancer

Rectum, rectosigmoid junction, and anus (male)

	Country	1953–1957	1958–1962	1963–1967	1968–1972	1973–1977	1978–1982	1983–1987
1.	Australia	6.4	6.1	5.9	6.1	6.2	6.3	6.3
2.	Austria		8.6	9.0	9.8	10.0	9.4	8.8
3.	Belgium	9.6[a)]	9.9	9.2	8.8	7.9	7.1	6.4[b)]
4.	Canada	7.8	7.2	7.0	7.0	6.4	5.9	5.2
5.	Chile		2.2	2.4	2.7	2.5	2.5	2.6
6.	Costa Rica			1.9	1.9	1.2	1.7	2.5
7.	Czechoslovakia	8.2	8.4	9.5	11.4	12.4	13.4	14.1
8.	Denmark	12.5	12.3	11.2	10.5	10.2	10.5	9.6
9.	Finland	4.6	4.6	5.3	5.7	5.8	5.9	5.7
10.	France	6.9	7.1	7.2	7.0	7.1	6.7	5.9
11.	Germany, Fed. Repub.	8.0	7.7	8.3	9.3	9.7	8.7	7.5
12.	Greece			0.6	0.8	0.7	0.9	0.8
13.	Hong Kong		3.9	4.4	4.9	4.9	5.6	5.7
14.	Hungary		6.0	7.1	7.8	9.1	11.0	12.3
15.	Ireland	8.5	7.4	7.4	8.0	8.3	7.8	7.1
16.	Israel	4.4	3.5	3.3	3.4	4.0	4.0	3.3
17.	Italy	4.0	4.5	5.4	6.0	6.2	6.0	5.9
18.	Japan	4.3	4.4	4.8	5.3	5.9	6.1	6.2
19.	Mexico		0.9	0.9	0.8	0.7	0.7[c)]	0.8[d)]
20.	Netherlands	7.3	7.1	6.9	6.9	7.0	6.3	5.6
21.	New Zealand	7.8	7.6	7.9	8.6	9.3	10.0	10.6
22.	Norway	5.1	4.6	5.4	6.2	7.0	8.1	8.2
23.	Poland		2.3[e)]	3.3	4.4	5.6	7.1	8.0
24.	Portugal		3.7	3.9	4.9	6.2	6.0	5.1
25.	Singapore			6.8	6.2	8.2	7.4	7.4
26.	Spain	2.2	2.7	3.0	3.5	4.2	4.4	4.2[f)]
27.	Sweden	6.3	6.8	6.3	6.4	6.9	6.1	5.4
28.	Switzerland	9.0	8.4	7.7	8.3	7.2	6.5	6.1
29.	U.K., England & Wales	11.1	10.0	9.4	9.4	9.1	8.7	8.2
30.	U.K., Northern Ireland	8.9	8.8	8.3	7.9	8.2	6.7	7.5
31.	U.K., Scotland	10.8	10.1	9.6	9.1	9.1	8.1	8.1
32.	U.S., White	6.8	6.1	5.4	5.0	4.2	3.4	2.9
33.	U.S., Nonwhite	5.2	4.7	4.6	4.5	4.1	3.3	2.8
34.	Yugoslavia			3.1	4.0	5.0	6.4	7.1

[a)] 1954–57, [b)] 1983, 84, 86, [c)] 1978, 81, 82, [d)] 1983, 85, 86, [e)] 1959–62, [f)] 1983–86.

by Site and Year (1953–57 to 1983–87)
Rectum, rectosigmoid junction, and anus (female)

Country	1953–1957	1958–1962	1963–1967	1968–1972	1973–1977	1978–1982	1983–1987
1. Australia	4.0	3.8	3.6	3.7	3.7	3.6	3.4
2. Austria		4.9	5.5	5.5	5.6	5.5	5.0
3. Belgium	6.0[a]	5.9	5.8	5.3	4.7	4.3	3.8[b]
4. Canada	4.7	4.7	4.5	4.1	3.5	3.4	2.8
5. Chile		2.1	2.3	2.4	2.1	2.2	2.1
6. Costa Rica			2.1	1.7	1.8	2.4	2.1
7. Czechoslovakia	4.6	4.8	5.2	6.6	6.7	7.0	6.9
8. Denmark	7.2	6.9	6.7	6.3	6.2	5.9	5.6
9. Finland	3.6	3.6	4.3	4.0	4.1	3.6	3.6
10. France	3.8	3.8	3.8	3.6	3.4	3.4	2.9
11. Germany, Fed. Repub.	4.6	4.8	5.2	5.8	5.8	5.2	4.6
12. Greece			0.6	0.6	0.7	0.6	0.7
13. Hong Kong		2.7	2.8	2.9	2.9	3.7	3.6
14. Hungary		4.6	4.8	5.4	5.7	6.9	7.0
15. Ireland	4.2	4.3	4.0	4.5	4.4	4.1	3.4
16. Israel	3.1	2.8	3.0	2.9	3.3	3.1	2.8
17. Italy	2.8	3.1	3.3	3.7	3.8	3.7	3.4
18. Japan	3.2	3.4	3.5	3.8	3.9	3.7	3.4
19. Mexico		1.0	1.1	0.9	0.7	0.7[c]	0.8[d]
20. Netherlands	5.1	4.7	4.6	4.4	4.0	3.6	3.1
21. New Zealand	4.8	5.2	5.1	5.1	6.1	6.3	5.6
22. Norway	3.1	3.0	3.4	4.0	4.5	4.9	4.9
23. Poland		1.7[e]	2.5	3.2	4.0	5.1	5.6
24. Portugal		2.6	2.8	3.5	4.0	3.2	2.8
25. Singapore			3.2	3.5	4.9	5.5	4.5
26. Spain	1.9	2.2	2.4	2.5	2.9	2.9	2.7[f]
27. Sweden	3.8	3.8	3.9	3.9	4.0	3.5	3.5
28. Switzerland	4.6	4.1	3.8	3.9	3.7	3.6	3.2
29. U.K., England & Wales	6.0	5.7	5.5	5.4	5.2	4.8	4.5
30. U.K., Northern Ireland	5.4	4.9	5.2	4.9	4.7	4.2	3.7
31. U.K., Scotland	5.7	5.8	5.7	5.3	5.1	4.6	5.0
32. U.S., White	4.6	4.0	3.4	2.9	2.5	2.0	1.7
33. U.S., Nonwhite	4.4	3.9	3.4	3.3	2.6	2.1	1.8
34. Yugoslavia			2.5	3.1	3.8	4.2	4.7

[a] 1954–57, [b] 1983, 84, 86, [c] 1978, 81, 82, [d] 1983, 85, 86, [e] 1959–62, [f] 1983–86.

TABLE I-7. Age-Adjusted Death Rates of Cancer

Liver and intrahepatic bile ducts (male)

Country	1953–1957	1958–1962	1963–1967	1968–1972	1973–1977	1978–1982	1983–1987
1. Australia				1.6	1.7	2.1	
2. Austria				4.2[a]	5.0	5.6	6.2
3. Belgium				4.9	4.5	3.6	3.4[b]
4. Canada				2.4[a]	2.3	2.3	2.7
5. Chile							4.9
6. Costa Rica							6.8
7. Czechoslovakia				6.6	5.9		
8. Denmark				3.3[a]	3.1	2.8	2.1
9. Finland				3.6[a]	3.8	3.7	3.8
10. France				7.3	7.1	7.4	8.6
11. Germany, Fed. Repub.				4.3	4.3	3.7	3.9
12. Greece				16.7	18.2	17.8	16.0
13. Hong Kong				36.3[a]	29.7	31.1	29.2
14. Hungary					7.9	8.1	8.0
15. Ireland				2.4	2.9	2.2	2.8
16. Israel				4.1[a]	4.1	3.4	
17. Italy				10.9	10.2	9.6	11.1
18. Japan				12.4	12.7	15.5	18.8
19. Mexico							1.3[c]
20. Netherlands				1.8[a]	2.3	1.8	1.7
21. New Zealand				2.0	2.1	2.4	2.5
22. Norway				1.9[a]	1.5	1.6	1.6
23. Poland							7.4
24. Portugal							3.6
25. Singapore				24.5[a]	26.5	23.6	24.5
26. Spain				10.0	10.0	9.3	9.0[d]
27. Sweden				2.7[a]	3.9	3.7	3.0
28. Switzerland				4.1[a]	4.2	3.9	5.2
29. U.K.,England & Wales				1.3	1.6	1.6	1.8
30. U.K.,Northern Ireland				0.5	1.4	2.1	2.1
31. U.K.,Scotland				1.9	1.9	2.1	2.5
32. U.S.,White		2.8	2.6			2.2[e]	2.4
33. U.S.,Nonwhite		4.9	5.5			4.9[e]	5.4
34. Yugoslavia				7.3	8.0	6.4	

[a] 1969–72, [b] 1983, 84, 86, [c] 1983, 85, 86, [d] 1983–86, [e] 1979–82.

by Site and Year (1953–57 to 1983–87)
Liver and intrahepatic bile ducts (female)

	Country	1953–1957	1958–1962	1963–1967	1968–1972	1973–1977	1978–1982	1983–1987
1.	Australia				0.7	0.8	0.9	
2.	Austria				1.7[a]	2.3	2.3	2.2
3.	Belgium				3.7	2.9	2.1	1.8[b]
4.	Canada				1.4[a]	1.3	1.2	1.3
5.	Chile							4.1
6.	Costa Rica							4.9
7.	Czechoslovakia				4.6	3.5		
8.	Denmark				2.1[a]	2.0	2.1	1.3
9.	Finland				1.9[a]	2.0	2.4	1.9
10.	France				4.0	3.1	2.4	2.1
11.	Germany, Fed. Repub.				3.1	2.7	2.0	1.6
12.	Greece				9.1	8.9	8.4	7.3
13.	Hong Kong				8.5[a]	7.5	7.6	7.3
14.	Hungary					4.7	4.1	3.8
15.	Ireland				2.0	2.2	1.3	1.9
16.	Israel				3.7[a]	2.5	2.3	
17.	Italy				7.7	6.7	5.5	5.2
18.	Japan				6.2	5.4	5.2	5.2
19.	Mexico							1.1[c]
20.	Netherlands				1.2[a]	1.4	1.0	0.8
21.	New Zealand				1.0	1.0	1.1	1.0
22.	Norway				1.0[a]	0.8	0.9	0.9
23.	Poland							6.0
24.	Portugal							1.9
25.	Singapore				8.3[a]	7.3	6.6	7.7
26.	Spain				9.6	8.3	6.3	4.9[d]
27.	Sweden				1.9[a]	2.5	2.2	1.8
28.	Switzerland				1.5[a]	1.5	1.1	1.3
29.	U.K., England & Wales				0.6	0.8	0.8	0.9
30.	U.K., Northern Ireland				0.4	0.8	1.3	1.5
31.	U.K., Scotland				0.9	0.8	1.0	1.1
32.	U.S., White		1.9	1.6			1.2[e]	1.2
33.	U.S., Nonwhite		2.6	2.3			1.9[e]	1.9
34.	Yugoslavia				5.1	5.3	3.9	

[a] 1969–72, [b] 1983, 84, 86, [c] 1983, 85, 86, [d] 1983–86, [e] 1979–82.

TABLE I-8. Age-Adjusted Death Rates of Cancer

Gallbladder and extrahepatic bile ducts (male)

	Country	1953–1957	1958–1962	1963–1967	1968–1972	1973–1977	1978–1982	1983–1987
1.	Australia				1.5	1.4	1.4	1.2
2.	Austria				3.2[a)]	3.0	3.2	2.6
3.	Belgium				1.9[a)]	1.8	1.8	1.8[b)]
4.	Canada		1.6	1.4	1.5	1.5	1.5	1.3
5.	Chile							
6.	Costa Rica							
7.	Czechoslovakia				2.7	3.0	3.3	2.2
8.	Denmark				1.7[a)]	1.6	1.6	1.4
9.	Finland		1.4	0.9	1.3	1.5	2.1	2.0
10.	France		0.9	0.9	1.0	1.1	1.2	1.4
11.	Germany, Fed. Repub.				2.8	2.7	2.6	2.5
12.	Greece				0.3	0.4	0.3	0.3
13.	Hong Kong				1.6[a)]	2.5	3.1[c)]	2.9
14.	Hungary					3.1	3.5	3.9
15.	Ireland				1.0	1.0	1.3	1.0
16.	Israel		1.6	1.8	1.7	1.7	1.3	1.0
17.	Italy		0.9	0.8	1.1	1.2	1.4	1.8
18.	Japan		1.5	2.3	2.9	3.6	4.3	5.3
19.	Mexico							
20.	Netherlands				2.3[a)]	2.2	2.3	1.9
21.	New Zealand				1.5	1.7	1.2	1.2
22.	Norway				1.0[a)]	0.9	1.0	1.1
23.	Poland							
24.	Portugal							1.0
25.	Singapore				0.8[a)]	0.8		0.8
26.	Spain				1.0	0.7	0.9	1.2[d)]
27.	Sweden		1.4	1.7[e)]	1.9	2.3	2.4	2.5
28.	Switzerland				1.6[a)]	1.7	1.8	1.7
29.	U.K., England & Wales		1.2	1.2	1.2	1.1	1.0	0.9
30.	U.K., Northern Ireland		1.1		1.0	1.2	0.9	0.9
31.	U.K., Scotland		1.3	1.6	1.3	1.2	1.2	0.9
32.	U.S., White		1.4	1.4	1.3	1.2	1.1	1.0
33.	U.S., Nonwhite		1.1	1.2	1.0	1.0	1.0	0.8
34.	Yugoslavia				0.9	0.9	1.2	1.5

[a)] 1969–72, [b)] 1983, 84, 86, [c)] 1978–81, [d)] 1983–86, [e)] 1963–66.

by Site and Year (1953–57 to 1983–87)
Gallbladder and extrahepatic bile ducts (female)

Country	1953–1957	1958–1962	1963–1967	1968–1972	1973–1977	1978–1982	1983–1987
1. Australia				2.0	1.9	1.6	1.6
2. Austria				5.8[a)]	5.2	5.0	4.3
3. Belgium				2.6[a)]	2.4	2.3	2.2[b)]
4. Canada		2.7	2.5	2.3	2.1	1.8	1.6
5. Chile							
6. Costa Rica							
7. Czechoslovakia				5.0	5.5	5.5	3.5
8. Denmark				2.9[a)]	2.8	2.5	2.4
9. Finland		1.8	1.7	2.5	3.2	3.5	3.5
10. France		1.4	1.4	1.5	1.6	1.7	1.8
11. Germany, Fed. Repub.				5.1	5.0	4.6	4.2
12. Greece				0.4	0.5	0.6	0.5
13. Hong Kong				1.0[a)]	1.7	2.1[c)]	2.1
14. Hungary					7.6	8.1	7.8
15. Ireland				1.9	2.0	1.7	1.4
16. Israel		4.9	4.5	4.5	3.8	2.7	2.0
17. Italy		1.3	1.3	1.7	1.7	2.1	2.4
18. Japan		1.5	2.3	3.1	3.8	4.5	5.3
19. Mexico							
20. Netherlands				4.3[a)]	3.7	3.5	2.8
21. New Zealand				2.0	1.8	1.7	1.4
22. Norway				1.3[a)]	1.2	1.2	1.3
23. Poland							
24. Portugal							1.2
25. Singapore				0.8[a)]	1.2		0.9
26. Spain				0.9	1.3	1.6	2.0[d)]
27. Sweden		2.5	3.4[e)]	3.8	4.0	4.4	4.3
28. Switzerland				3.0[a)]	3.0	2.9	2.5
29. U.K., England & Wales		1.6	1.5	1.4	1.3	1.1	1.0
30. U.K., Northern Ireland		2.2		1.7	1.5	1.3	1.2
31. U.K., Scotland		1.8	1.8	1.5	1.5	1.3	1.0
32. U.S., White		2.5	2.2	1.8	1.6	1.4	1.2
33. U.S., Nonwhite		1.5	1.6	1.3	1.3	1.2	1.1
34. Yugoslavia				1.8	1.9	2.5	2.5

[a)] 1969–72, [b)] 1983,84,86, [c)] 1978–81, [d)] 1983–86, [e)] 1963–66.

TABLE I-9. Age-Adjusted Death Rates of Cancer

Pancreas (male)

Country	1953–1957	1958–1962	1963–1967	1968–1972	1973–1977	1978–1982	1983–1987
1. Australia	6.0	6.7	7.2	7.8	8.0	7.6	7.0
2. Austria		7.1	7.4	8.1	8.3	8.7	8.9
3. Belgium	3.6[a]	4.7	5.5	6.4	7.5[b]	7.9[c]	7.5[d]
4. Canada	7.1	7.9	8.4	9.1	8.9	9.0	8.6
5. Chile		3.1	4.0				
6. Costa Rica							
7. Czechoslovakia		5.2	6.6	7.3	8.2	8.8	10.0
8. Denmark	6.0	7.2	7.9	9.3	9.3	9.2	9.1
9. Finland	5.2	7.3	7.9	9.9	9.9	9.5	9.8
10. France		4.5	5.2	5.9	6.6	7.0	7.1
11. Germany, Fed. Repub.	3.8	4.9	5.9	6.6	6.9	7.8	8.2
12. Greece				3.2	4.0	4.8	5.6
13. Hong Kong				4.1	4.1	4.5	4.1
14. Hungary					7.9	9.1	9.8
15. Ireland	5.3	6.0	7.4	8.3	8.8	8.7	9.0
16. Israel	4.8	5.6	6.6	7.8	8.2	7.8	7.5
17. Italy	2.8	3.5	4.0	4.9	5.6	6.3	7.0
18. Japan	1.9	3.0	4.1	5.4	6.0	7.0	8.0
19. Mexico							
20. Netherlands	4.2	5.8	6.7	8.1	8.8	9.3	8.8
21. New Zealand	6.6	7.6	8.1	7.7	8.4	7.7	7.2
22. Norway	5.4	5.8	6.8	7.6	7.7	8.1	8.0
23. Poland			3.8				7.8
24. Portugal							5.4
25. Singapore				2.3	3.0	3.8	5.1
26. Spain		1.9	2.6	3.0	3.6	4.3	5.0[e]
27. Sweden	6.3	7.2	8.2	9.1	9.4	9.2	8.6
28. Switzerland	4.9	5.2	5.9	6.5	7.6	7.6	7.7
29. U.K., England & Wales	6.4	6.9	7.5	8.1	8.1	8.2	7.7
30. U.K., Northern Ireland	6.0	6.6	6.7	8.1	8.3	8.2	6.9
31. U.K., Scotland	6.6	7.5	8.8	9.3	8.8	8.3	7.6
32. U.S., White	7.4	8.0	8.4	8.5	8.3	7.9	7.4
33. U.S., Nonwhite	7.8	9.0	9.9	10.4	10.1	9.8	9.6
34. Yugoslavia			2.9	3.6	4.5	4.9	6.0

[a] 1954–57, [b] 1973–76, [c] 1979–82, [d] 1983, 84, 86, [e] 1983–86.

by Site and Year (1953–57 to 1983–87)
Pancreas (female)

Country	1953–1957	1958–1962	1963–1967	1968–1972	1973–1977	1978–1982	1983–1987
1. Australia	3.5	3.6	4.0	4.4	4.6	4.4	4.6
2. Austria		4.5	4.8	5.3	5.3	5.6	5.8
3. Belgium	2.5[a]	3.0	3.3	3.5	4.0[b]	4.5[c]	4.3[d]
4. Canada	4.6	4.6	4.9	5.3	5.5	5.5	5.6
5. Chile		2.9	3.4				
6. Costa Rica							
7. Czechoslovakia		3.2	3.8	4.3	4.8	5.0	5.5
8. Denmark	4.2	4.6	5.6	5.7	6.1	7.1	6.9
9. Finland	3.4	4.2	5.2	5.5	6.1	6.5	6.3
10. France		2.6	2.8	3.1	3.1	3.3	3.5
11. Germany, Fed. Repub.	2.5	3.2	3.8	4.0	4.2	4.8	5.2
12. Greece				1.8	2.2	2.7	3.1
13. Hong Kong				2.2	2.3	2.8	2.8
14. Hungary					5.2	5.8	5.8
15. Ireland	4.1	5.2	5.0	5.7	6.2	6.0	5.5
16. Israel	4.7	4.0	4.7	5.8	5.8	5.4	5.1
17. Italy	1.7	2.1	2.4	2.7	3.2	3.5	4.1
18. Japan	1.3	1.9	2.6	3.2	3.5	4.0	4.5
19. Mexico							
20. Netherlands	3.0	3.8	4.4	4.9	5.3	5.5	5.5
21. New Zealand	4.5	3.8	4.8	4.2	5.0	4.8	4.7
22. Norway	3.1	3.6	3.7	4.6	4.7	5.0	5.4
23. Poland			2.8				4.7
24. Portugal							2.9
25. Singapore				1.0	1.9	2.2	3.3
26. Spain		1.4	1.8	2.0	2.3	2.4	2.8[e]
27. Sweden	4.3	4.7	5.6	5.8	6.5	6.6	6.6
28. Switzerland	3.3	3.4	4.0	4.3	4.6	4.8	5.1
29. U.K., England & Wales	3.9	4.3	4.5	4.7	5.0	5.0	5.1
30. U.K., Northern Ireland	4.1	4.5	4.3	5.0	5.4	5.6	5.4
31. U.K., Scotland	4.6	5.1	5.3	5.4	5.5	5.9	5.5
32. U.S., White	4.5	4.7	4.9	5.0	5.1	5.1	5.1
33. U.S., Nonwhite	4.5	5.7	6.0	6.3	6.6	6.7	6.9
34. Yugoslavia			1.8	2.3	2.6	2.9	3.4

[a] 1954–57, [b] 1973–76, [c] 1979–82, [d] 1983,84,86, [e] 1983–86.

TABLE I-10. Age-Adjusted Death Rates of Cancer

Larynx (male)

	Country	1953–1957	1958–1962	1963–1967	1968–1972	1973–1977	1978–1982	1983–1987
1.	Australia	1.7	1.8	1.9	2.0	2.3	2.2	2.2
2.	Austria		3.6	3.9	3.2	3.6	3.8	3.5
3.	Belgium	3.3[a]	4.0	4.8	4.6	4.6	4.7	4.6[b]
4.	Canada	1.7	1.7	2.0	2.1	2.3	2.5	2.5
5.	Chile		1.4	1.8	1.9	2.3	2.2	2.2
6.	Costa Rica			1.4	1.6	2.3	1.8	3.1
7.	Czechoslovakia	2.5	2.8	3.2	3.5	4.3	4.5	5.2
8.	Denmark	1.0	1.2	1.2	1.7	1.6	2.2	2.6
9.	Finland	2.8	2.8	3.2	3.0	2.3	2.2	1.5
10.	France	8.6	9.6	11.0	11.2	11.9	11.1	9.5
11.	Germany, Fed. Repub.	1.9	2.0	2.1	2.3	2.3	2.5	2.7
12.	Greece			4.4	4.2	4.1	3.9	3.5
13.	Hong Kong		1.8	1.8	2.4	3.9	3.7	3.0
14.	Hungary		4.0	4.2	5.1	5.6	6.1	7.3
15.	Ireland	2.8	2.4	2.1	2.1	2.1	2.5	2.4
16.	Israel	2.0	1.9	2.1	1.9	2.1	1.9	1.2
17.	Italy	3.7	4.5	5.5	6.5	6.6	6.6	6.3
18.	Japan	1.7	1.6	1.5	1.5	1.4	1.2	1.0
19.	Mexico		1.8	2.1	2.1	2.2	2.2[c]	2.4[d]
20.	Netherlands	1.5	1.7	1.6	1.8	1.9	1.9	1.7
21.	New Zealand	2.1	1.3	1.5	1.6	1.8	1.6	1.7
22.	Norway	0.5	0.5	0.7	1.1	1.0	1.0	1.1
23.	Poland		1.9[e]	3.0	3.5	4.4	5.8	7.0
24.	Portugal		5.1	5.4	5.3	5.3	5.5	5.5
25.	Singapore			3.5	3.6	4.3	4.5	3.9
26.	Spain	6.0	6.5	6.9	7.1	7.5	7.6	7.3[f]
27.	Sweden	0.5	0.6	0.6	0.7	0.9	0.8	0.8
28.	Switzerland	3.6	3.2	3.3	3.3	3.0	3.0	2.4
29.	U.K., England & Wales	2.4	2.2	1.9	1.8	1.7	1.7	1.7
30.	U.K., Northern Ireland	1.7	1.6	1.7	1.8	1.7	1.7	1.6
31.	U.K., Scotland	2.3	2.0	2.1	2.0	1.8	1.7	1.8
32.	U.S., White	2.1	2.1	2.1	2.2	2.2	2.0	1.8
33.	U.S., Nonwhite	2.0	2.4	2.7	3.0	3.4	3.5	3.4
34.	Yugoslavia			3.8	4.6	5.2	6.1	6.2

[a] 1954–57, [b] 1983, 84, 86, [c] 1978, 81, 82, [d] 1983, 85, 86, [e] 1959–62, [f] 1983–86.

by Site and Year (1953–57 to 1983–87)
Larynx (female)

	Country	1953–1957	1958–1962	1963–1967	1968–1972	1973–1977	1978–1982	1983–1987
1.	Australia	0.3	0.2	0.2	0.2	0.2	0.3	0.2
2.	Austria		0.2	0.2	0.2	0.2	0.2	0.2
3.	Belgium	0.3[a]	0.3	0.4	0.3	0.3	0.4	0.4[b]
4.	Canada	0.3	0.3	0.2	0.3	0.3	0.3	0.4
5.	Chile		0.3	0.3	0.3	0.4	0.3	0.3
6.	Costa Rica			0.4	0.2	0.5	0.6	0.6
7.	Czechoslovakia	0.3	0.2	0.2	0.2	0.2	0.2	0.2
8.	Denmark	0.2	0.2	0.2	0.2	0.3	0.4	0.4
9.	Finland	0.3	0.2	0.1	0.1	0.1	0.1	0.1
10.	France	0.4	0.4	0.4	0.4	0.4	0.4	0.4
11.	Germany, Fed. Repub.	0.2	0.2	0.2	0.2	0.2	0.2	0.2
12.	Greece			0.4	0.4	0.5	0.2	0.3
13.	Hong Kong		0.2	0.3	0.2	0.4	0.4	0.3
14.	Hungary		0.4	0.4	0.5	0.4	0.4	0.5
15.	Ireland	1.0	1.1	1.0	1.1	0.8	0.6	0.5
16.	Israel	0.3	0.3	0.2	0.3	0.4	0.2	0.2
17.	Italy	0.3	0.3	0.3	0.3	0.3	0.3	0.3
18.	Japan	0.5	0.4	0.3	0.3	0.2	0.1	0.1
19.	Mexico		0.7	0.7	0.6	0.6	0.6[c]	0.5[d]
20.	Netherlands	0.3	0.2	0.2	0.2	0.1	0.1	0.2
21.	New Zealand	0.2	0.2	0.1	0.2	0.3	0.3	0.3
22.	Norway	0.1	0.0	0.0	0.1	0.1	0.1	0.1
23.	Poland		0.3[e]	0.3	0.3	0.3	0.4	0.5
24.	Portugal		0.4	0.4	0.5	0.5	0.4	0.3
25.	Singapore			0.3	0.4	0.4	0.4	0.5
26.	Spain	0.4	0.4	0.4	0.4	0.3	0.2	0.2[f]
27.	Sweden	0.1	0.1	0.1	0.1	0.1	0.1	0.1
28.	Switzerland	0.2	0.1	0.2	0.1	0.2	0.2	0.2
29.	U.K., England & Wales	0.5	0.4	0.3	0.3	0.3	0.4	0.3
30.	U.K., Northern Ireland	0.9	0.7	0.7	0.4	0.6	0.5	0.4
31.	U.K., Scotland	0.6	0.5	0.4	0.3	0.4	0.4	0.4
32.	U.S., White	0.2	0.2	0.2	0.3	0.3	0.3	0.4
33.	U.S., Nonwhite	0.3	0.3	0.4	0.5	0.5	0.6	0.6
34.	Yugoslavia			0.5	0.5	0.6	0.5	0.5

[a] 1954–57, [b] 1983, 84, 86, [c] 1978, 81, 82, [d] 1983, 85, 86, e) 1959–62, [f] 1983–86.

TABLE I-11. Age-Adjusted Death Rates of Cancer

Trachea, bronchus, and lung (male)

	Country	1953–1957	1958–1962	1963–1967	1968–1972	1973–1977	1978–1982	1983–1987
1.	Australia	20.9	27.8	36.2	43.0	46.9	48.3	46.3
2.	Austria		48.8	51.3	51.6	51.2	49.1	47.6
3.	Belgium	28.8[a)]	37.7	49.2	60.0	69.9	77.8	79.0[b)]
4.	Canada	20.5	25.9	33.0	40.6	47.5	53.0	55.8
5.	Chile		13.0	15.1	18.2	19.4	20.7	21.8
6.	Costa Rica			7.0	8.6	10.6	14.4	15.7
7.	Czechoslovakia	34.2	47.1	58.6	61.7	65.8	69.3	73.3
8.	Denmark	21.4	29.2	37.2	43.4	46.8	53.4	54.8
9.	Finland	47.7	58.2	62.0	67.8	65.4	64.4	56.8
10.	France	16.7	21.9	27.7	31.1	36.8	42.1	44.9
11.	Germany, Fed. Repub.	27.4	35.4	42.0	44.9	47.4	49.0	49.0
12.	Greece			30.6	33.1	40.8	44.8	48.0
13.	Hong Kong		20.8	29.9	39.0	47.6	55.4	55.9
14.	Hungary		28.0	35.7	41.4	47.7	58.8	69.2
15.	Ireland	19.6	25.8	31.2	39.3	45.4	46.8	50.3
16.	Israel	16.9	18.1	21.5	22.8	25.1	24.8	23.8
17.	Italy	15.1	21.5	29.6	38.2	44.9	52.9	57.9
18.	Japan	5.8	9.8	13.2	16.3	19.8	24.2	27.7
19.	Mexico		5.8	7.2	7.7	9.7	12.5[c)]	14.9[d)]
20.	Netherlands	31.9	42.4	54.5	65.1	72.7	77.6	76.3
21.	New Zealand	25.7	30.6	37.3	45.0	49.0	48.8	49.0
22.	Norway	8.5	12.0	14.7	19.0	22.1	26.4	29.5
23.	Poland		18.1[e)]	28.1	36.7	45.6	54.6	64.7
24.	Portugal		8.7	10.9	13.5	15.5	20.1	23.5
25.	Singapore			31.0	37.5	47.6	55.1	55.3
26.	Spain	11.8	16.1	19.3	22.7	28.6	34.4	39.3[f)]
27.	Sweden	10.8	14.6	16.9	20.4	24.1	24.6	24.2
28.	Switzerland	27.2	31.4	37.0	41.8	47.4	48.8	48.3
29.	U.K., England & Wales	52.9	63.2	70.0	74.0	73.6	69.9	64.2
30.	U.K., Northern Ireland	30.7	36.2	42.5	49.8	54.3	54.8	56.4
31.	U.K., Scotland	54.4	67.1	78.0	82.6	84.0	83.5	78.5
32.	U.S., White	25.8	31.9	38.5	46.3	51.2	54.7	55.3
33.	U.S., Nonwhite	22.8	31.3	41.6	53.8	62.2	68.3	68.8
34.	Yugoslavia			22.5	27.3	32.8	39.3	44.0

[a)] 1954–57, [b)] 1983, 84, 86, [c)] 1978, 81, 82, [d)] 1983, 85, 86, [e)] 1959–62, [f)] 1983–86.

by Site and Year (1953–57 to 1983–87)
Trachea, bronchus, and lung (female)

Country	1953–1957	1958–1962	1963–1967	1968–1972	1973–1977	1978–1982	1983–1987
1. Australia	3.3	3.5	4.4	6.0	7.6	9.7	11.4
2. Austria		5.9	6.0	6.3	6.7	7.4	8.4
3. Belgium	3.6[a)]	4.0	4.4	4.6	5.7	6.2	6.8[b)]
4. Canada	3.6	3.8	5.0	6.6	9.5	13.4	17.7
5. Chile		4.6	5.3	5.3	5.0	5.4	5.9
6. Costa Rica			3.9	5.0	5.0	6.5	5.9
7. Czechoslovakia	5.4	5.4	5.8	5.6	5.7	6.7	7.8
8. Denmark	4.4	5.3	6.9	8.8	11.0	14.9	20.7
9. Finland	4.0	3.6	4.0	4.2	4.5	5.6	6.2
10. France	3.4	3.4	3.8	3.4	3.5	3.8	4.4
11. Germany, Fed. Repub.	4.1	4.5	5.1	4.7	5.1	5.8	7.0
12. Greece			5.9	5.8	6.4	6.4	6.4
13. Hong Kong		10.0	15.6	19.3	22.5	23.6	23.9
14. Hungary		6.5	7.3	7.6	8.6	10.0	12.0
15. Ireland	5.6	6.1	7.4	10.5	13.4	15.6	17.6
16. Israel	6.4	7.0	7.0	7.9	7.6	8.0	7.8
17. Italy	3.2	3.8	4.5	4.7	5.4	6.0	6.9
18. Japan	2.1	3.7	4.6	5.3	6.0	7.0	7.7
19. Mexico		3.4	4.0	4.0	4.4	4.7[c)]	5.8[d)]
20. Netherlands	3.1	3.3	3.5	3.8	4.5	6.1	8.2
21. New Zealand	3.3	4.4	5.3	8.1	11.1	13.4	14.8
22. Norway	2.4	2.6	2.8	3.7	4.5	5.7	8.1
23. Poland		3.6[e)]	4.3	5.1	5.6	6.8	8.2
24. Portugal		2.3	2.5	2.9	3.3	3.6	3.8
25. Singapore			11.4	12.1	14.9	17.4	18.9
26. Spain	2.9	3.5	3.8	4.0	4.0	3.8	3.6[f)]
27. Sweden	3.7	3.9	4.1	4.8	6.0	7.3	8.6
28. Switzerland	3.2	3.0	3.4	3.5	4.4	5.2	6.5
29. U.K., England & Wales	6.7	8.1	10.2	12.5	14.9	17.3	19.3
30. U.K., Northern Ireland	5.5	5.9	6.7	9.3	11.6	13.8	15.4
31. U.K., Scotland	7.7	9.0	11.3	14.3	17.8	23.2	26.3
32. U.S.,White	4.1	4.7	6.2	9.4	12.9	17.3	21.5
33. U.S., Nonwhite	4.2	5.0	6.6	9.7	12.7	16.3	19.3
34. Yugoslavia			4.0	4.7	5.5	6.4	7.2

a) 1954–57, b) 1983, 84, 86, c) 1978, 81, 82, d) 1983, 85, 86, e) 1959–62, f) 1983–86.

Table I-12. Age-Adjusted Death Rates of Cancer

Skin (male)

	Country	1953–1957	1958–1962	1963–1967	1968–1972	1973–1977	1978–1982	1983–1987
1.	Australia	3.8	4.2	4.5	4.7	5.2	5.9	6.2
2.	Austria		1.7	2.0	2.1	2.2	2.4	3.1
3.	Belgium	1.6[a]	1.6	1.6	1.5	1.4	1.6	1.5[b]
4.	Canada	1.8	1.8	1.9	1.8	1.8	1.9	2.2
5.	Chile		0.8	1.1	1.4	1.1	0.8	0.8
6.	Costa Rica			1.6	1.8	0.9	0.7	0.7
7.	Czechoslovakia	1.9	2.1	2.5	2.3	2.6	3.0	3.3
8.	Denmark	2.0	2.0	2.0	2.6	2.6	2.7	3.2
9.	Finland	1.7	1.9	2.1	2.6	2.8	2.6	2.5
10.	France	2.0	2.0	1.9	1.7	1.7	1.7	1.7
11.	Germany, Fed. Repub.	1.5	1.7	2.0	1.9	1.9	2.0	2.1
12.	Greece			1.0	0.9	1.0	1.0	1.1
13.	Hong Kong		0.5	0.6	0.6	0.8	0.4	0.5
14.	Hungary		2.5	2.3	2.6	2.9	2.8	2.9
15.	Ireland	2.7	3.0	2.5	2.5	2.2	2.2	2.8
16.	Israel	1.5	1.2	1.4	1.8	2.3	2.5	2.2
17.	Italy	1.9	1.7	1.7	1.7	1.4	1.9	2.0
18.	Japan	1.0	1.0	0.9	0.8	0.8	0.6	0.5
19.	Mexico		0.7	0.6	0.7	0.8	0.5[c]	0.4[d]
20.	Netherlands	1.6	1.7	1.6	1.8	1.9	2.1	2.4
21.	New Zealand	3.3	2.7	3.2	4.1	4.8	5.9	6.3
22.	Norway	1.7	1.8	2.2	2.7	3.6	3.3	3.8
23.	Poland		0.9[e]	1.7	1.9	2.0	2.1	2.5
24.	Portugal		1.4	1.7	1.8	1.9	1.3	1.0
25.	Singapore			1.2	1.2	1.4	0.7	1.0
26.	Spain	1.6	1.6	1.6	1.2	1.4	1.4	2.1[f]
27.	Sweden	1.4	1.8	1.9	2.2	2.4	2.8	3.0
28.	Switzerland	2.2	2.4	2.5	2.6	3.2	3.2	3.8
29.	U.K., England & Wales	1.7	1.5	1.5	1.6	1.7	1.8	2.0
30.	U.K., Northern Ireland	1.6	1.9	1.7	2.2	1.7	1.5	1.7
31.	U.K., Scotland	2.2	2.2	1.7	1.9	2.1	1.9	1.8
32.	U.S., White	2.5	2.5	2.7	2.5	2.9	3.2	3.6
33.	U.S., Nonwhite	1.1	1.1	1.2	1.0	0.9	0.9	1.3
34.	Yugoslavia			1.4	1.5	1.7	1.6	2.1

[a] 1954–57, [b] 1983, 84, 86, [c] 1978, 81, 82, [d] 1983, 85, 86, [e] 1959–62, [f] 1983–86.

by Site and Year (1953–57 to 1983–87)
Skin (female)

	Country	1953–1957	1958–1962	1963–1967	1968–1972	1973–1977	1978–1982	1983–1987
1.	Australia	2.3	2.3	2.6	2.6	2.7	2.7	2.9
2.	Austria		1.6	1.6	1.7	1.5	1.7	1.8
3.	Belgium	1.3[a]	1.1	1.1	1.0	1.0	1.0	1.0[b]
4.	Canada	1.2	1.2	1.3	1.3	1.2	1.2	1.3
5.	Chile		0.6	0.9	1.0	1.0	0.5	0.7
6.	Costa Rica			1.3	0.7	0.9	0.3	0.3
7.	Czechoslovakia	1.7	1.7	1.8	1.6	1.7	2.0	2.1
8.	Denmark	1.6	1.8	1.9	2.0	2.2	2.1	2.2
9.	Finland	1.4	1.4	1.4	1.7	1.6	1.4	1.4
10.	France	1.7	1.6	1.4	1.3	1.3	1.2	1.2
11.	Germany, Fed. Repub.	1.6	1.5	1.5	1.4	1.4	1.4	1.4
12.	Greece			0.9	0.8	0.9	0.8	0.8
13.	Hong Kong		0.3	0.4	0.4	0.5	0.3	0.3
14.	Hungary		2.0	1.9	2.0	2.2	2.0	2.0
15.	Ireland	2.1	1.8	2.1	2.1	1.8	2.2	2.2
16.	Israel	1.2	1.5	1.6	1.3	1.4	1.9	1.8
17.	Italy	1.3	1.2	1.2	1.1	1.0	1.2	1.3
18.	Japan	0.7	0.7	0.6	0.6	0.5	0.4	0.3
19.	Mexico		0.7	0.7	0.8	0.6	0.4[c]	0.3[d]
20.	Netherlands	1.4	1.2	1.3	1.3	1.3	1.4	1.5
21.	New Zealand	1.8	2.2	2.4	2.5	3.2	3.2	3.6
22.	Norway	1.5	1.3	1.6	1.8	2.0	1.9	2.3
23.	Poland		0.7[e]	1.5	1.6	1.6	1.6	1.8
24.	Portugal		1.1	1.3	1.4	1.3	0.9	0.6
25.	Singapore			1.2	0.8	0.7	0.7	0.6
26.	Spain	1.2	1.2	1.1	0.8	0.9	0.8	1.0[f]
27.	Sweden	1.0	1.2	1.3	1.5	1.5	1.9	1.8
28.	Switzerland	1.8	1.9	1.8	1.7	1.9	2.0	2.3
29.	U.K., England & Wales	1.3	1.2	1.2	1.3	1.5	1.5	1.5
30.	U.K., Northern Ireland	1.6	1.4	1.4	1.5	1.3	1.7	1.6
31.	U.K., Scotland	1.4	1.5	1.4	1.6	1.6	1.6	1.6
32.	U.S., White	1.6	1.6	1.6	1.5	1.6	1.7	1.7
33.	U.S., Nonwhite	0.8	0.8	0.8	0.7	0.5	0.6	0.5
34.	Yugoslavia			1.1	1.2	1.2	1.2	1.5

[a] 1954–57, [b] 1983, 84, 86, [c] 1978, 81, 82, [d] 1983, 85, 86, [e] 1959–62, [f] 1983–86.

TABLE I-13. Age-Adjusted Death Rates of Cancer by Site and Year (1953–57 to 1983–87)
Breast (female)

Country	1953–1957	1958–1962	1963–1967	1968–1972	1973–1977	1978–1982	1983–1987
1. Australia	20.1	19.1	19.5	20.0	20.1	19.5	20.6
2. Austria		15.7	17.4	18.4	19.7	19.8	21.9
3. Belgium	20.1[a]	20.6	21.4	23.0	23.5	25.8	26.3[b]
4. Canada	22.9	23.3	24.0	23.9	23.8	23.1	23.9
5. Chile		9.4	9.9	12.2	11.8	12.0	12.7
6. Costa Rica			8.2	8.7	8.7	9.9	12.3
7. Czechoslovakia	12.4	13.3	14.9	16.1	17.4	19.1	19.9
8. Denmark	24.4	24.3	24.7	25.9	26.3	25.4	27.4
9. Finland	12.4	13.5	14.1	14.7	15.5	15.2	16.4
10. France	14.8	15.7	17.0	17.4	18.4	18.7	19.3
11. Germany, Fed. Repub.	15.7	16.4	18.0	19.4	20.5	21.1	22.5
12. Greece			8.0	10.4	12.1	14.6	15.2
13. Hong Kong		8.6	8.9	9.0	9.4	8.6	8.7
14. Hungary		12.6	14.2	16.6	18.9	20.6	21.4
15. Ireland	19.7	20.0	21.7	23.8	26.0	26.6	26.1
16. Israel	19.9	21.7	22.3	25.3	24.5	22.5	23.5
17. Italy	13.9	14.6	16.2	17.7	18.6	19.2	20.4
18. Japan	3.8	3.8	3.9	4.3	4.9	5.4	5.8
19. Mexico		3.9	4.5	4.8	5.7	6.1[c]	7.1[d]
20. Netherlands	23.2	24.3	26.1	27.0	26.6	26.2	26.4
21. New Zealand	21.9	22.2	23.5	24.2	24.9	25.5	26.3
22. Norway	17.4	17.1	17.2	18.2	18.0	18.3	18.1
23. Poland		6.4[e]	10.5	11.7	13.2	14.6	15.1
24. Portugal		11.5	12.5	13.5	14.0	15.0	16.3
25. Singapore			10.3	10.1	10.2	13.5	13.2
26. Spain	6.1	7.9	9.5	10.6	12.6	13.7	15.0[f]
27. Sweden	19.0	19.3	18.7	19.2	19.6	18.5	18.0
28. Switzerland	22.2	21.8	22.6	23.8	24.0	24.1	25.2
29. U.K., England & Wales	23.5	23.9	24.8	26.4	27.6	28.2	29.2
30. U.K., Northern Ireland	19.3	18.7	21.5	24.3	25.3	25.9	26.2
31. U.K., Scotland	23.2	23.6	23.6	26.2	26.3	27.9	27.8
32. U.S., White	22.1	21.7	22.1	22.5	22.6	22.2	22.4
33. U.S., Nonwhite	19.4	19.5	20.7	21.2	21.3	20.9	21.8
34. Yugoslavia			7.8	9.6	11.1	12.7	14.1

[a] 1954–57, [b] 1983, 84, 86, [c] 1978, 81, 82, [d] 1983, 85, 86, [e] 1959–62, [f] 1983–86.

Table I-14. Age-Adjusted Death Rates of Cancer by Site and Year (1953–57 to 1983–87)

Uterus

Country	1953–1957	1958–1962	1963–1967	1968–1972	1973–1977	1978–1982	1983–1987
1. Australia	11.1	9.9	8.7	8.0	6.9	5.8	5.5
2. Austria		19.6	18.1	17.0	13.9	11.3	9.7
3. Belgium	14.9[a)]	14.3	12.4	10.7	8.3	7.8	6.9[b)]
4. Canada	13.7	12.1	10.8	9.2	7.2	6.1	5.3
5. Chile		20.2	20.9	22.2	20.3	17.6	15.8
6. Costa Rica			26.8	20.0	16.6	15.0	15.5
7. Czechoslovakia	16.4	14.3	12.8	11.9	11.1	11.2	11.8
8. Denmark	18.4	18.6	17.7	14.7	12.8	11.6	9.8
9. Finland	12.0	11.2	10.3	8.5	6.5	5.4	4.5
10. France	12.9	12.3	11.3	10.2	9.3	7.8	6.6
11. Germany, Fed. Repub.	13.8	12.8	12.9	11.9	10.3	8.4	7.1
12. Greece			6.4	5.9	6.0	5.3	4.6
13. Hong Kong		15.7	12.4	10.7	9.1	6.8	6.4
14. Hungary		21.3	19.0	16.6	16.4	14.5	12.8
15. Ireland	9.2	7.9	8.0	8.1	7.2	6.3	6.0
16. Israel	8.0	6.7	5.9	5.5	5.1	4.3	4.2
17. Italy	13.7	13.7	13.2	12.1	10.4	8.7	7.0
18. Japan	19.1	16.0	13.6	11.3	8.9	6.9	5.2
19. Mexico		19.9	20.9	19.4	18.9	17.6[c)]	18.5[d)]
20. Netherlands	10.9	10.6	10.3	9.5	7.9	6.4	5.5
21. New Zealand	11.0	10.7	9.8	8.8	8.4	8.1	7.7
22. Norway	10.6	9.7	9.0	9.0	8.1	8.1	7.0
23. Poland		12.5[e)]	16.0	15.3	13.4	12.6	12.5
24. Portugal		14.1	13.2	13.3	10.9	9.0	7.8
25. Singapore			14.7	12.4	11.0	10.2	10.1
26. Spain	8.9	9.7	9.9	9.0	8.4	6.9	5.9[f)]
27. Sweden	10.7	11.1	9.8	9.7	8.2	6.8	5.6
28. Switzerland	13.4	13.1	12.3	11.5	9.4	8.3	7.0
29. U.K., England & Wales	11.0	10.8	10.1	9.5	8.7	8.2	7.7
30. U.K.,Northern Ireland	10.6	9.5	7.9	8.8	7.5	6.7	6.1
31. U.K., Scotland	12.9	11.5	10.5	9.1	8.8	7.6	7.8
32. U.S., White	13.9	11.9	10.1	8.2	6.7	5.7	5.0
33. U.S., Nonwhite	32.6	27.2	23.5	18.8	14.8	11.7	9.8
34. Yugoslavia			11.2	11.1	10.6	9.8	9.2

[a)] 1954–57, [b)] 1983, 84, 86, [c)] 1978, 81, 82, [d)] 1983, 85, 86, [e)] 1959–62, [f)] 1983–86.

Table I-15. Age-Adjusted Death Rates of Cancer by Site and Year (1953–57 to 1983–87)
Ovary and other uterine adnexa

Country	1953–1957	1958–1962	1963–1967	1968–1972	1973–1977	1978–1982	1983–1987
1. Australia	6.2	6.0	6.5	6.3	6.4	6.0	5.8
2. Austria				9.2[a]	8.9	8.7	8.2
3. Belgium	5.0[b]	5.6	5.8	7.1	7.1	7.0	7.2[c]
4. Canada	7.1	7.2	7.5	7.6	7.2	6.8	6.3
5. Chile		1.8	2.5				
6. Costa Rica							
7. Czechoslovakia		6.4	6.7	7.4	7.7	8.1	8.2
8. Denmark	10.4	10.8	11.3	12.1	10.7	10.8	9.8
9. Finland	4.8	5.6	6.1	6.6	6.9	6.4	6.3
10. France		3.5	3.9	4.3	4.9	5.5	5.8
11. Germany, Fed. Repub.				7.7	8.0	7.9	7.9
12. Greece				1.3	1.8	2.6	3.0
13. Hong Kong				3.5	3.4	3.0	3.1
14. Hungary					7.0	7.2	7.2
15. Ireland	4.4	4.8	5.4	6.0	7.4	6.9	8.1
16. Israel		6.6	6.8	7.9	7.6	7.1	6.2
17. Italy	2.4	3.0	3.2	3.6	3.8	4.2	4.8
18. Japan	1.2	1.5	1.8	2.1	2.5	3.0	3.2
19. Mexico							
20. Netherlands	7.5	7.8	8.2	9.3	9.3	8.2	8.0
21. New Zealand	6.6	7.7	7.9	8.3	7.7	7.8	7.0
22. Norway	8.1	8.0	8.3	8.8	8.4	8.2	8.9
23. Poland							6.4
24. Portugal							3.0
25. Singapore				2.5	2.8	4.0	3.8
26. Spain		0.7	0.9	1.1	1.8	2.4	2.9[d]
27. Sweden	8.2	8.9	9.3	9.6	9.5	9.0	8.1
28. Switzerland	8.1	7.9	8.3	8.3	8.3	8.1	7.0
29. U.K., England & Wales	8.0	8.1	8.4	9.0	8.7	8.7	8.7
30. U.K., Northern Ireland	5.6	5.7	5.3	6.7	6.7	6.4	7.6
31. U.K., Scotland	7.0	7.4	8.0	8.6	8.4	8.0	8.1
32. U.S., White	7.5	7.5	7.5	7.6	7.3	6.8	6.5
33. U.S., Nonwhite	5.6	6.0	6.1	6.3	5.7	5.2	4.8
34. Yugoslavia			2.7	3.3	3.7	4.2	4.3

[a] 1969–72, [b] 1954–57, [c] 1983, 84, 86, [d] 1983–86.

TABLE I-16. Age-Adjusted Death Rates of Cancer by Site and Year (1953–57 to 1983–87)

Prostate

	Country	1953–1957	1958–1962	1963–1967	1968–1972	1973–1977	1978–1982	1983–1987
1.	Australia	15.1	14.7	14.5	15.4	15.6	15.1	16.0
2.	Austria		13.0	13.6	14.0	14.8	15.3	15.6
3.	Belgium	12.9[a]	14.3	15.7	15.2	16.1	17.5	17.4[b]
4.	Canada	12.9	13.4	13.0	13.9	14.3	14.5	15.7
5.	Chile		8.7	9.1	10.6	11.8	11.0	12.4
6.	Costa Rica			9.3	9.4	9.4	10.6	14.4
7.	Czechoslovakia	7.7	8.3	8.9	9.7	10.9	11.6	12.8
8.	Denmark	13.5	14.2	14.3	12.9	13.5	15.9	17.8
9.	Finland	9.9	11.9	11.3	13.4	15.3	16.3	16.9
10.	France	11.9	14.7	15.6	14.9	15.0	15.3	16.5
11.	Germany, Fed. Repub.	11.2	11.7	12.9	14.0	15.9	15.9	16.3
12.	Greece			5.2	5.8	6.6	7.2	7.9
13.	Hong Kong		1.5	2.1	2.4	2.1	2.4	2.7
14.	Hungary		10.5	12.7	14.5	15.9	15.8	15.6
15.	Ireland	8.0	9.7	11.2	12.7	13.6	14.0	15.4
16.	Israel	7.1	7.5	7.8	8.0	7.5	8.6	8.4
17.	Italy	6.8	8.2	9.4	10.4	10.5	10.8	11.6
18.	Japan	0.9	1.5	1.8	2.0	2.4	2.8	3.3
19.	Mexico		3.5	4.6	5.1	5.9	6.8[c]	8.9[d]
20.	Netherlands	12.6	13.3	14.3	15.0	15.4	16.0	17.0
21.	New Zealand	14.3	13.6	14.0	14.9	16.9	16.0	17.2
22.	Norway	14.4	14.9	16.5	17.0	18.2	19.9	20.8
23.	Poland		3.7[e]	7.4	8.3	8.0	8.4	9.2
24.	Portugal		9.7	11.6	13.2	13.4	13.8	12.5
25.	Singapore			2.3	2.5	1.9	2.9	4.2
26.	Spain	6.8	9.4	11.0	11.9	12.4	12.6	12.7[f]
27.	Sweden	13.1	16.9	17.7	19.0	21.6	19.6	18.9
28.	Switzerland	14.5	15.7	16.3	18.3	19.4	19.8	21.7
29.	U.K., England & Wales	11.4	11.9	12.2	11.8	12.1	12.5	14.8
30.	U.K., Northern Ireland	11.1	11.7	11.8	12.5	13.2	12.9	13.7
31.	U.K., Scotland	11.4	12.0	12.6	11.0	11.8	12.1	13.0
32.	U.S., White	13.9	13.1	12.8	12.8	13.4	13.8	14.2
33.	U.S., Nonwhite	21.3	22.4	22.4	24.5	24.8	26.0	26.5
34.	Yugoslavia			5.9	6.9	8.3	10.4	8.3

[a] 1954–57, [b] 1983, 84, 86, [c] 1978, 81, 82, [d] 1983, 85, 86, [e] 1959–62, [f] 1983–86.

TABLE I-17. Age-Adjusted Death Rates of Cancer

Bladder (male)

	Country	1953–1957	1958–1962	1963–1967	1968–1972	1973–1977	1978–1982	1983–1987
1.	Australia		4.9	4.9	5.3	5.0	5.1	4.8
2.	Austria				7.3[a]	6.9	6.7	6.4
3.	Belgium		5.5	6.3	7.1	8.1	8.6	8.4[b]
4.	Canada		5.5	5.4	5.6[a]	5.3	5.0	4.7
5.	Chile							2.7
6.	Costa Rica							2.6
7.	Czechoslovakia				5.9	6.2	7.0	7.2
8.	Denmark		6.5	7.5	7.9[a]	8.3	9.1	9.7
9.	Finland		4.5	4.5	5.2[a]	5.0	4.8	4.4
10.	France			5.3[c]	5.6	6.1	6.7	6.8
11.	Germany, Fed. Repub.				7.0	7.2	7.3	7.2
12.	Greece				5.1	5.3	6.2	6.7
13.	Hong Kong				3.9[a]	5.3	4.5	4.2
14.	Hungary					6.3	6.9	7.1
15.	Ireland		3.3	3.5	3.8	4.3	4.4	4.5
16.	Israel		4.7	5.6	6.2[a]	6.8	6.1	5.4
17.	Italy		4.9	5.6	6.5	7.4	8.2	9.1
18.	Japan	1.6	2.0	2.1	2.3	2.4	2.5	2.3
19.	Mexico							1.4[d]
20.	Netherlands		5.0	6.2	6.8[a]	7.0	7.4	7.4
21.	New Zealand		5.2	5.0	5.1	5.6	5.5	4.6
22.	Norway		3.7	4.5	5.0[a]	5.5	5.7	5.8
23.	Poland							7.1
24.	Portugal							4.8
25.	Singapore				2.8[a]	4.6	2.9	3.1
26.	Spain				5.3	7.0	7.3	7.7[e]
27.	Sweden		3.2	3.9	4.6[a]	4.8	4.4	4.2
28.	Switzerland		4.6	5.0	5.7[a]	6.0	6.6	6.6
29.	U.K., England & Wales	6.8	7.1	7.6	8.0	7.9	7.6	7.5
30.	U.K., Northern Ireland		4.2	5.0	4.7	5.1	5.7	5.2
31.	U.K., Scotland		6.9	7.0	8.1	8.0	8.0	7.4
32.	U.S., White	5.4	5.3	5.1	5.1	5.2	4.7	4.1
33.	U.S., Nonwhite	4.1	4.3	4.4	4.3	3.9	3.5	3.0
34.	Yugoslavia				3.6	3.8	4.1	4.3

[a] 1969–72, [b] 1983, 84, 86, [c] 1964–67, [d] 1983, 1985, 1986, [e] 1983–86.

by Site and Year (1953–57 to 1983–87)
Bladder (female)

	Country	1953–1957	1958–1962	1963–1967	1968–1972	1973–1977	1978–1982	1983–1987
1.	Australia		1.5	1.6	1.6	1.6	1.5	1.4
2.	Austria				1.6[a]	1.7	1.8	1.7
3.	Belgium		1.7	1.8	1.7	1.8	1.9	2.0[b]
4.	Canada		1.9	1.9	1.6[a]	1.6	1.4	1.3
5.	Chile							1.0
6.	Costa Rica							0.7
7.	Czechoslovakia				1.1	1.2	1.2	1.4
8.	Denmark		2.3	2.4	2.2[a]	2.7	2.4	2.5
9.	Finland		1.0	1.2	1.0[a]	1.2	1.0	0.8
10.	France			1.3[c]	1.3	1.3	1.3	1.3
11.	Germany, Fed. Repub.				1.5	1.7	1.7	1.7
12.	Greece				1.2	1.0	1.1	1.4
13.	Hong Kong				1.6[a]	1.9	1.7	1.3
14.	Hungary					1.1	1.3	1.4
15.	Ireland		1.5	1.5	1.4	1.7	1.3	1.5
16.	Israel		1.4	1.6	1.3[a]	1.4	1.3	1.3
17.	Italy		1.2	1.2	1.2	1.3	1.4	1.4
18.	Japan	0.8	0.9	1.0	1.0	0.9	0.8	0.7
19.	Mexico							0.5[d]
20.	Netherlands		1.7	1.9	1.8[a]	1.7	1.6	1.7
21.	New Zealand		1.5	1.4	1.7	1.7	1.4	1.4
22.	Norway		1.8	1.7	1.8[a]	1.8	1.8	1.8
23.	Poland							1.0
24.	Portugal							1.1
25.	Singapore				1.0[a]	1.1	1.0	1.3
26.	Spain				0.9	1.1	1.1	1.1[e]
27.	Sweden		1.4	1.3	1.5[a]	1.5	1.4	1.2
28.	Switzerland		1.6	1.5	1.5[a]	1.7	1.6	1.8
29.	U.K., England & Wales	2.0	2.0	2.0	2.1	2.2	2.2	2.2
30.	U.K., Northern Ireland		1.8	1.8	1.5	1.7	1.7	1.5
31.	U.K., Scotland		2.2	2.5	2.4	2.6	3.0	2.4
32.	U.S., White	2.1	1.8	1.7	1.5	1.4	1.3	1.2
33.	U.S., Nonwhite	2.7	2.7	2.6	2.3	2.1	1.8	1.5
34.	Yugoslavia				0.8	0.9	1.0	1.1

[a] 1969–72, [b] 1983, 84, 86, [c] 1964–67, [d] 1983, 1985, 1986, [e] 1983–86.

TABLE I-18. Age-Adjusted Death Rates of Cancer

Thyroid gland (male)

Country	1953–1957	1958–1962	1963–1967	1968–1972	1973–1977	1978–1982	1983–1987
1. Australia		0.3	0.3	0.3	0.3	0.2	0.3
2. Austria		1.2	1.1	1.1	1.0	0.9	0.7
3. Belgium		0.4	0.4	0.5	0.3	0.3	0.5[a]
4. Canada		0.4	0.4	0.4	0.3	0.3	0.3
5. Chile		0.4	0.4				
6. Costa Rica							
7. Czechoslovakia		0.5	0.6	0.5	0.6	0.6	0.5
8. Denmark		0.6	0.4	0.5	0.5	0.5	0.5
9. Finland		0.5	0.6	0.6	0.6	0.6	0.5
10. France		0.3	0.3	0.4	0.4	0.4	0.4
11. Germany, Fed. Repub.		0.6	0.5	0.6	0.6	0.6	0.6
12. Greece				0.1	0.2	0.2	0.3
13. Hong Kong				0.6	0.4	0.4[b]	0.4
14. Hungary					0.6	0.6	0.7
15. Ireland		0.4	0.3	0.3	0.4	0.4	0.4
16. Israel		0.5	0.5	0.6	0.6	0.6	0.6
17. Italy		0.4	0.5	0.5[c]	0.6	0.5	0.5
18. Japan	0.1	0.2	0.3	0.3	0.3	0.3	0.3
19. Mexico							
20. Netherlands		0.4	0.3	0.5	0.5	0.4	0.4
21. New Zealand		0.4	0.4	0.5	0.4	0.4	0.3
22. Norway		0.5	0.5	0.6	0.4	0.4	0.4
23. Poland			0.4				
24. Portugal							0.2
25. Singapore				0.4	0.5		0.7
26. Spain		0.1	0.2	0.2	0.2	0.2	0.2[d]
27. Sweden		0.5	0.5	0.6	0.6	0.5	0.4
28. Switzerland		1.4	1.2	1.2	1.0	0.9	0.7
29. U.K., England & Wales	0.3	0.3	0.3	0.3	0.3	0.3	0.3
30. U.K., Northern Ireland		0.5	0.3	0.4	0.3	0.3	0.5
31. U.K., Scotland		0.4	0.5	0.4	0.3	0.3	0.3
32. U.S., White	0.4	0.4	0.3	0.3	0.3	0.3	
33. U.S., Nonwhite	0.3	0.3	0.3	0.3	0.3	0.2	
34. Yugoslavia			0.2	0.3	0.4	0.5	0.4

[a] 1983,84,86, [b] 1978–81, [c] 1969–72, [d] 1983–86.

by Site and Year (1953–57 to 1983–87)
Thyroid gland (female)

Country	1953–1957	1958–1962	1963–1967	1968–1972	1973–1977	1978–1982	1983–1987
1. Australia		0.6	0.5	0.5	0.5	0.4	0.4
2. Austria		1.7	1.5	1.4	1.3	1.1	1.0
3. Belgium		0.7	0.6	0.6	0.6	0.7	0.5[a]
4. Canada		0.7	0.6	0.6	0.5	0.4	0.3
5. Chile		0.8	0.8				
6. Costa Rica							
7. Czechoslovakia		1.0	0.9	0.9	0.9	0.9	0.7
8. Denmark		0.9	0.9	0.8	0.8	0.6	0.6
9. Finland		0.9	1.0	1.1	0.9	1.0	0.7
10. France		0.5	0.6	0.6	0.6	0.6	0.6
11. Germany, Fed. Repub.		0.9	0.8	0.9	0.9	0.9	0.8
12. Greece				0.2	0.3	0.4	0.4
13. Hong Kong				0.8	0.6	0.7[b]	0.7
14. Hungary					0.9	0.9	0.8
15. Ireland		1.0	0.9	1.2	0.7	0.7	0.7
16. Israel		1.3	1.2	1.1	1.2	0.8	0.7
17. Italy		0.7	0.7	0.8[c]	0.8	0.7	0.7
18. Japan	0.3	0.4	0.5	0.6	0.6	0.6	0.5
19. Mexico							
20. Netherlands		0.7	0.7	0.7	0.7	0.6	0.5
21. New Zealand		0.7	0.8	0.7	0.7	0.5	0.4
22. Norway		0.9	0.7	0.7	0.7	0.7	0.6
23. Poland			0.6				
24. Portugal							0.3
25. Singapore				1.1	1.0		0.9
26. Spain		0.3	0.3	0.3	0.4	0.4	0.4[d]
27. Sweden		1.0	0.9	0.8	0.8	0.8	0.5
28. Switzerland		1.6	1.4	1.4	1.2	1.0	0.8
29. U.K., England & Wales	0.7	0.6	0.6	0.6	0.6	0.5	0.4
30. U.K., Northern Ireland		0.9	1.0	0.8	0.9	0.6	0.6
31. U.K., Scotland		0.8	0.9	0.8	0.6	0.5	0.4
32. U.S., White	0.7	0.6	0.5	0.4	0.4	0.3	
33. U.S., Nonwhite	0.6	0.7	0.6	0.5	0.4	0.4	
34. Yugoslavia			0.6	0.6	0.6	0.7	0.6

[a] 1983, 84, 86, [b] 1978–81, [c] 1969–72, [d] 1983–86.

TABLE I-19. Age-Adjusted Death Rates of Cancer

Leukaemia (male)

Country	1953–1957	1958–1962	1963–1967	1968–1972	1973–1977	1978–1982	1983–1987
1. Australia	5.3	6.2	6.4	6.6	6.4	6.3	6.3
2. Austria		6.1	5.7	6.2	6.0	6.0	5.7
3. Belgium	4.8[a]	6.3	6.2	6.2	6.3	6.5	5.9[b]
4. Canada	6.0	6.6	6.9	7.0	7.1	6.8	6.6
5. Chile		3.7	4.0	4.2	4.0	4.1	4.1
6. Costa Rica			4.4	3.8	5.2	5.8	6.0
7. Czechoslovakia	5.2	6.0	6.4	6.7	6.9	7.1	6.6
8. Denmark	7.3	8.2	8.3	7.6	6.8	7.0	7.2
9. Finland	5.4	6.0	7.0	7.1	6.8	6.5	5.8
10. France	5.6	6.2	6.6	6.7	7.0	6.9	6.8
11. Germany, Fed. Repub.	5.4	5.8	6.1	6.1	6.4	6.3	5.9
12. Greece			7.3	7.1	7.0	6.5	6.1
13. Hong Kong		2.8	3.3	3.2	3.6	4.1	3.8
14. Hungary		5.5	6.2	6.1	6.4	6.6	7.4
15. Ireland	4.1	5.0	5.5	6.1	5.5	5.7	5.5
16. Israel	6.8	7.8	7.4	6.9	6.7	6.1	5.7
17. Italy	4.9	5.9	6.5	7.0	6.8	6.8	6.7
18. Japan	2.7	3.3	3.8	3.9	4.3	4.4	4.5
19. Mexico		1.7	2.1	2.3	2.7	3.1[c]	3.7[d]
20. Netherlands	5.9	6.7	7.1	6.8	6.5	6.3	5.8
21. New Zealand	6.6	6.6	6.7	6.8	7.0	6.4	6.1
22. Norway	6.7	7.0	7.0	6.9	6.1	6.1	5.6
23. Poland		4.3[e]	5.1	5.5	5.7	5.8	5.7
24. Portugal		4.2	5.1	5.4	5.5	5.4	5.2
25. Singapore			4.1	3.3	4.0	3.8	4.4
26. Spain	2.6	3.6	4.1	4.4	4.7	4.9	5.2[f]
27. Sweden	6.6	7.3	7.1	6.9	6.7	6.4	5.0
28. Switzerland	5.9	6.4	6.3	6.8	6.2	5.9	6.2
29. U.K., England & Wales	5.0	5.4	5.6	5.7	5.6	5.6	5.5
30. U.K., Northern Ireland	4.7	5.6	5.9	5.9	6.3	6.1	5.1
31. U.K., Scotland	5.1	5.2	5.3	5.6	5.2	5.1	4.8
32. U.S., White	7.4	7.8	7.8	7.5	7.1	6.9	6.5
33. U.S., Nonwhite	5.1	5.1	5.7	5.8	5.7	5.6	5.4
34. Yugoslavia			4.4	4.4	4.4	3.4	3.9

[a] 1954–57, [b] 1983, 84, 86, [c] 1978, 81, 82, [d] 1983, 85, 86, [e] 1959–62, [f] 1983–86.

by Site and Year (1953–57 to 1983–87)

Leukaemia (female)

Country	1953–1957	1958–1962	1963–1967	1968–1972	1973–1977	1978–1982	1983–1987
1. Australia	4.1	4.5	4.3	4.4	4.2	4.0	3.9
2. Austria		4.2	4.5	4.3	4.2	4.0	3.7
3. Belgium	4.1[a]	4.3	4.4	4.3	3.8	4.2	4.0[b]
4. Canada	4.3	4.6	4.6	4.6	4.3	4.2	4.1
5. Chile		3.1	3.0	3.5	3.3	3.4	3.5
6. Costa Rica			3.3	3.8	4.4	5.2	4.4
7. Czechoslovakia	3.7	3.9	4.3	4.2	4.5	4.6	4.4
8. Denmark	5.6	5.2	5.1	4.8	4.6	4.5	4.5
9. Finland	3.8	4.8	5.2	5.3	4.4	4.0	4.0
10. France	4.1	4.5	4.6	4.3	4.4	4.4	4.1
11. Germany, Fed. Repub.	3.8	4.4	4.4	4.4	4.3	4.2	3.8
12. Greece			5.0	4.7	4.4	4.1	3.9
13. Hong Kong		2.1	3.0	2.6	2.8	3.2	2.8
14. Hungary		3.9	4.2	4.2	4.4	4.5	4.5
15. Ireland	3.2	3.4	3.7	3.6	3.4	3.6	3.7
16. Israel	5.8	5.9	5.9	5.3	5.0	4.7	4.1
17. Italy	3.7	4.3	4.7	4.8	4.6	4.4	4.3
18. Japan	1.9	2.6	2.9	3.0	3.1	3.0	2.9
19. Mexico		1.3	1.9	2.1	2.4	2.7[c]	3.0[d]
20. Netherlands	4.5	5.0	5.0	4.9	4.2	4.1	3.7
21. New Zealand	5.2	5.4	5.1	4.8	4.3	3.9	4.6
22. Norway	5.0	4.8	4.8	4.7	4.1	3.9	3.5
23. Poland		3.1[e]	3.7	3.8	3.8	3.8	3.7
24. Portugal		3.2	4.0	4.4	3.9	4.1	3.5
25. Singapore			2.3	3.2	2.9	3.6	3.2
26. Spain	1.9	2.8	3.3	3.4	3.4	3.4	3.4[f]
27. Sweden	4.7	5.2	5.1	4.9	4.7	4.3	3.6
28. Switzerland	4.1	4.5	4.5	4.6	4.0	4.0	3.6
29. U.K., England & Wales	3.7	3.9	3.9	3.9	3.6	3.6	3.5
30. U.K., Northern Ireland	2.9	4.0	3.6	3.6	3.2	3.8	3.3
31. U.K., Scotland	3.2	3.8	3.9	3.5	3.4	3.2	3.2
32. U.S., White	5.1	5.1	5.0	4.7	4.3	4.2	4.0
33. U.S., Nonwhite	3.2	3.8	3.8	3.8	3.7	3.7	3.6
34. Yugoslavia			3.1	3.2	3.1	2.4	2.5

[a] 1954–57, [b] 1983, 84, 86, [c] 1978, 81, 82, [d] 1983, 85, 86, [e] 1959–62, [f] 1983–86.

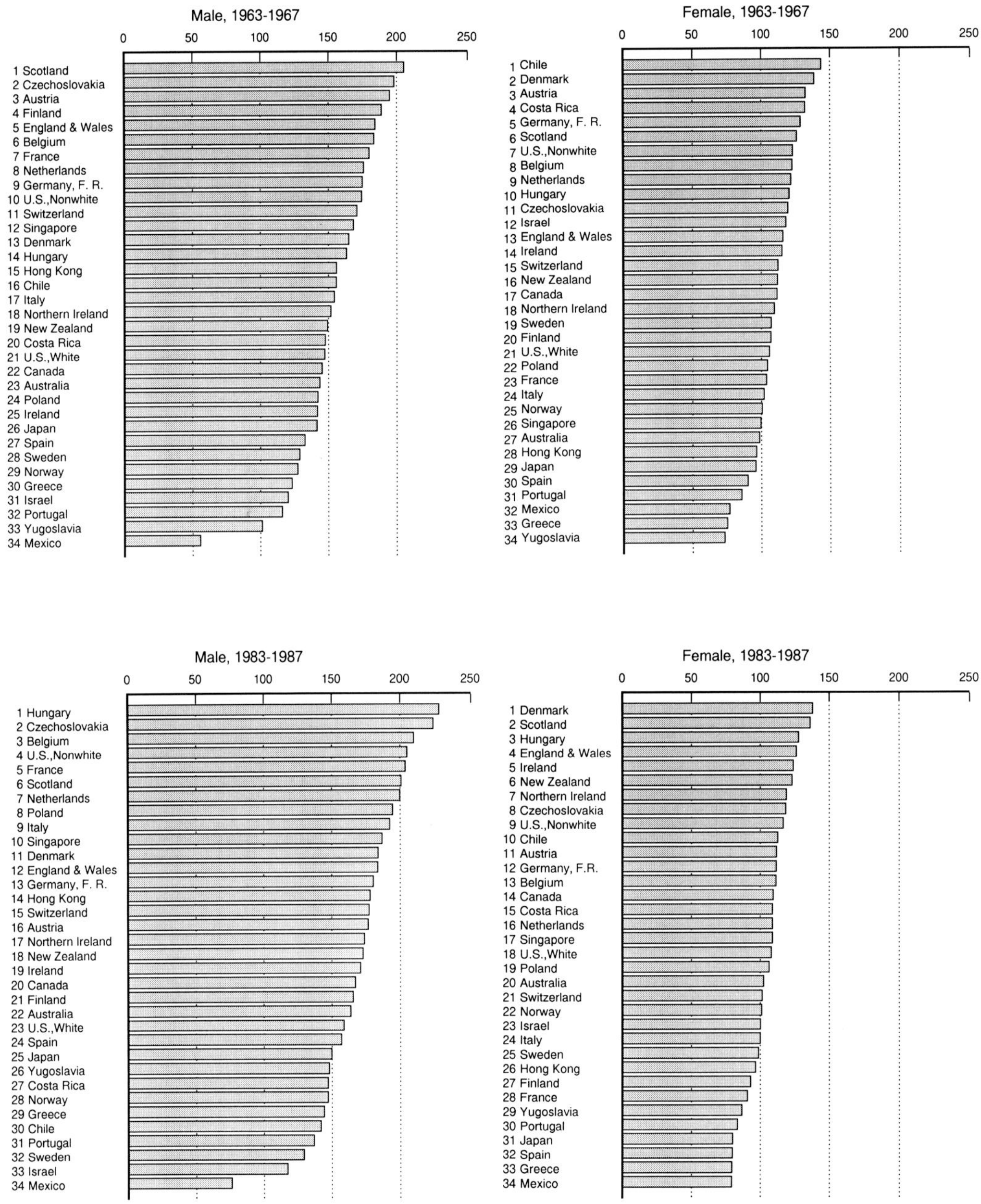

FIG. 1-1. Age-adjusted death rates of cancer by site in 1963–1967 (above) and in 1983–1987 (below). All sites.

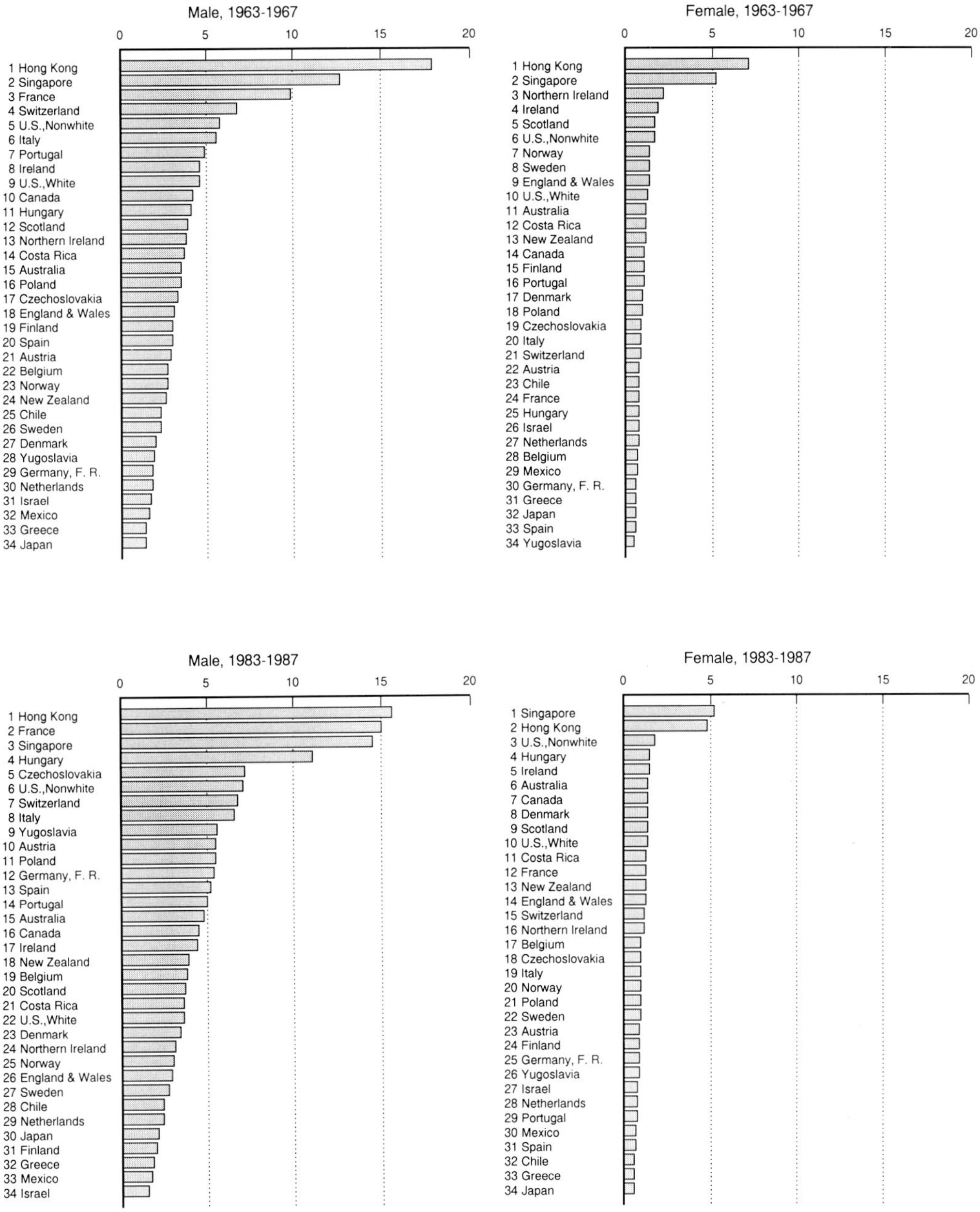

FIG. 1-2. Age-adjusted death rates of cancer by site in 1963–1967 (above) and in 1983–1987 (below). Lip, oral cavity, and pharynx.

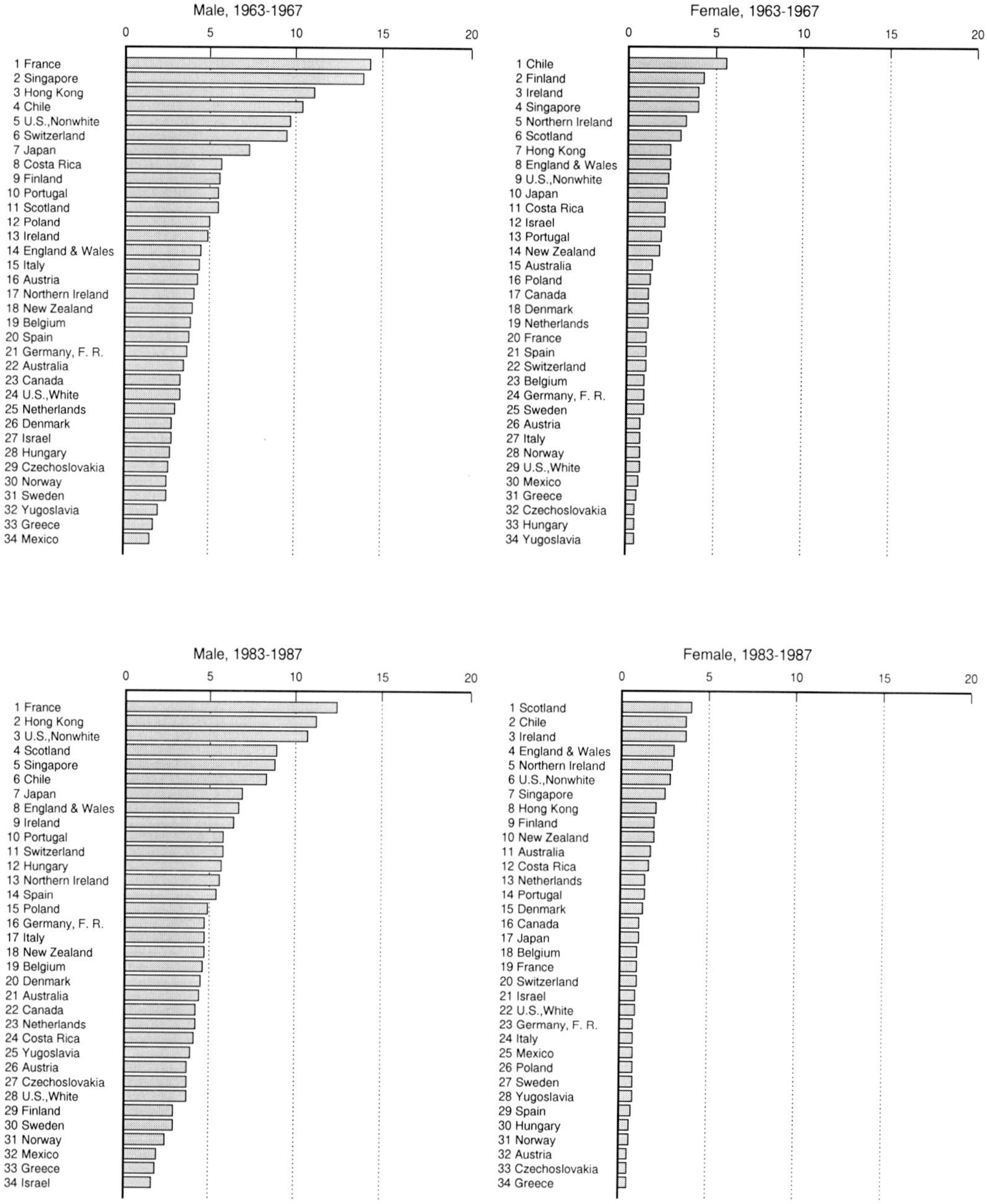

FIG. 1-3. Age-adjusted death rates of cancer by site in 1963–1967 (above) and in 1983–1987 (below). Esophagus.

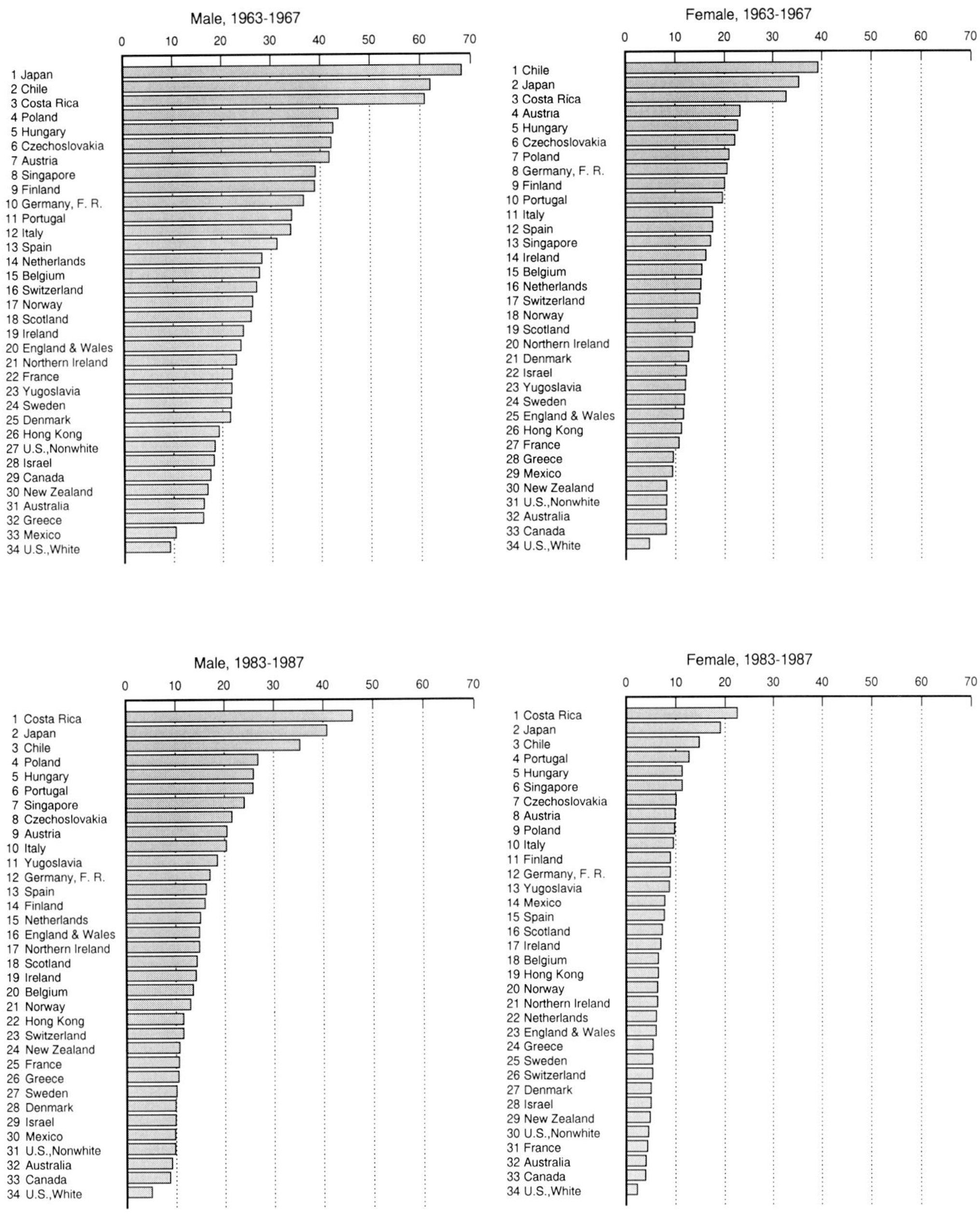

FIG. 1-4. Age-adjusted death rates of cancer by site in 1963–1967 (above) and in 1983–1987 (below). Stomach.

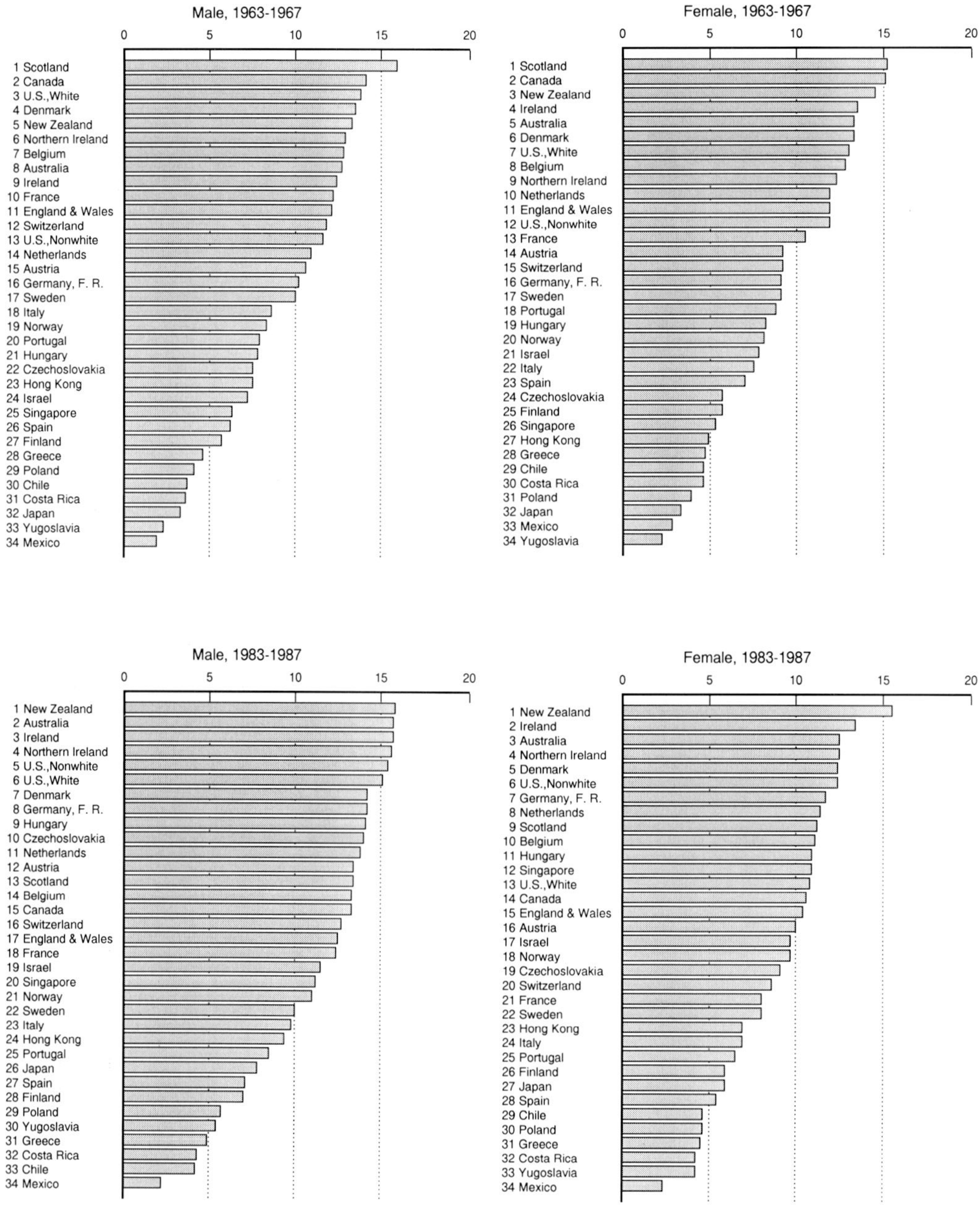

FIG. 1-5. Age-adjusted death rates of cancer by site in 1963–1967 (above) and in 1983–1987 (below). Intestine, except rectum.

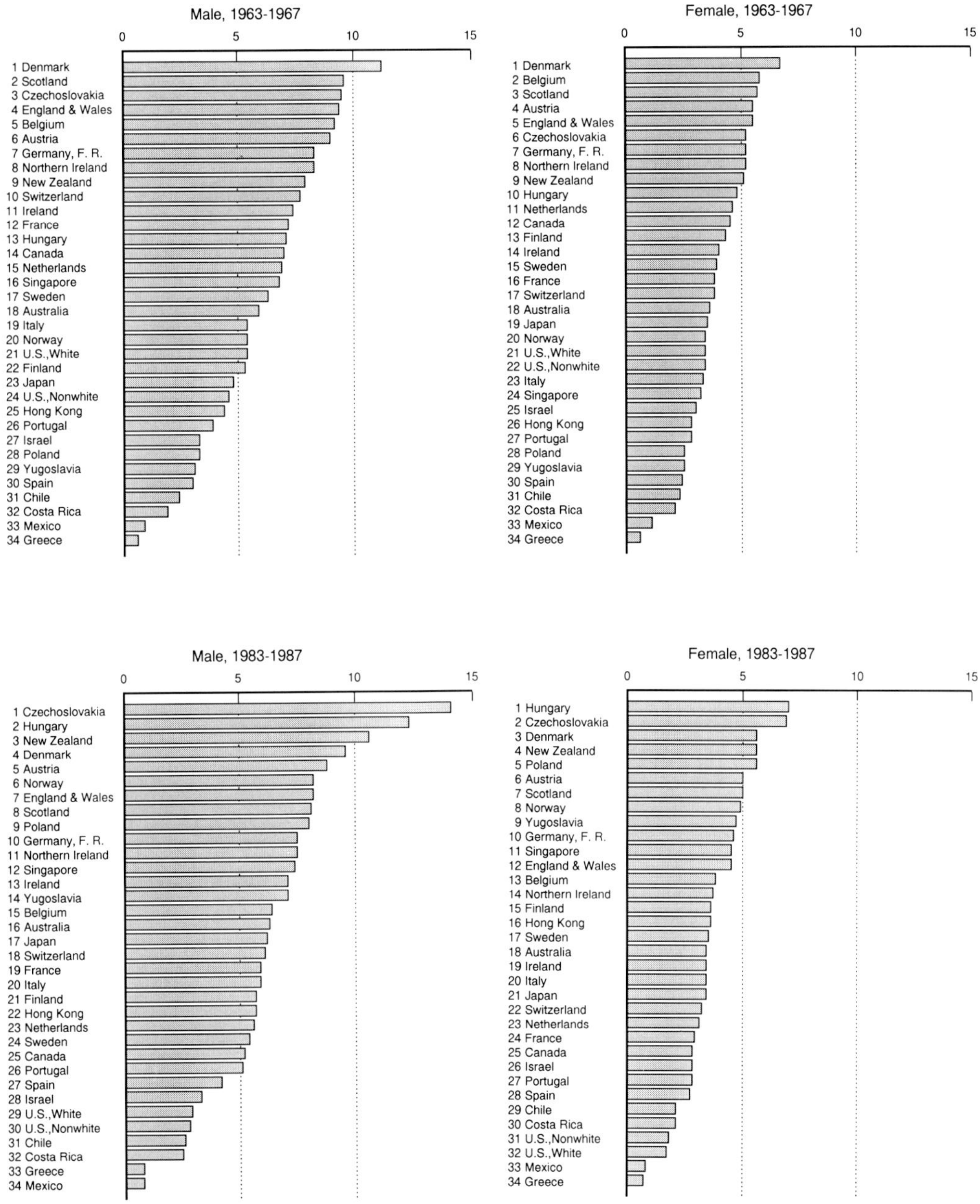

FIG. 1-6. Age-adjusted death rates of cancer by site in 1963–1967 (above) and in 1983–1987 (below). Rectum, rectosigmoid junction, and anus.

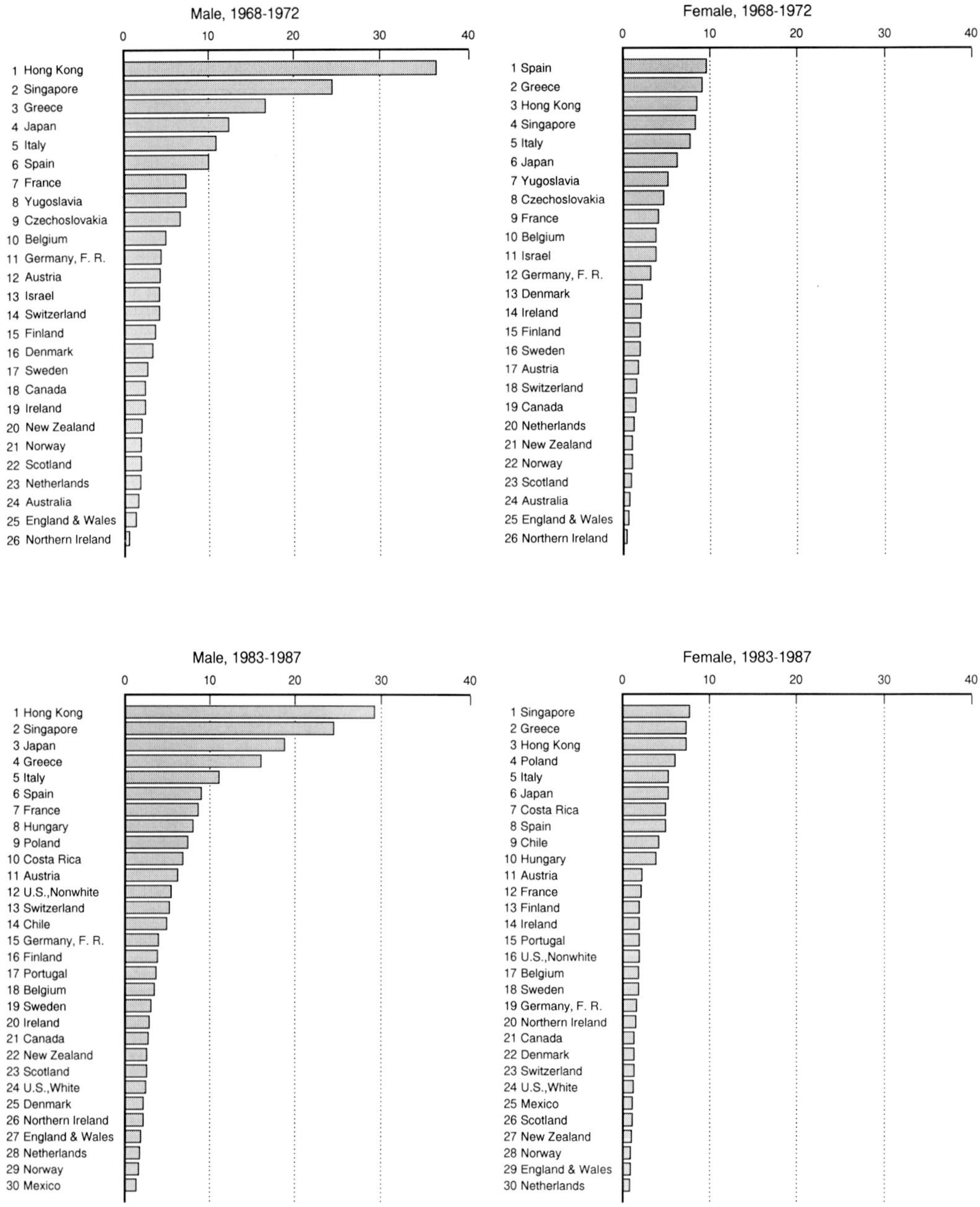

FIG. 1-7. Age-adjusted death rates of cancer by site in 1968–1972 (above) and in 1983–1987 (below). Liver and intrahepatic bile ducts.

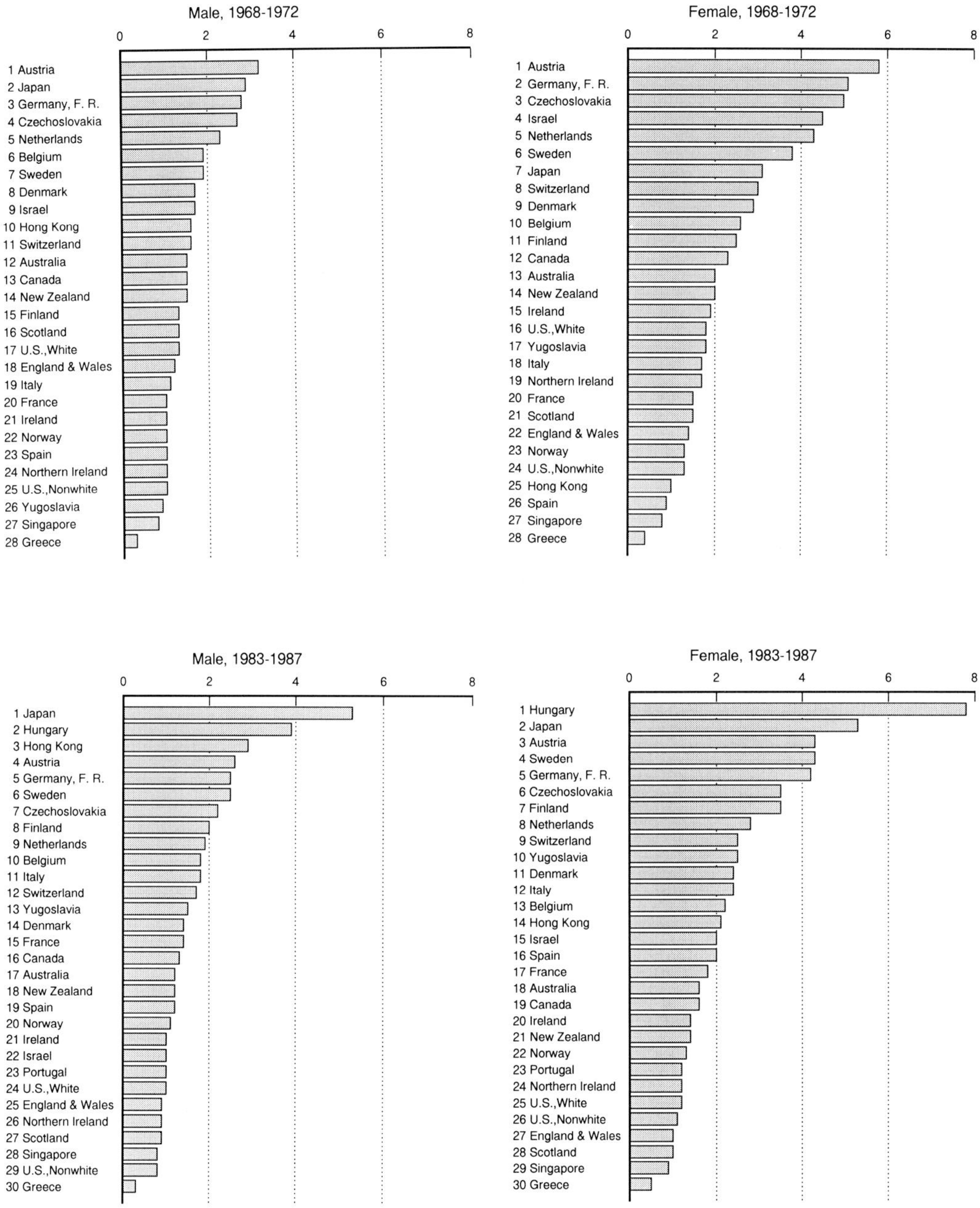

FIG. 1-8. Age-adjusted death rates of cancer by site in 1968–1972 (above) and in 1983–1987 (below). Gallbladder and extrahepatic bile ducts.

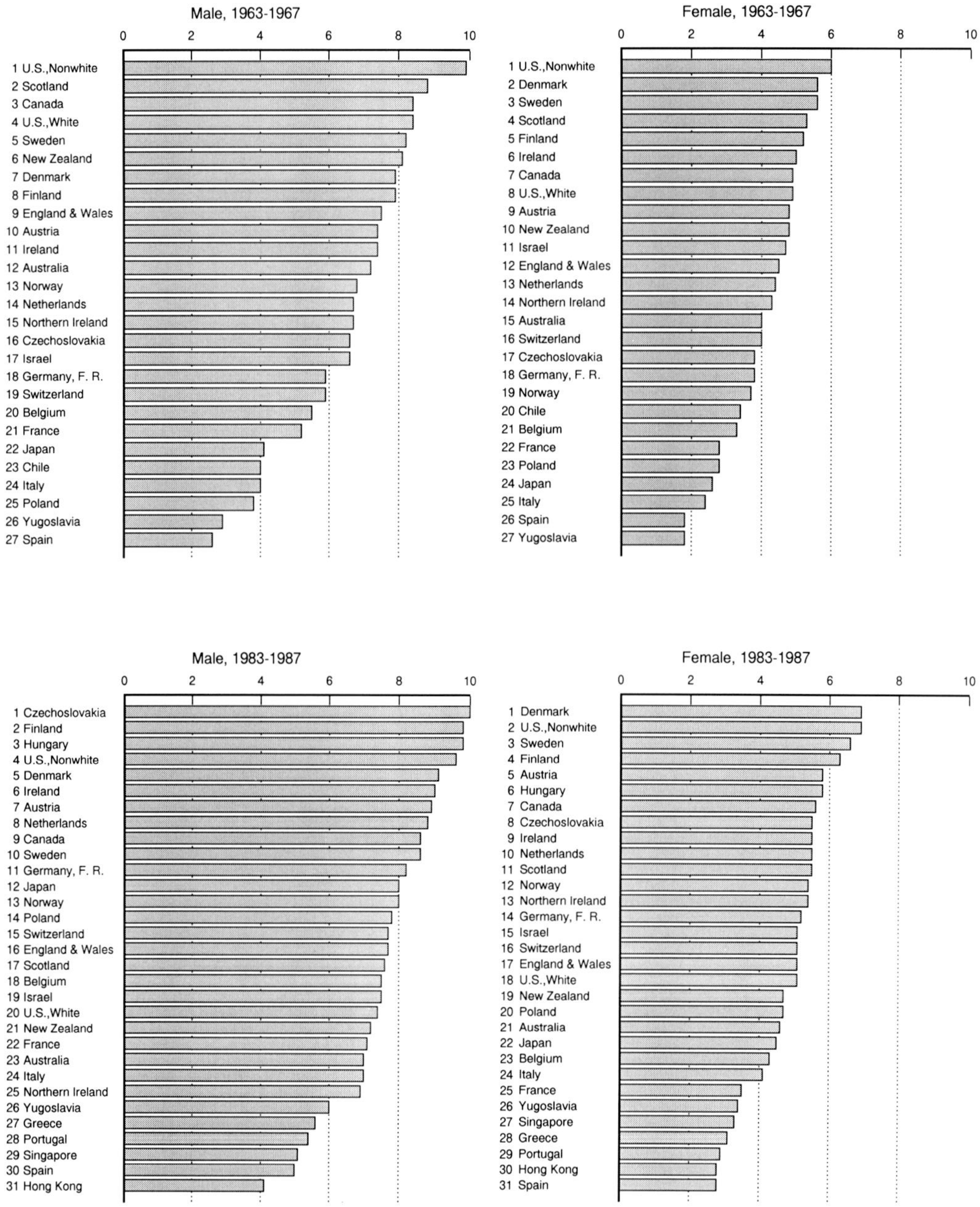

FIG. 1-9. Age-adjusted death rates of cancer by site in 1963–1967 (above) and in 1983–1987 (below). Pancreas.

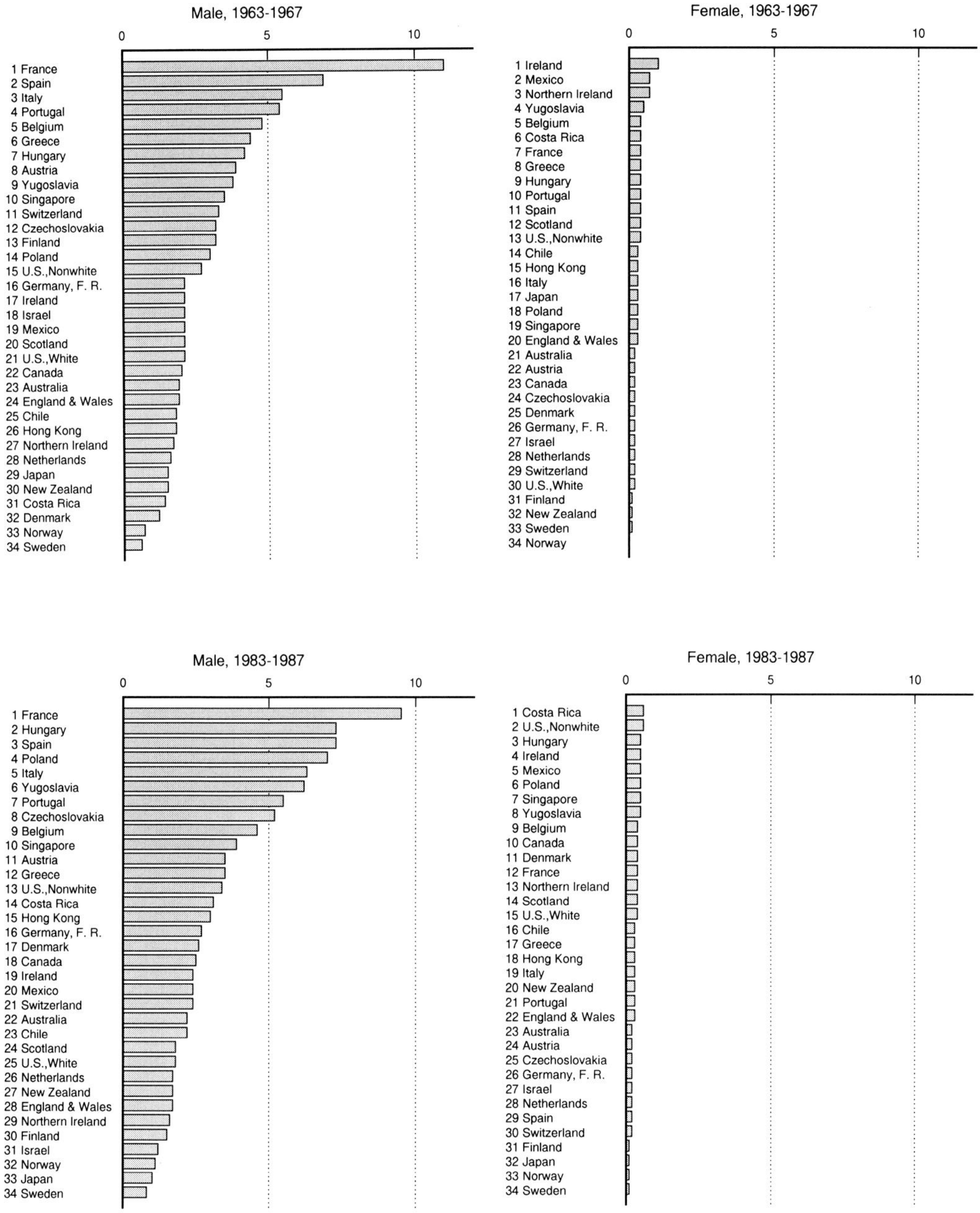

FIG. 1-10. Age-adjusted death rates of cancer by site in 1963–1967 (above) and in 1983–1987 (below). Larynx.

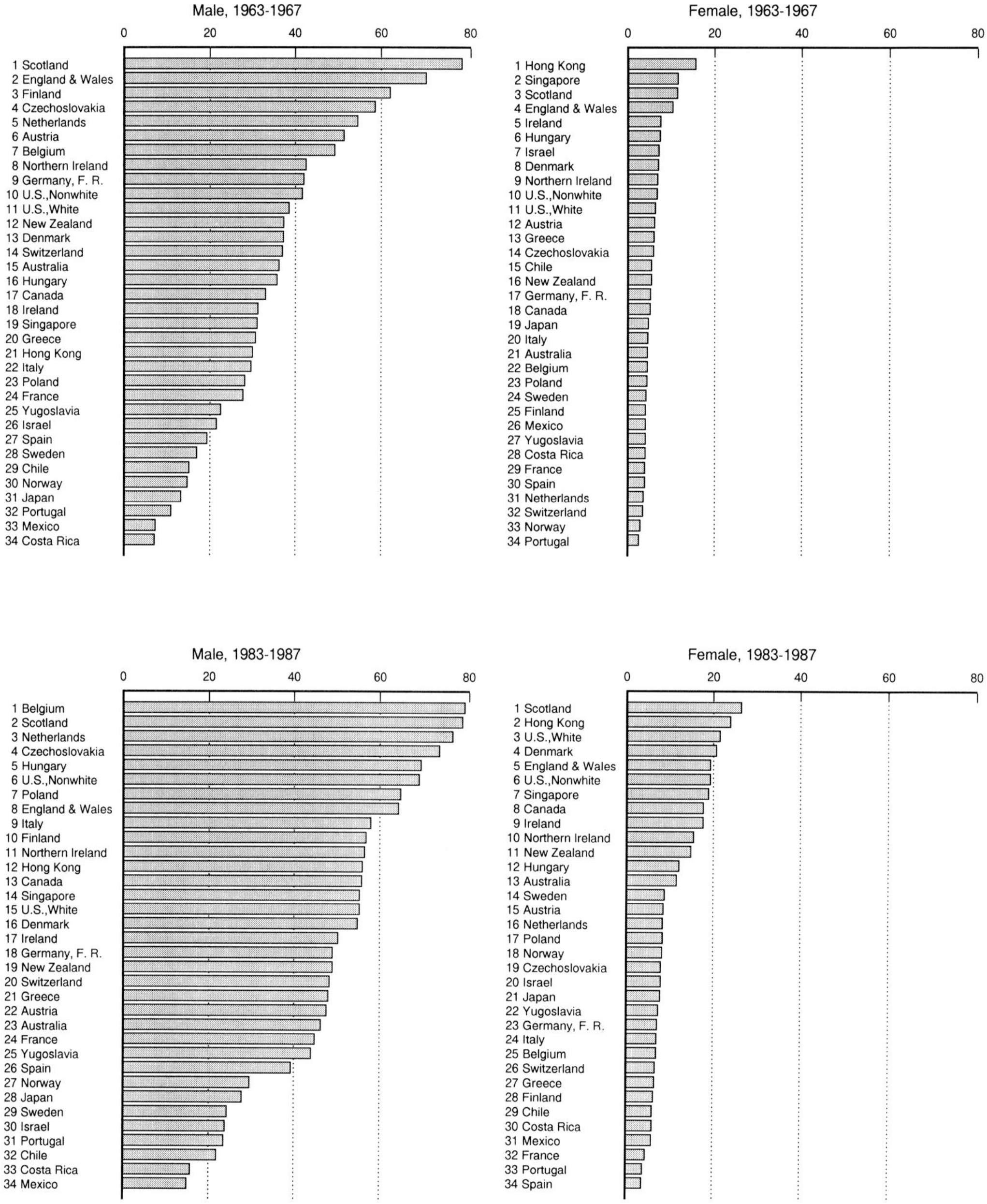

FIG. 1-11. Age-adjusted death rates of cancer by site in 1963–1967 (above) and in 1983–1987 (below). Trachea, bronchus, and lung.

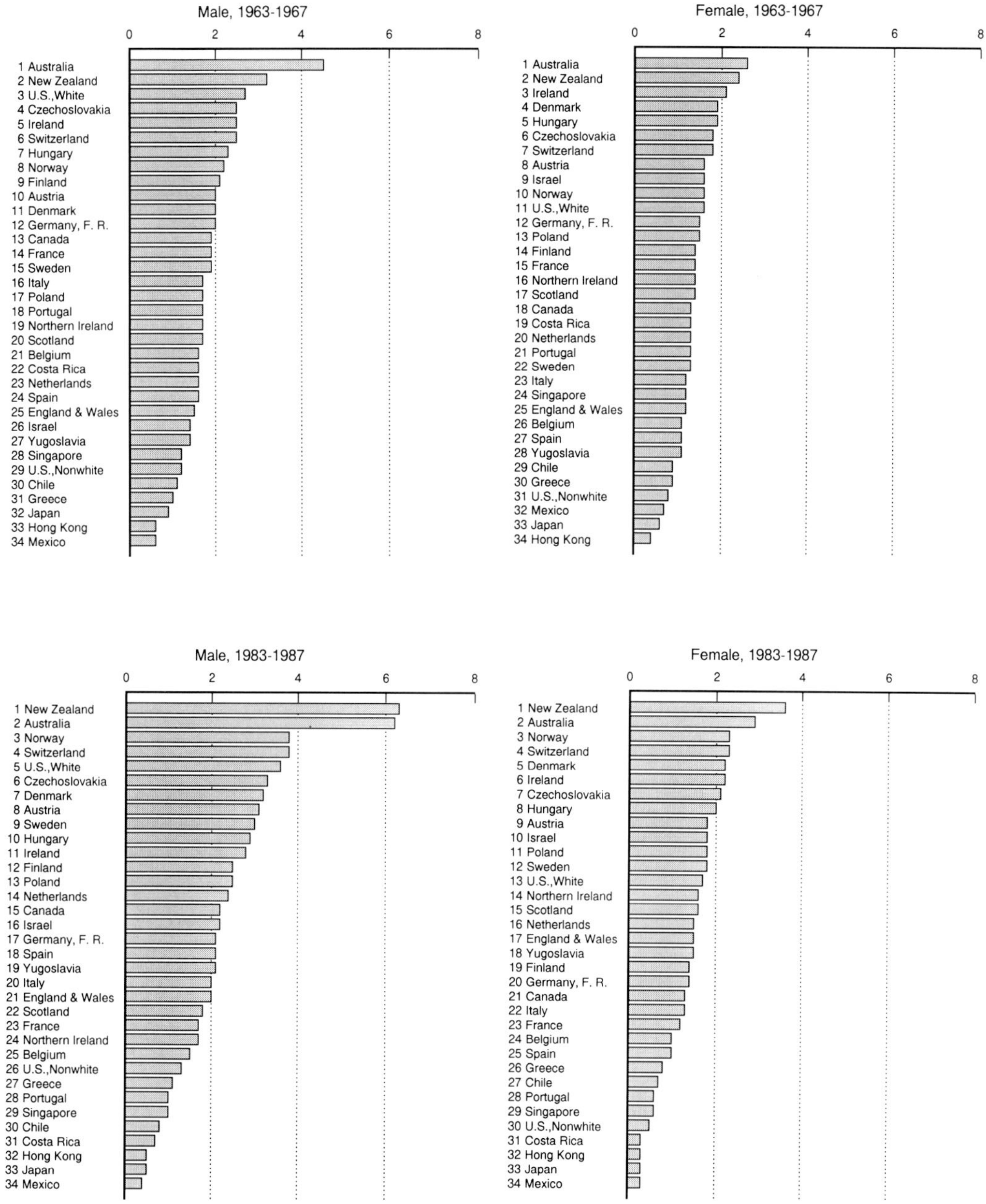

FIG. 1-12. Age-adjusted death rates of cancer by site in 1963–1967 (above) and in 1983–1987 (below). Skin.

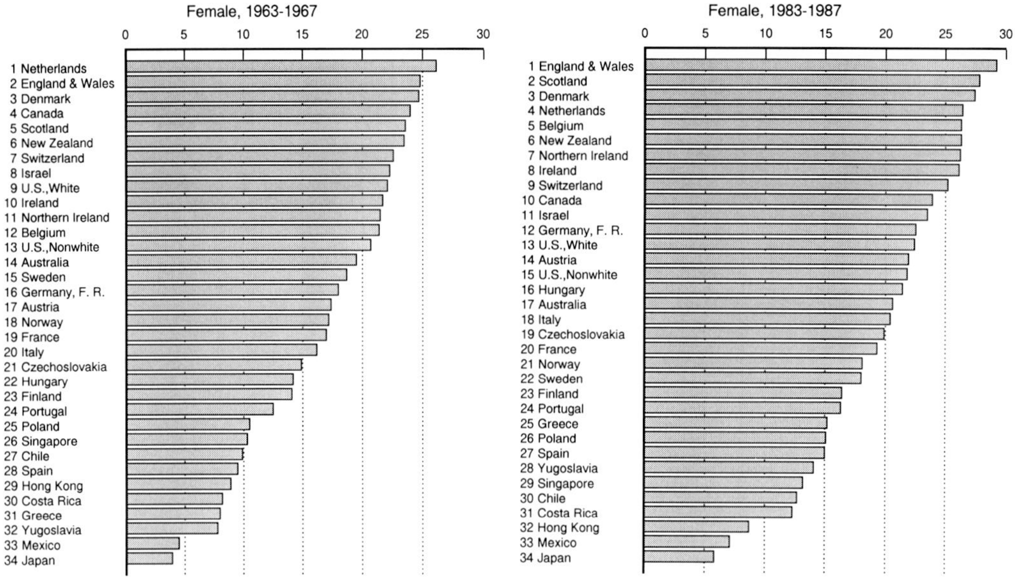

FIG. 1-13. Age-adjusted death rates of cancer by site in 1963–1967 (left) and in 1983–1987 (right). Breast.

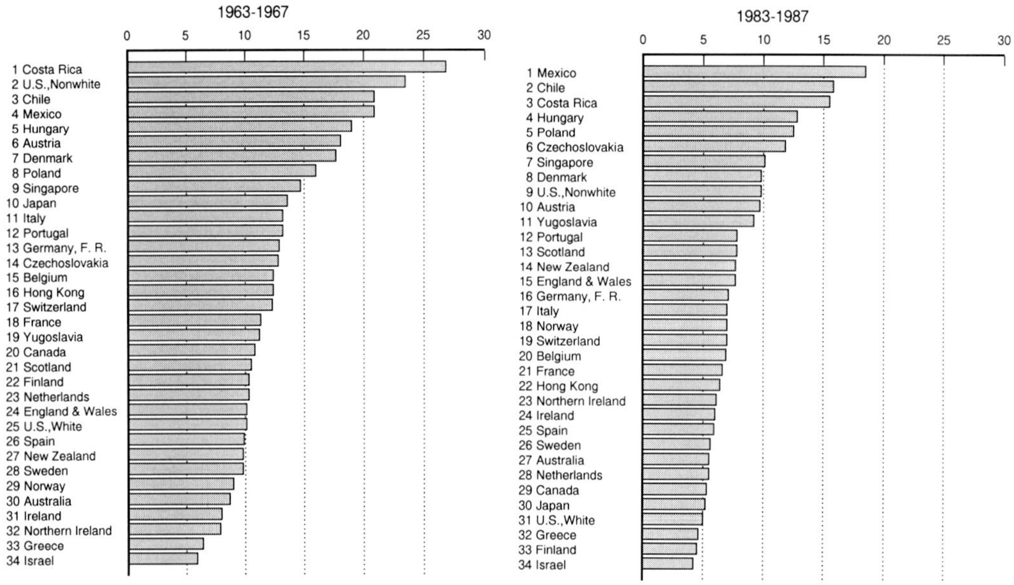

FIG. 1-14. Age-adjusted death rates of cancer by site in 1963–1967 (left) and in 1983–1987 (right). Uterus.

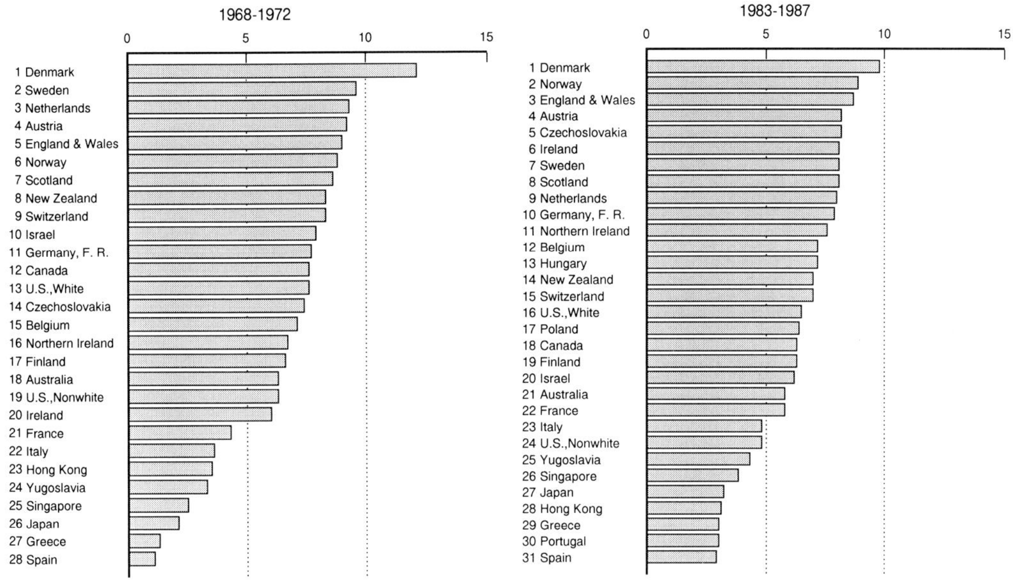

FIG. 1-15. Age-adjusted death rates of cancer by site in 1968–1972 (left) and in 1983–1987 (right). Ovary and other uterine adnexa.

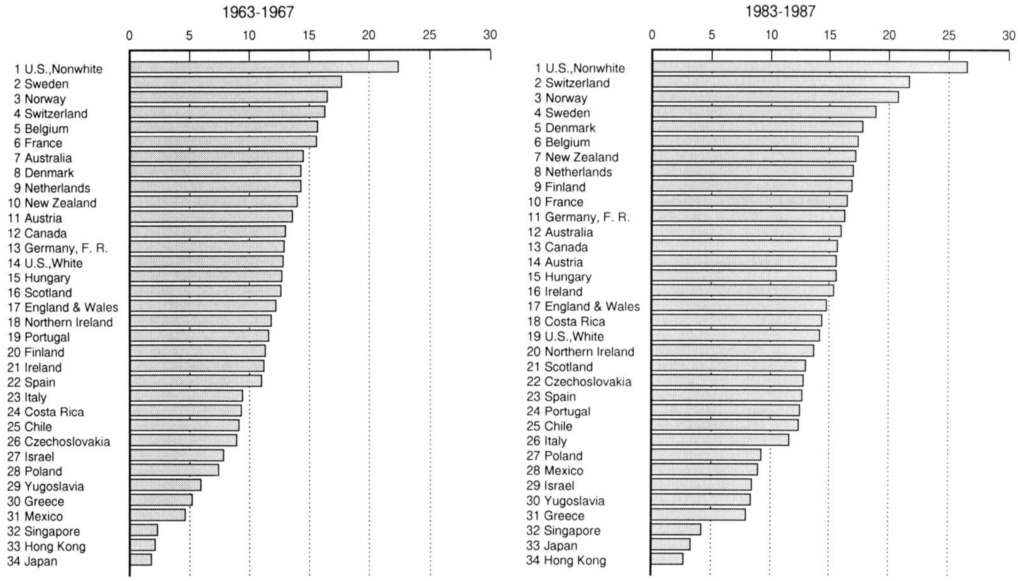

FIG. 1-16. Age-adjusted death rates of cancer by site in 1963–1967 (left) and in 1983–1987 (right) Prostate.

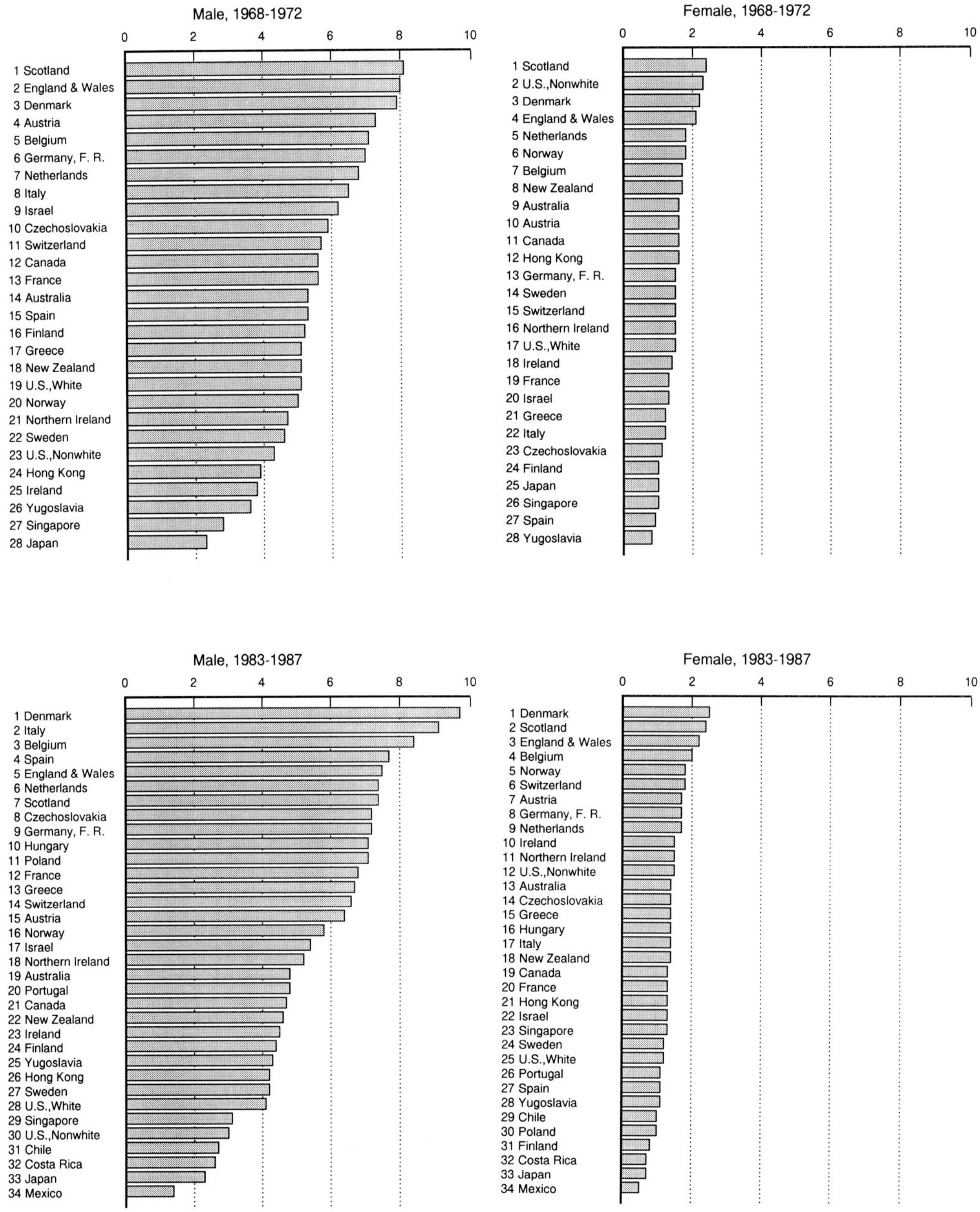

FIG. 1-17. Age-adjusted death rates of cancer by site in 1968–1972 (above) and in 1983–1987 (below). Bladder.

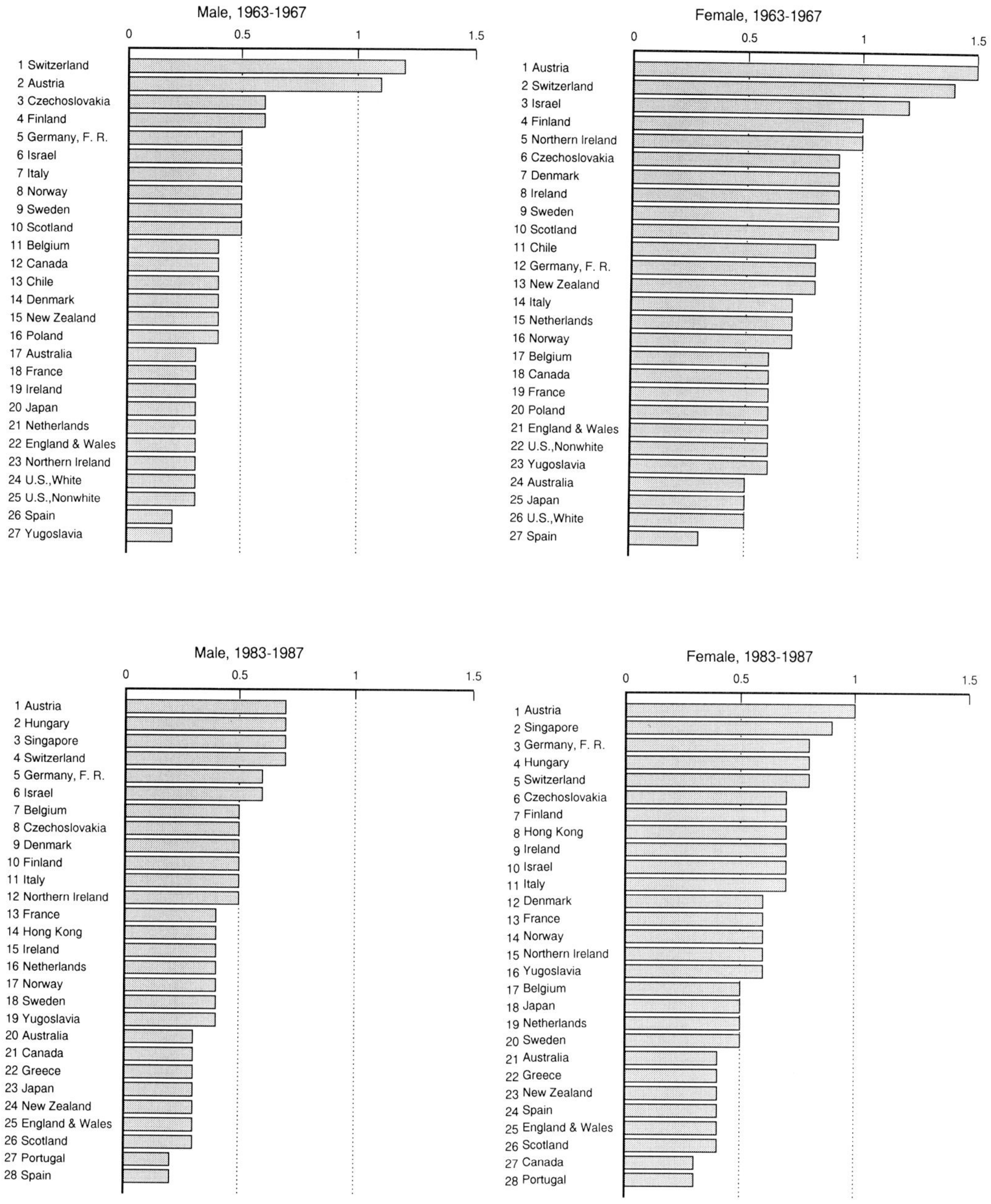

FIG. 1-18. Age-adjusted death rates of cancer by site in 1963–1967 (above) and in 1983–1987 (below). Thyroid gland.

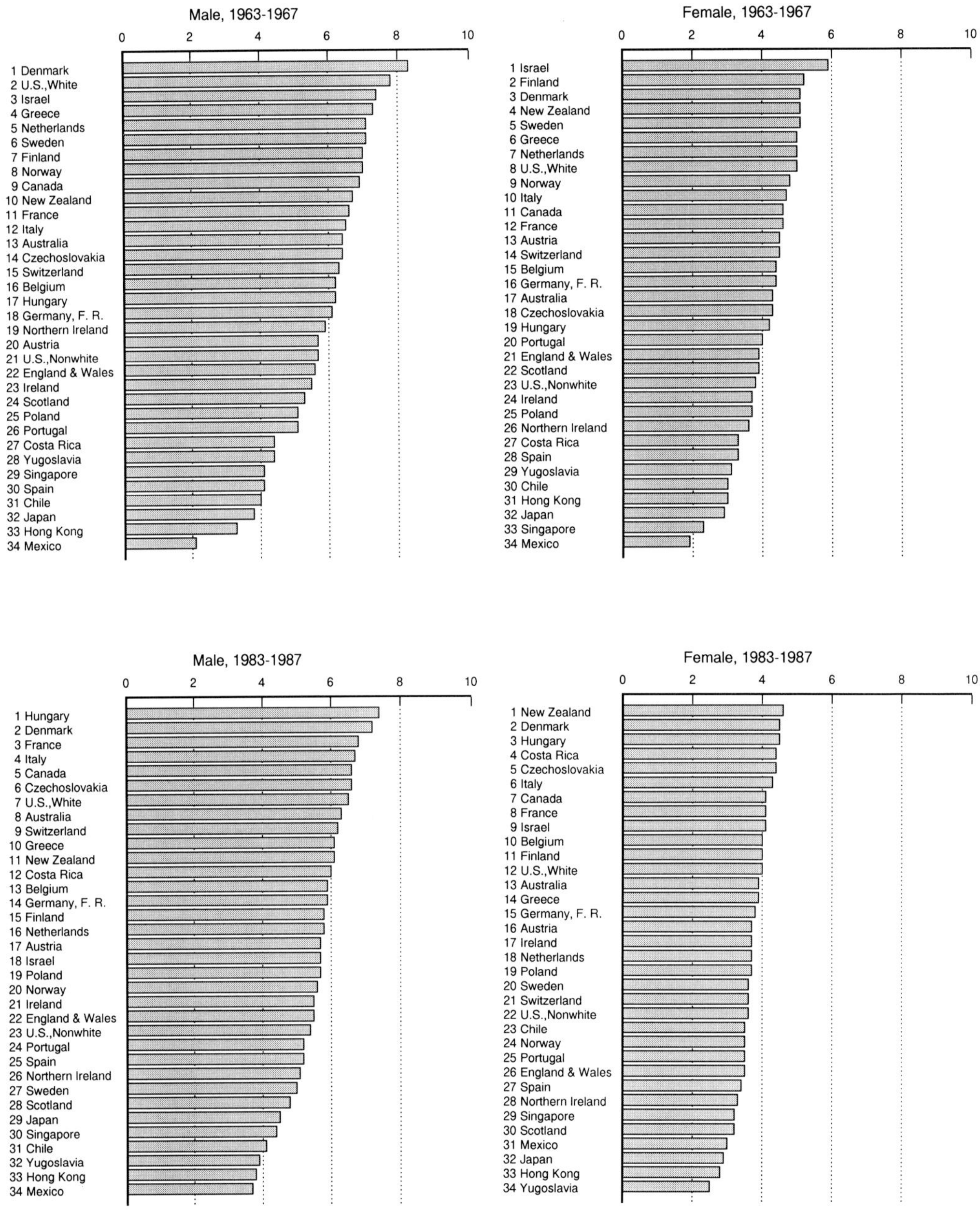

FIG. 1-19. Age-adjusted death rates of cancer by site in 1963–1967 (above) and in 1983–1987 (below). Leukaemia.

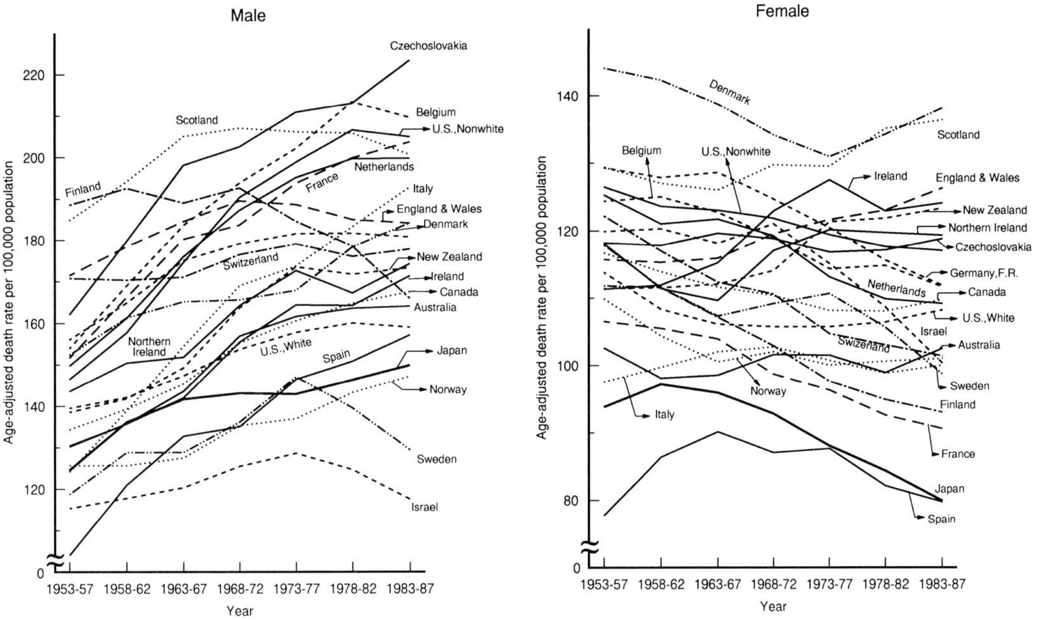

FIG. 2-1. Trends in the age-adjusted death rate of cancer by site from 1953–1957 to 1983–1987. All sites.

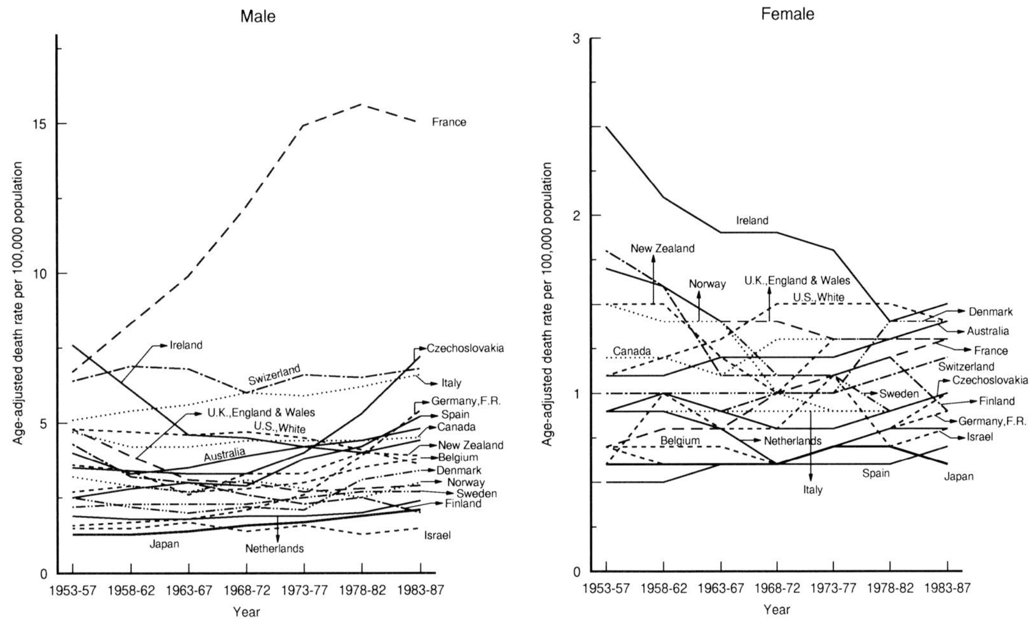

FIG. 2-2. Trends in the age-adjusted death rate of cancer by site from 1953–1957 to 1983–1987. Lip, oral cavity, and pharynx.

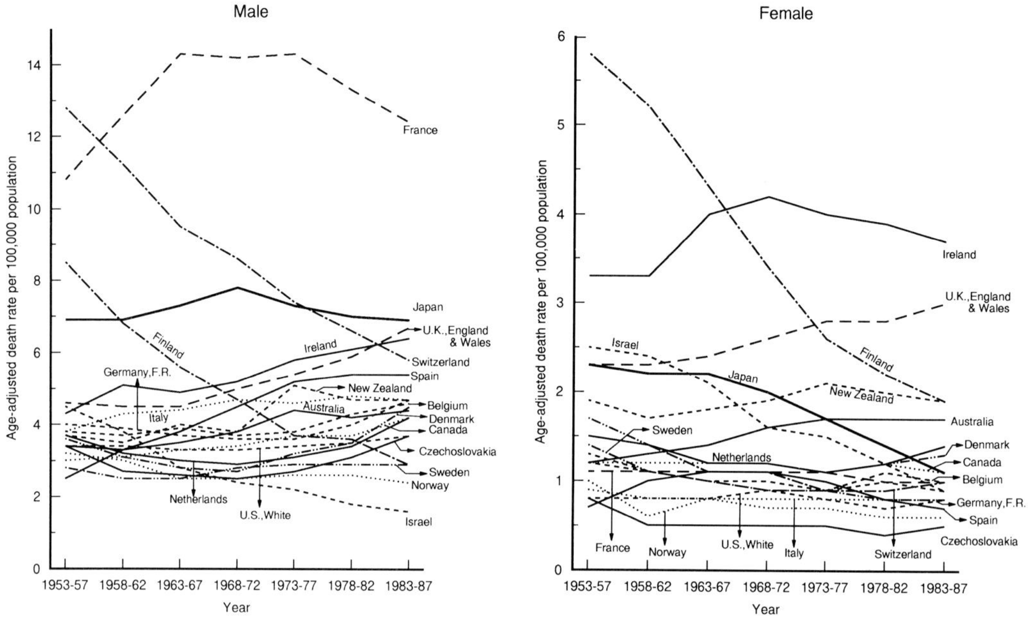

FIG. 2-3. Trends in the age-adjusted death rate of cancer by site from 1953–1957 to 1983–1987. Esophagus.

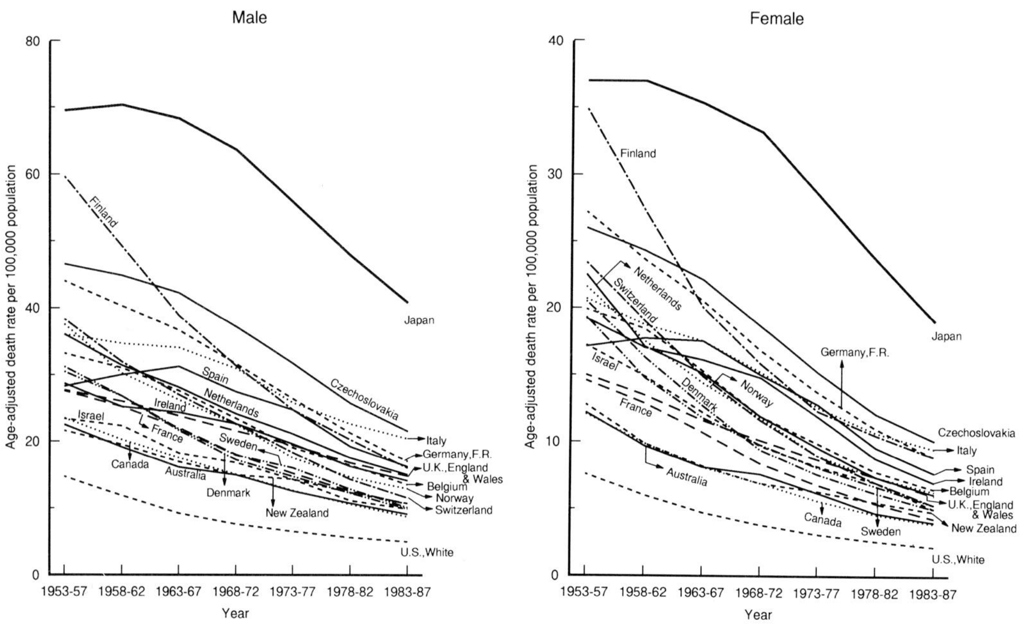

FIG. 2-4. Trends in the age-adjusted death rate of cancer by site from 1953–1957 to 1983–1987. Stomach.

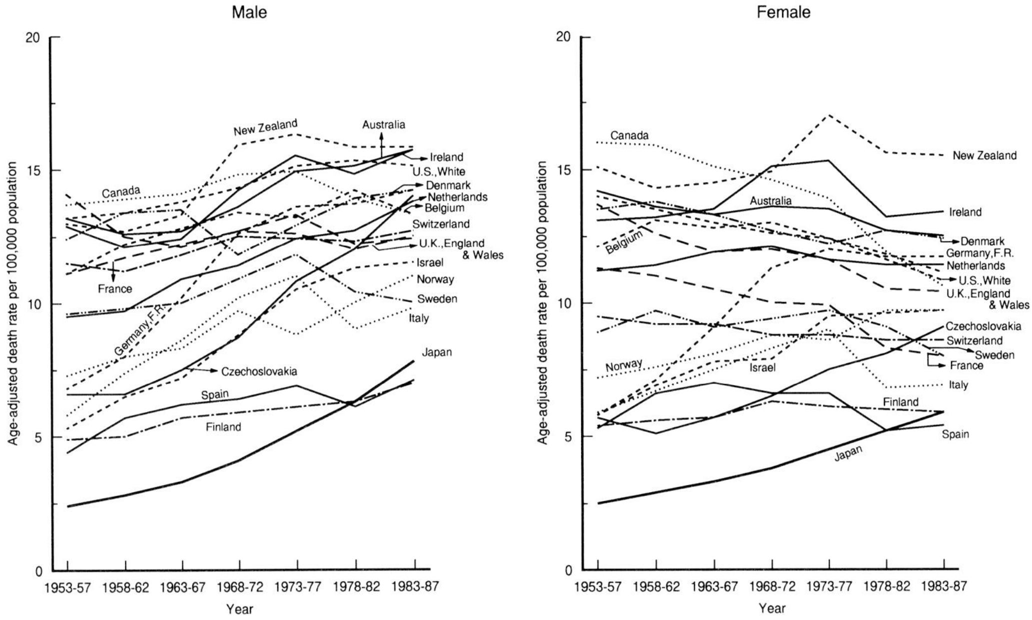

FIG. 2-5. Trends in the age-adjusted death rate of cancer by site from 1953–1957 to 1983–1987. Intestine, except rectum.

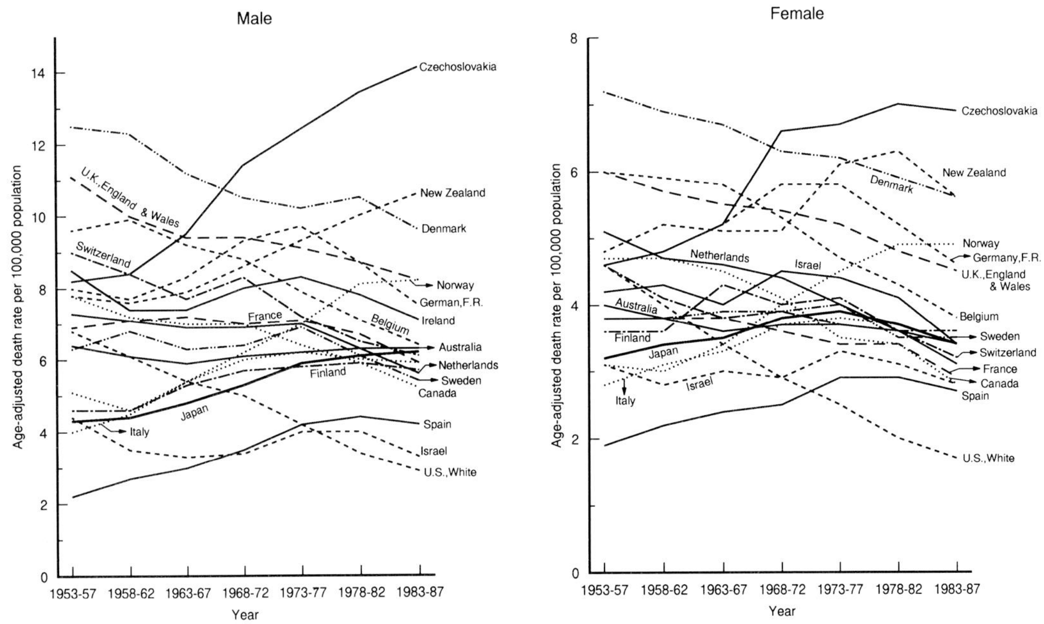

FIG. 2-6. Trends in the age-adjusted death rate of cancer by site from 1953–1957 to 1983–1987. Rectum, rectosigmoid junction, and anus.

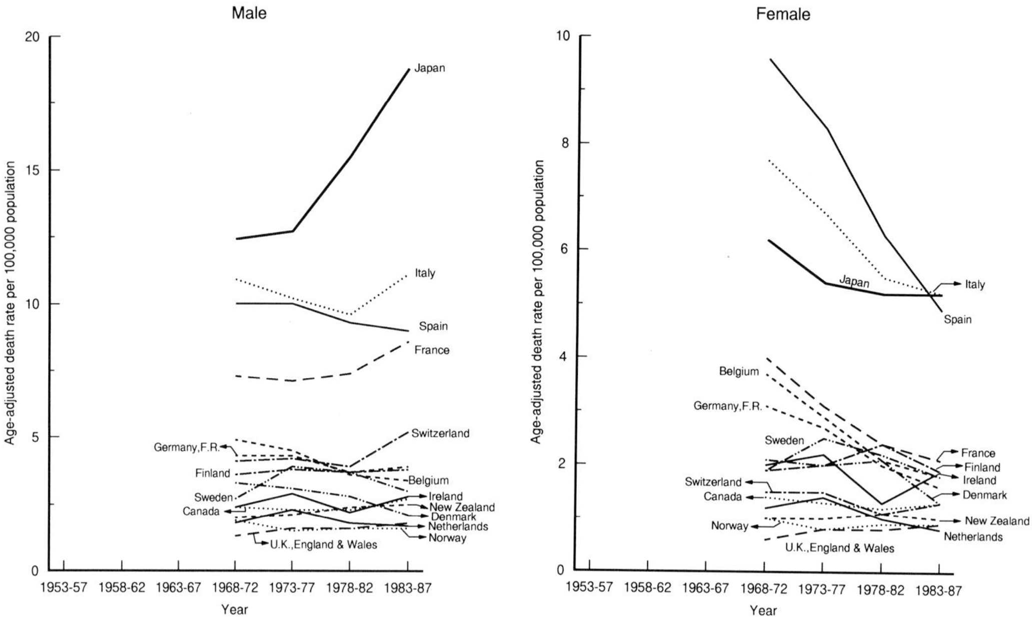

FIG. 2-7. Trends in the age-adjusted death rate of cancer by site from 1953–1957 to 1983–1987. Liver and intrahepatic bile ducts.

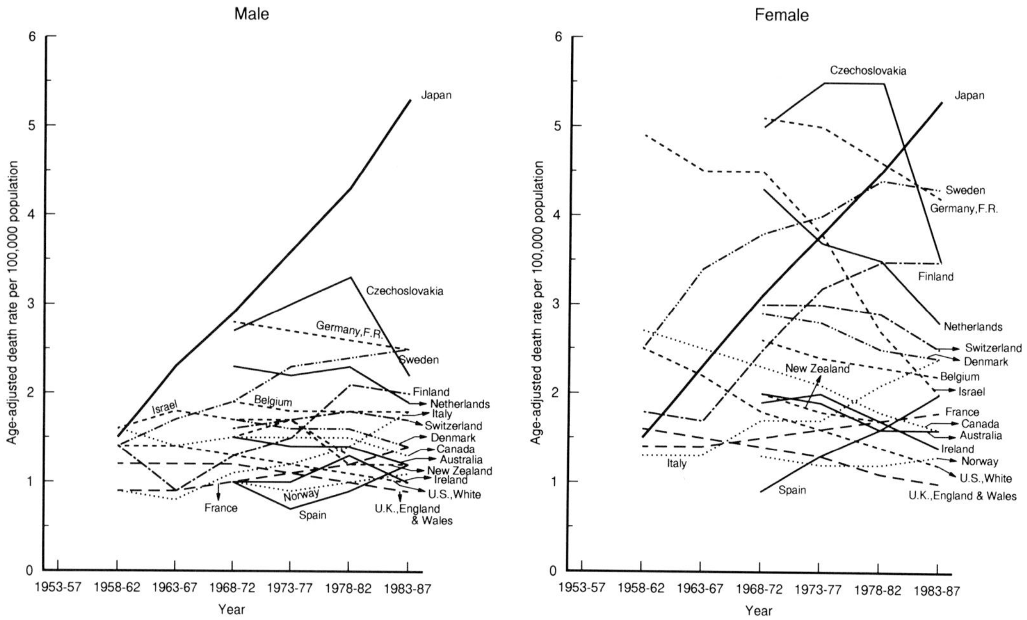

FIG. 2-8. Trends in the age-adjusted death rate of cancer by site from 1953–1957 to 1983–1987. Gallbladder and extrahepatic bile ducts.

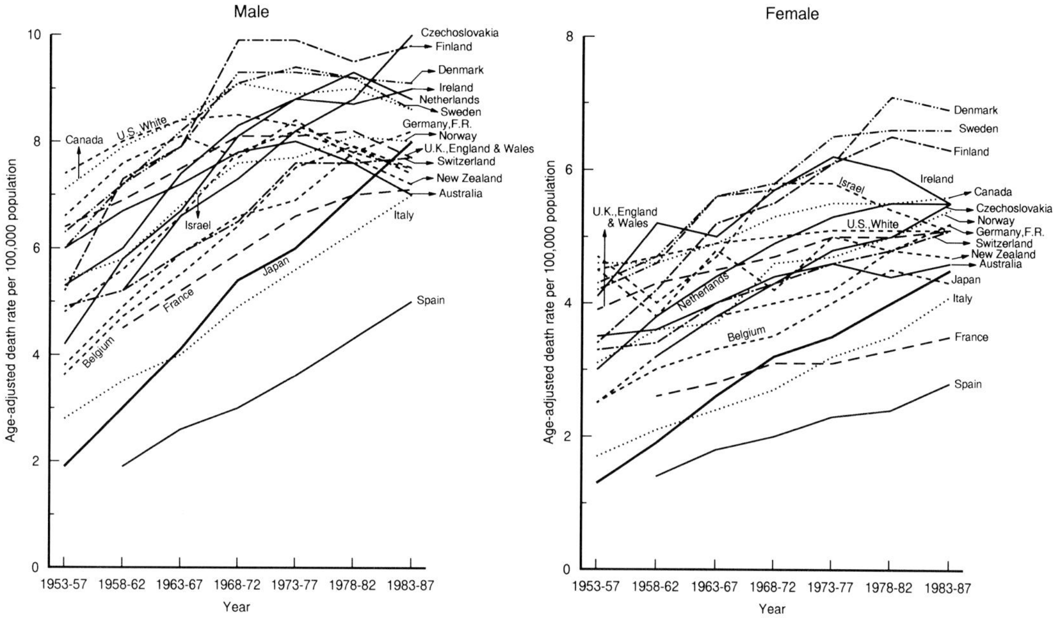

FIG. 2-9. Trends in the age-adjusted death rate of cancer by site from 1953–1957 to 1983–1987. Pancreas.

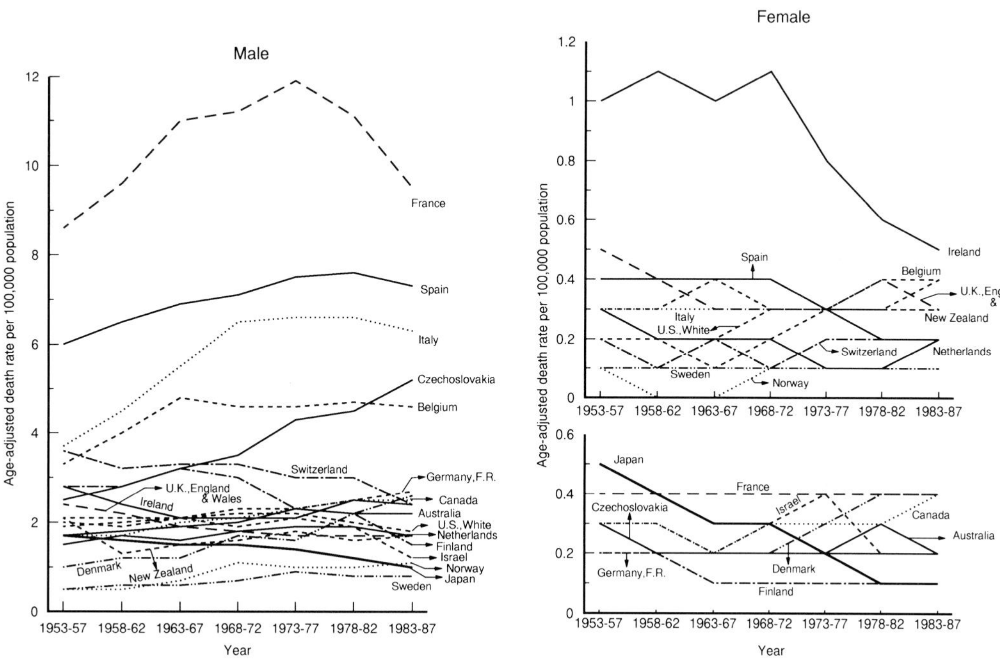

FIG. 2-10. Trends in the age-adjusted death rate of cancer by site from 1953–1957 to 1983–1987. Larynx.

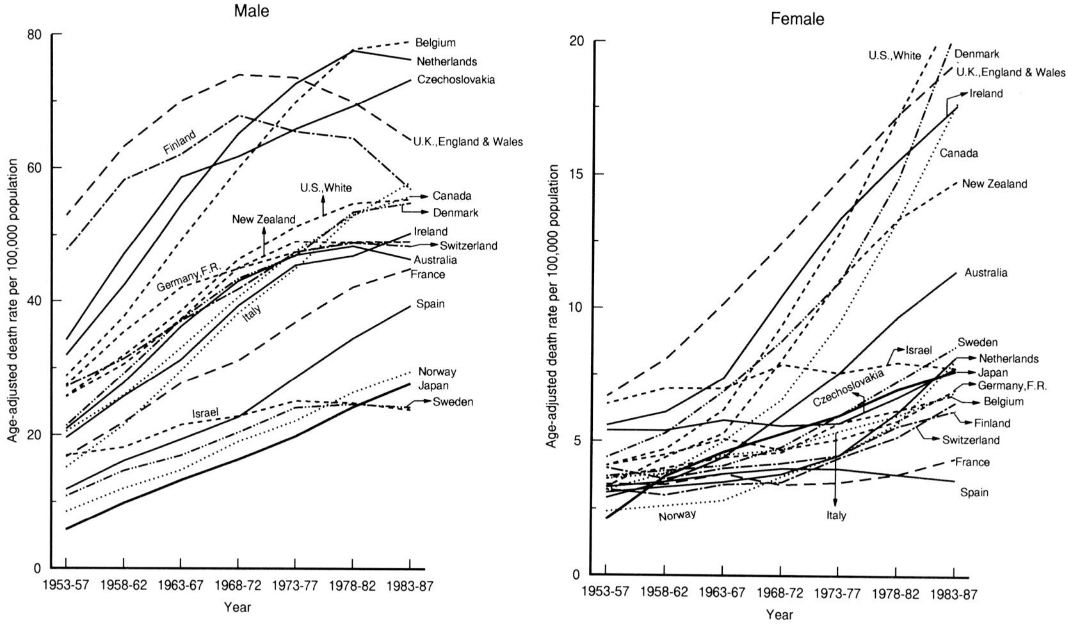

FIG. 2-11. Trends in the age-adjusted death rate of cancer by site from 1953–1957 to 1983–1987. Trachea, bronchus, and lung.

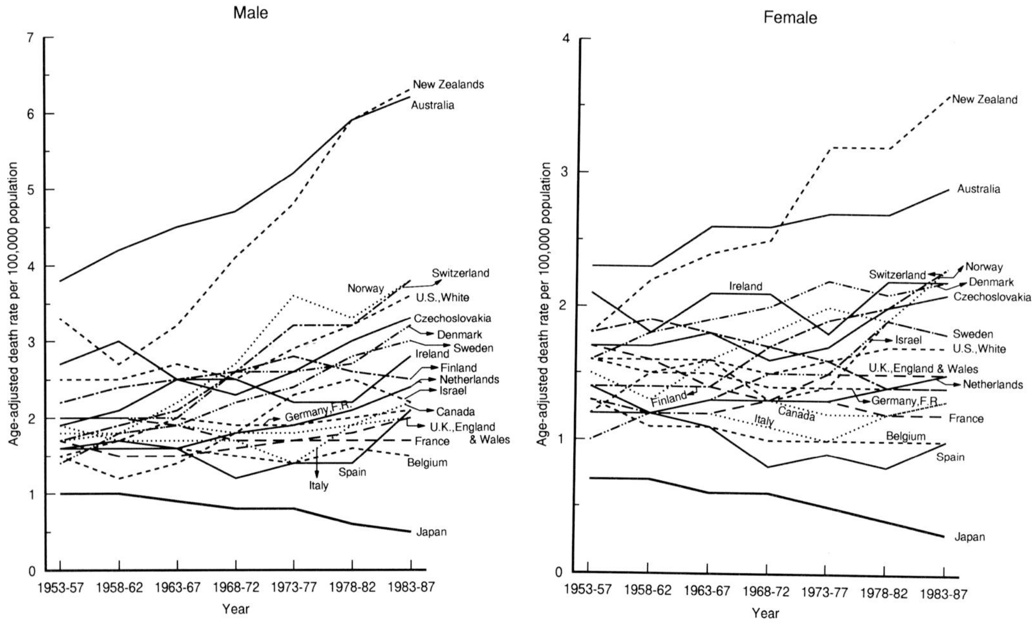

FIG. 2-12. Trends in the age-adjusted death rate of cancer by site from 1953–1957 to 1983–1987. Skin.

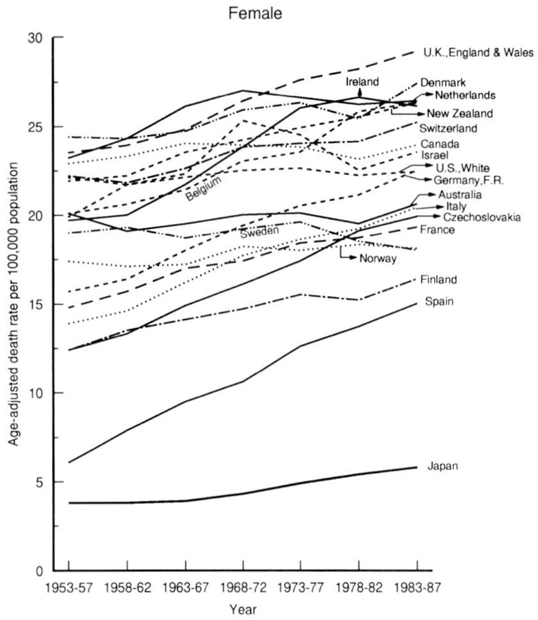

FIG. 2-13. Trends in the age-adjusted death rate of cancer by site from 1953–1957 to 1983–1987. Breast.

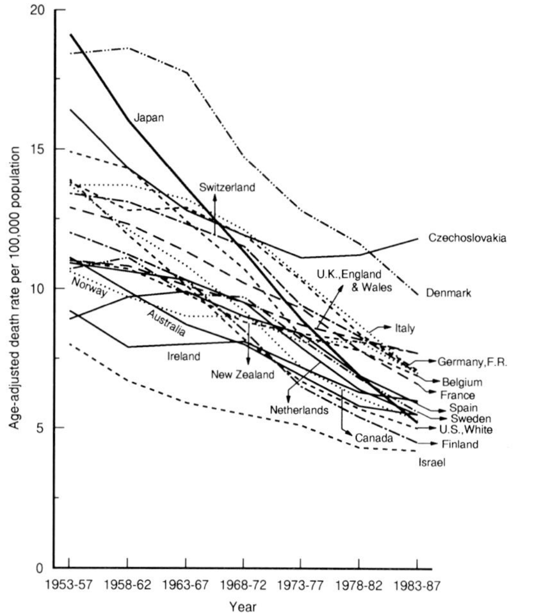

FIG. 2-14. Trends in the age-adjusted death rate of cancer by site from 1953–1957 to 1983–1987. Uterus.

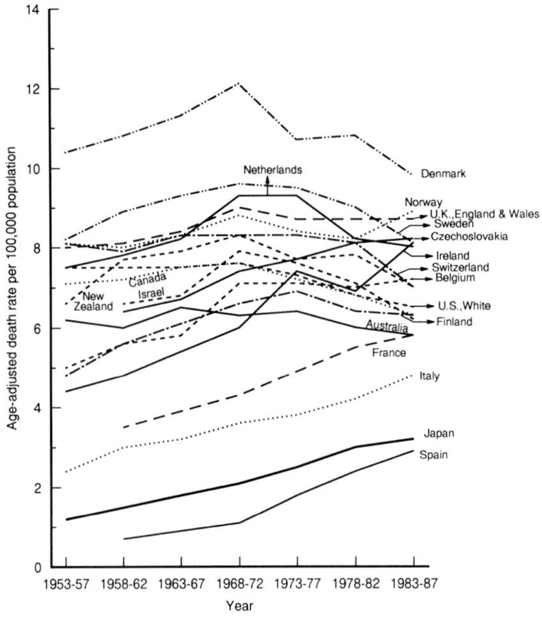

FIG. 2-15. Trends in the age-adjusted death rate of cancer by site from 1953–1957 to 1983–1987. Ovary and other uterine adnexa.

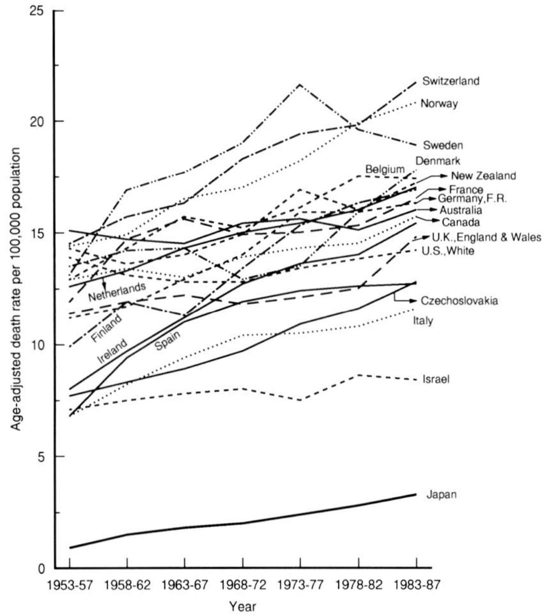

FIG. 2-16. Trends in the age-adjusted death rate of cancer by site from 1953–1957 to 1983–1987. Prostate.

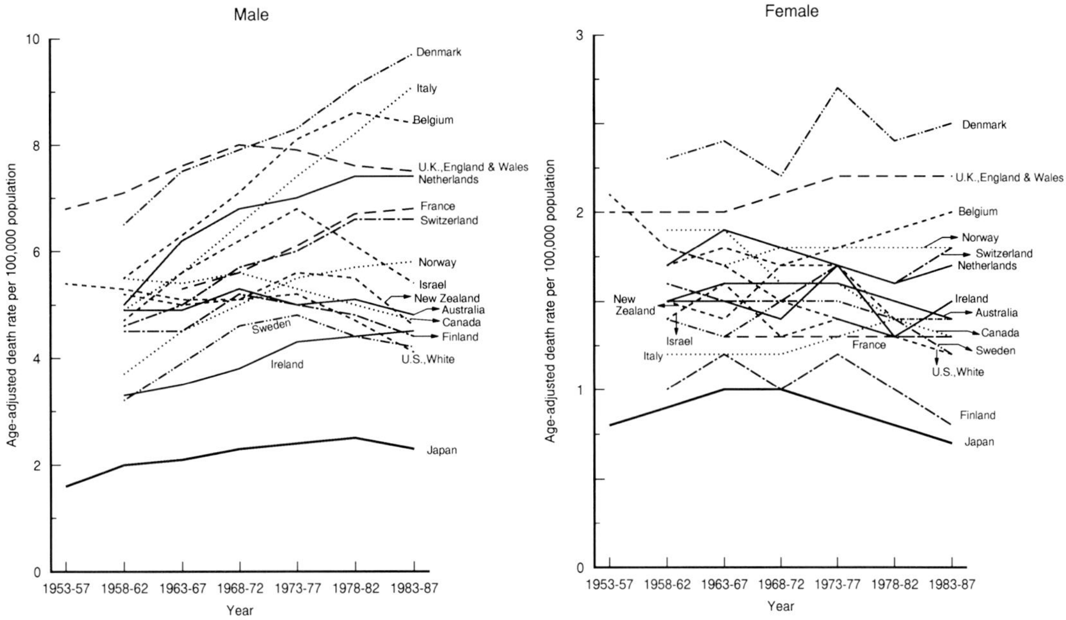

FIG. 2-17. Trends in the age-adjusted death rate of cancer by site from 1953–1957 to 1983–1987. Bladder.

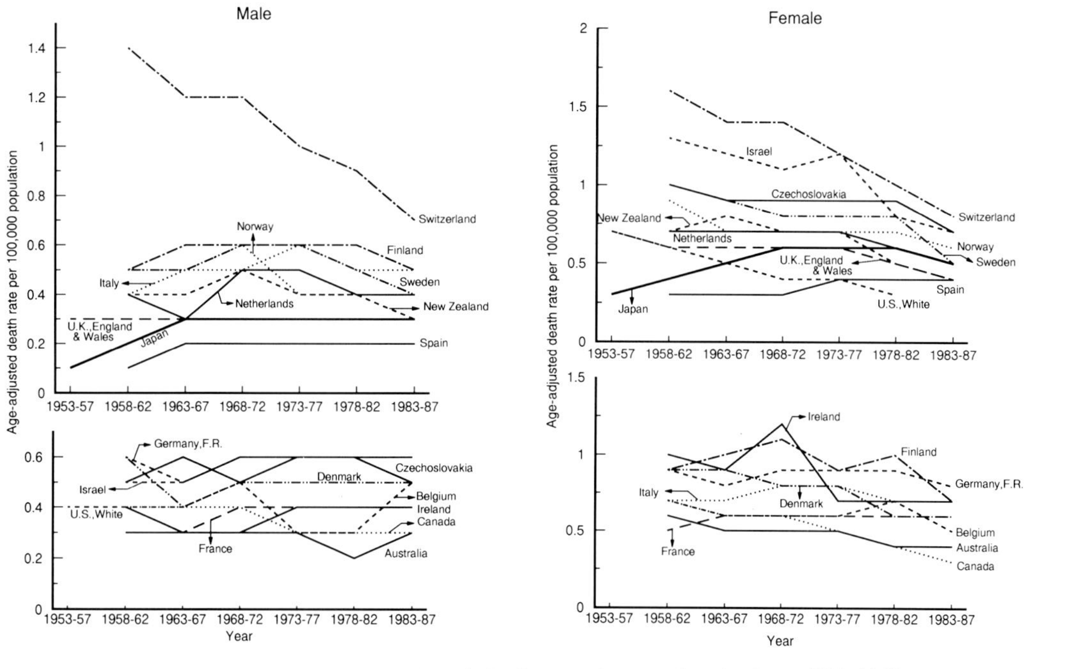

FIG. 2-18. Trends in the age-adjusted death rate of cancer by site from 1953–1957 to 1983–1987. Thyroid gland.

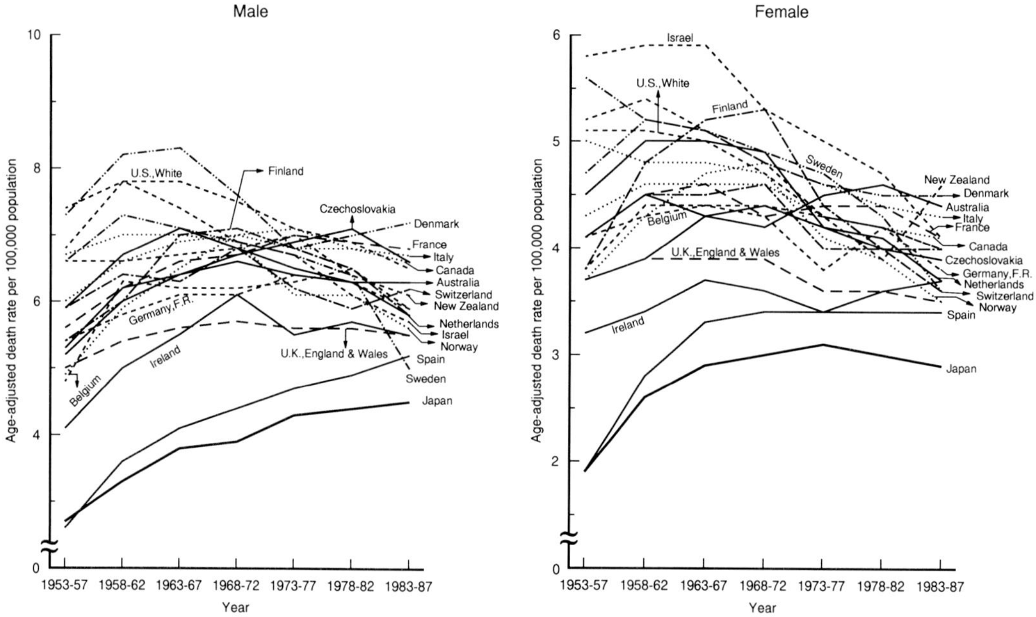

FIG. 2-19. Trends in the age-adjusted death rate of cancer by site from 1953–1957 to 1983–1987. Leukaemia.